2011
YEAR BOOK OF
**DIAGNOSTIC
RADIOLOGY**®

The 2011 Year Book Series

Year Book of Anesthesiology and Pain Management™: Drs Chestnut, Abram, Black, Gravlee, Lien, Mathru, and Roizen

Year Book of Cardiology®: Drs Gersh, Cheitlin, Elliott, Gold, Graham, and Thourani

Year Book of Critical Care Medicine®: Drs Dellinger, Parrillo, Balk, Dorman, Dries, and Zanotti-Cavazzoni

Year Book of Dermatology and Dermatologic Surgery™: Dr Del Rosso

Year Book of Diagnostic Radiology®: Drs Osborn, Abbara, Elster, Manaster, Oestreich, Offiah, Rosado de Christenson, Stephens, and Walker

Year Book of Emergency Medicine®: Drs Hamilton, Bruno, Handly, Mullin, Quintana, and Ramoska

Year Book of Endocrinology®: Drs Schott, Apovian, Clarke, Eugster, Ludlam, Meikle, Ovalle, Schinner, Schteingart, and Toth

Year Book of Gastroenterology™: Drs Talley, DeVault, Harnois, Pearson, Picco, Scolapio, Smith, and Vege

Year Book of Hand and Upper Limb Surgery®: Drs Yao and Steinmann

Year Book of Medicine®: Drs Barker, Garrick, Gersh, Khardori, LeRoith, Seo, Talley, and Thigpen

Year Book of Neonatal and Perinatal Medicine®: Drs Fanaroff, Benitz, Donn, Neu, Papile, Polin, and van Marter

Year Book of Neurology and Neurosurgery®: Drs Klimo and Rabinstein

Year Book of Obstetrics, Gynecology, and Women's Health®: Drs Dungan and Shulman

Year Book of Oncology®: Drs Arceci, Bauer, Gordon, Lawton, and Thigpen

Year Book of Ophthalmology®: Drs Rapuano, Cohen, Flanders, Hammersmith, Milman, Myers, Nelson, Penne, Pyfer, Sergott, Shields, and Vander

Year Book of Orthopedics®: Drs Morrey, Beauchamp, Huddleston, Swiontkowski, and Trigg

Year Book of Otolaryngology-Head and Neck Surgery®: Drs Sindwani, Balough, Franco, Gapany, and Mitchell

Year Book of Pathology and Laboratory Medicine®: Drs Raab, Parwani, Bejarano, and Bissell

Year Book of Pediatrics®: Dr Stockman

Year Book of Plastic and Aesthetic Surgery™: Drs Miller, Gosain, Gurtner, Gutowski, Ruberg, Salisbury, and Smith

Year Book of Psychiatry and Applied Mental Health®: Drs Talbott, Ballenger, Buckley, Frances, Krupnick, and Mack

Year Book of Pulmonary Disease®: Drs Barker, Jones, Maurer, Raza, Tanoue, and Willsie

Year Book of Sports Medicine®: Drs Shephard, Cantu, Feldman, Jankowski, Khan, Lebrun, Nieman, Pierrynowski, and Rowland

Year Book of Surgery®: Drs Copeland, Behrns, Daly, Eberlein, Fahey, Huber, Klodell, Mozingo, and Pruett

Year Book of Urology®: Drs Andriole and Coplen

Year Book of Vascular Surgery®: Drs Moneta, Gillespie, Starnes, and Watkins

2011

The Year Book of DIAGNOSTIC RADIOLOGY®

Editor-in-Chief
Anne G. Osborn, MD
University Distinguished Professor and Professor of Radiology, University of Utah School of Medicine, Salt Lake City, Utah

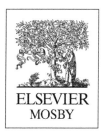

ELSEVIER
MOSBY

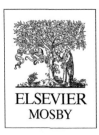

ELSEVIER
MOSBY

Vice President, Continuity: Kimberly Murphy
Editor: Teia Stone
Supervisor, Electronic Year Books: Donna M. Skelton
Electronic Article Manager: Mike Sheets
Illustrations and Permissions Coordinator: Dawn Vohsen

Composition by TNQ Books and Journals Pvt Ltd, India

Editorial Office:
Elsevier
Suite 1800
1600 John F. Kennedy Blvd.
Philadelphia, PA 19103-2899

International Standard Serial Number: 0098-1672
International Standard Book Number: 978-0-323-08411-6

Printed and bound by CPI Group (UK) Ltd, Croydon, CR0 4YY

Transferred to Digital Print 2011

Associate Editors

Suhny Abbara, MD
Associate Professor, Harvard Medical School; Director, Cardiovascular Imaging, Massachusetts General Hospital, Boston, Massachusetts

Allen D. Elster, MD, FACR
Professor and Chair, Division of Radiologic Sciences, Director of Radiologic Sciences, Wake Forest Baptist Health, Winston-Salem, North Carolina

B. J. Manaster, MD, PhD
Professor of Radiology, University of Utah School of Medicine, Salt Lake City, Utah

Alan E. Oestreich, MD
Professor Emeritus of Radiology, University of Cincinnati College of Medicine; Pediatric Radiologist Emeritus, Cincinnati Children's Hospital Medical Center, Cincinnati, Ohio; Professor of Radiology and Pediatrics, University of Kentucky, Lexington, Kentucky

Amaka C. Offiah, BSc, MBBS, MRCP, FRCR, PhD
HEFCE Clinical Senior Lecturer, Academic Unit of Child Health, Sheffield Children's NHS Foundation Trust, Western Bank, Sheffield, United Kingdom

Melissa L. Rosado de Christenson, MD, FACR
Section Chief, Thoracic Imaging, St. Luke's Hospital of Kansas City; Professor of Radiology, University of Missouri–Kansas City, Kansas City, Missouri

Tanya W. Stephens, MD
Associate Professor, Department of Diagnostic Radiology, Division of Diagnostic Imaging, The University of Texas M.D. Anderson Cancer Center, Houston, Texas

T. Gregory Walker, MD
Associate Radiologist, Harvard Medical School; Associate Director Fellowship, Section of Vascular Imaging and Intervention, Massachusetts General Hospital, Boston, Massachusetts

Contributors

Deanna L. Lane, MD

Assistant Professor, Department of Diagnostic Radiology, Division of Diagnostic Imaging, The University of Texas M.D. Anderson Cancer Center, Houston, Texas

Huong Le-Petross, MD

Associate Professor, Department of Diagnostic Radiology, Division of Diagnostic Imaging, The University of Texas M.D. Anderson Cancer Center, Houston, Texas

Table of Contents

Journals Represented

Journals represented in this YEAR BOOK are listed below.

AJNR American Journal of Neuroradiology
AJR American Journal of Roentgenology
American Journal of Emergency Medicine
American Journal of Kidney Diseases
American Journal of Medical Genetics Part A
American Journal of Public Health
American Journal of Sports Medicine
American Journal of Surgery
American Surgeon
Annals of Internal Medicine
Annals of Neurology
Annals of Surgical Oncology
Annals of the Rheumatic Diseases
Annals of Vascular Surgery
British Journal of Radiology
Cancer
Cardiovascular and Intervenlional Radiology
Clinical Genetics
Clinical Nuclear Medicine
Clinical Orthopaedics and Related Research
Clinical Radiology
European Journal of Paediatric Neurology
European Journal of Radiology
Foot and Ankle International
Heart
Hormone Research in Paediatrics
Journal of Bone Mineral Research
Journal of Burn Care & Research
Journal of Cardiovascular Computed Tomography
Journal of Computed Assisted Tomography
Journal of Emergency Medicine
Journal of Laryngology & Otology
Journal of Neurology, Neurosurgery & Psychiatry
Journal of Pediatric Orthopaedics
Journal of Pediatric Surgery
Journal of Plastic, Reconstructive & Aesthetic Surgery
Journal of Pediatrics
Journal of the American Academy of Child & Adolescent Psychiatry
Journal of the American College of Radiology
Journal of the American College of Surgeons
Journal of the American Medical Association
Journal of the American Society of Echocardiography
Journal of the National Cancer Institute
Journal of Thoracic Imaging
Journal of Trauma
Journal of Urology
Journal of Vascular and Interventional Radiology

Journal of Vascular Surgery
Kidney International
Neuroradiology
Neurosurgery
New England Journal of Medicine
Pediatric Neurology
Pediatric Radiology
Plastic and Reconstructive Surgery
RadioGraphics
Radiology
Scandinavian Journal of Urology and Nephrology
Seminars In Nuclear Medicine
Skeletal Radiology
Spine
Stroke
Surgery
Ulusal Travma ve Acil Cerrahi Dergisi

STANDARD ABBREVIATIONS

The following terms are abbreviated in this edition: acquired immunodeficiency syndrome (AIDS), cardiopulmonary resuscitation (CPR), central nervous system (CNS), cerebrospinal fluid (CSF), computed tomography (CT), deoxyribonucleic acid (DNA), electrocardiography (ECG), health maintenance organization (HMO), human immunodeficiency virus (HIV), intensive care unit (ICU), intramuscular (IM), intravenous (IV), magnetic resonance (MR) imaging (MRI), ultrasound (US), and ribonucleic acid (RNA).

NOTE

The YEAR BOOK OF DIAGNOSTIC RADIOLOGY® is a literature survey service providing abstracts of articles published in the professional literature. Every effort is made to assure the accuracy of the information presented in these pages. Neither the editors nor the publisher of the YEAR BOOK OF DIAGNOSTIC RADIOLOGY® can be responsible for errors in the original materials. The editors' comments are their own opinions. Mention of specific products within this publication does not constitute endorsement.

To facilitate the use of the YEAR BOOK OF DIAGNOSTIC RADIOLOGY® as a reference tool, all illustrations and tables included in this publication are now identified as they appear in the original article. This change is meant to help the reader recognize that any illustration or table appearing in the YEAR BOOK OF DIAGNOSTIC RADIOLOGY® may be only one of many in the original article. For this reason, figure and table numbers will often appear to be out of sequence within the YEAR BOOK OF DIAGNOSTIC RADIOLOGY®.

Introduction

As we say here in Utah, "Oh, my heck!" Was 2010-2011 a fascinating year or what?! It's remarkable for what is happening all over the world. And not just our own little world of medical imaging, although that's been fascinating to watch as well. Radiology has been thrust to the forefront of the public consciousness and not for reasons we would have anticipated at the beginning of 2010. As I write, we are captivated by images of the Fukushima nuclear disaster and horrified by its consequences and human impact on both a local and worldwide stage. Radiologists are being questioned everywhere about what does it really mean? Will my children's milk be safe? What is radiation sickness?

It's a sobering reminder that the very name of our beloved profession—radiology—is sometimes linked in the public mind with radiation and its potentially deleterious effects. It strikes close to home when newspapers pick up and disseminate stories about shocking overdoses delivered by some CT angiograms, shown together with graphic pictures of scalp burns and hair loss in the affected areas. This sobering development, together with the world's second-worst nuclear disaster, reminds us that radiation has its downside. Allen Elster, in his fascinating overview of the world of safety, quality, and clinical practice management, addresses some of these concerns. Articles that discuss just "how low is low" dose and what are the exposure risks from everyday sources such as airport scanners are included for your interest and education.

The border line between radiology as diagnosis and radiology as minimally invasive treatment becomes more and more blurred every year. Greg Walker looks at optimizing less-invasive ways of treating diseases and the healthy dialogue about just what are the best treatment regimens. He too has selected articles that discuss cumulative radiation exposure as well as the economic costs of less-invasive versus traditional treatments (hint: less-invasive doesn't always mean less expensive …).

In her final year as our musculoskeletal systems editor, B. J. Manaster has selected a spectrum of articles that she describes as "some that may be groundbreaking, some that may remind us of how to improve our value to our colleagues, and some that are simply beautiful reviews of difficult topics." Nicely stated, B. J.—we will miss you and your pithy comments. And I can promise all our readers that her selections are very valuable in today's changing clinical environment. Just a taste of what awaits you: B. J. selected an article describing diabetic myopathy. So, the worldwide epidemic of diabetes affects more than the blood vessels, eye, and brain? Fascinating stuff!

Pediatric radiology articles selected by Drs Offiah and Oestreich were aimed at what all of us need to know in an era of increasing subspecialization (and sub- sub- specialization). Think about it for a moment! What percentage of your own practice is pediatric imaging? Betcha for almost everyone it's around 10%—at least. Not an insignificant number—and attention to the most vulnerable segments of our populations (the young and the elderly) is a must in our specialty.

Tanya Stephens is the self-described "new kid on the block," in our great cadre of YEAR BOOK associate editors in Diagnostic Radiology. She is heading up our breast imaging section and dived right into the deep end of the pool! She has included articles that frame some of the controversial—and VERY public—issues surrounding breast disease and women's health. Welcome aboard, Tanya! And thanks for your kind words about me. Sorta made me blush ...

Every time we do whole-body trauma imaging, the brain, C-T-L spine(s) land in my reading queue. And there are LOTS of these cases. I've had to relearn some stuff about thoracic and abdominal pathology as there is indeed "life outside the neural foramina." Melissa Rosado de Christenson reminds us of a number of important new issues in chest imaging. And what in the world do "we" do with those incidentalomas we find in the lungs on our T-spine CTs (reminder: ALWAYS look at the lung with lung windows, not just the bones ...)? Are they really incidental?

Last—but by no means least—is cardiovascular imaging. Dr Abbara points out that cardiac CT has been used as the "poster child" for radiation reduction strategies and has gone from (in my words) 'worst to first' in terms of lowest radiation dose imaging. And he tackles the tough issues of outcomes. In an inevitable era of belt-tightening in medical costs, that will become more and more pertinent for us to consider. How do we justify (or not) what we do? If it doesn't make a difference, why should we do it? Just because we can?

So, a gourmet buffet of delightful, delicious, and highly educational articles from the worldwide radiology literature awaits you, our colleagues. Sit back, dig in, and prepare to be astonished and intrigued at how much has happened in our universe of diagnostic imaging in the last year. Enjoy!

Anne G. Osborn, MD
Editor-in-Chief

1 Thoracic Radiology

Introduction

I am delighted to present the final selections of thoracic imaging articles from the 2010 literature. The featured articles largely represent the radiology literature in the United States. However, articles from the European and medical literature are also included.

I want to call the reader's attention to the article by Ahn and colleagues addressing the significance of perifissural nodules seen at CT, an issue encountered by all radiologists engaged in thoracic imaging. In addition to recommending the article by Eisenberg and colleagues, I also urge the readers to review their institution's policy with regard to management recommendations for incidentally discovered small solid nodules. Are we appropriately implementing the Fleischner guidelines in our practices?

The continuing controversy regarding the use of CT pulmonary angiography for the diagnosis of pulmonary embolism in the pregnant patient is highlighted by the articles by Stein and colleagues and Shakir and colleagues. These authors present practical approaches to the diagnosis of pulmonary thromboembolic disease in this patient population. With the introduction of the Image Wisely Campaign, we are urged to raise our level of awareness regarding radiation exposure to the population. The articles by Mamlouk and colleagues and Leipsic and colleagues provide insight into this important issue.

Additional important topics addressed by this year's selections include the use of daily radiography in the ICU, the importance of extracardiac findings in patients undergoing cardiac CT, radiologic predictors of outcomes in patients with H1N1 pulmonary infection, and the challenges of accurately diagnosing interstitial lung disease.

I hope the YEAR BOOK readers find these articles useful in addressing issues that arise in the daily practice of thoracic imaging.

Melissa L. Rosado de Christenson, MD

Lung Cancer

Lung Cancer Detected at Cardiac CT: Prevalence, Clinicoradiologic Features, and Importance of Full–Field-of-View Images
Kim TJ, Han DH, Jin KN, et al (Seoul Natl Univ Bundang Hosp, Bundang-gu, Seongnam-si, Korea; Catholic Univ of Korea, Seoul)
Radiology 255:369-376, 2010

Purpose.—To retrospectively evaluate the prevalence and clinicoradiologic features of lung cancer detected at cardiac computed tomography (CT) and compare the detection rates at different field-of-view (FOV) settings.

Materials and Methods.—The institutional review board approved this retrospective study and waived the requirement for patient consent. Patients with lung cancer initially detected at cardiac CT were identified by means of a retrospective search of a lung cancer registry patient database between January 2004 and December 2007. Patients known to have lung cancer at the time of cardiac CT were excluded. The prevalence and clinical and radiologic features of lung cancer were evaluated. The rates of lung cancer detection at three FOVs—limited and full FOV at cardiac scanning and full FOV at thoracic scanning—were compared by using McNemar testing.

Results.—The prevalence of lung cancer detected at CT was 0.31% (36 of 11 654 patients, 16 [44%] never smokers) and was higher in patients suspected or known to have coronary artery disease (0.43% [24 of 5615 patients]) than in asymptomatic screening-examined patients (0.20% [12 of 5924 patients]) (*P* =.0457). Adenocarcinoma was the most common (in 31 [86%] of 36 patients) histologic subtype. Of 34 non–small cell lung cancers, 23 (68%)—including 16 stage IA cancers—were resectable. Four (11%) and 19 (53%) of the 36 CT-depicted cancers were visible in limited and full FOV at cardiac scanning, respectively, and 17 (47%) were visible in full FOV at thoracic scanning only.

Conclusion.—The prevalence of lung cancer at cardiac CT was 0.31%; and 68% of these malignancies were at a resectable stage. Use of a limited FOV at cardiac scanning led to a large majority (89% [32 of 36 cancers]) of the lung cancers detected at full thoracic scanning being missed; thus, inclusion of the entire chest at cardiac CT is advisable.

▶ There are conflicting views regarding the importance of reporting and evaluating incidental findings encountered during cardiac CT. Some maintain that documenting such findings is an important part of image interpretation and that incidental findings deemed to be potentially significant should be evaluated. Others maintain that incidental extracardiac findings only add to the increasing costs of medical care and increase patient anxiety without added benefits. Although many incidental findings encountered during cardiac CT have no clinical significance, few studies have focused on the prevalence of lung cancer in the patient population imaged with cardiac CT. To this end, the authors performed a retrospective review of the prevalence and clinical and imaging features of lung cancers detected during dedicated cardiac CT using different field-of-view (FOV) settings.

They determined that 11 679 patients underwent 12 268 cardiac CT examinations at their institution between January 2004 and December 2007. They performed a computer search of their database of patients with lung cancer from January 2004 to June 2008 and found 5914 patients with primary lung cancer. They then determined that there were 61 patients with lung cancer who also underwent cardiac CT and identified a subgroup of 36 patients who underwent cardiac CT at their institution, in whom lung cancer was initially detected at cardiac CT and in whom the diagnosis was confirmed by biopsy or surgery. These 36 patients formed the basis of the study.

In each case, thoracic extracardiac findings reported by the cardiac radiologist were ultimately confirmed by a thoracic radiologist, and a series of incidental indeterminate nodules underwent imaging follow-up or histopathologic diagnosis. The cardiac CT studies were performed with either a 16-detector row or a 64-detector row multidetector CT and were followed by delayed thoracic CT scanning without intravenous contrast from the thoracic inlet to the lung base. Demographic factors were recorded, and the CT characteristics of the lung cancers were identified.

The indications for cardiac CT included asymptomatic screening for coronary artery disease (CAD) in 51% of patients, suspected CAD in 42%, evaluation of known CAD in 6%, and evaluation of other cardiovascular diseases in 1%. In 35 of the 36 cases, the lung cancer was detected on the initial examination. The prevalence of lung cancer on an individual patient basis was 0.31%, and it was 0.43% in the patients with suspected or known CAD. The most frequent histologic diagnosis was adenocarcinoma (found in 86% of patients), and 68% of patients had resectable disease. The lesions had a mean maximal diameter of 23 mm ± 10.5, and most occurred in the right upper lobe. Four lung cancers (11%) were detected with the limited FOV used for cardiac CT, 53% were visible on full FOV cardiac CT (Fig 2 in the original article), and 47% were only visible with full FOV thoracic CT.

The authors postulate that the low prevalence of lung cancer in the study population may relate to the high proportion of young asymptomatic nonsmokers evaluated (44%) and note that a higher prevalence of lung cancer occurred in the population with known or suspected CAD. The authors add that the larger and more conspicuous lesions may have been suspected of representing lung cancer by the cardiac radiologist and that additional less-suspicious lung nodules might have existed, which could have also represented undiagnosed early lung cancer, but were not evaluated.

The data suggest that all the cardiac CT data contained in the larger FOV images should be reviewed in all patients undergoing dedicated cardiac CT. In this study, 89% of lung cancers would have been missed with only limited FOV cardiac imaging (Fig 2 in the original article). The authors add that at the very least, the cardiac CT report should document whether the entire lung or only portions of the lung were evaluated. They suggest that in patients with risk factors for lung cancer, low-dose thoracic CT for extracardiac evaluation might be performed before cardiac CT with an acceptable added radiation exposure.

The authors list several limitations to their study:

• The lung cancer prevalence may have been underestimated, as some indeterminate pulmonary nodules may not have been evaluated.

• The patient population may not be representative of the population undergoing cardiac CT.

• The study was retrospective, and the study design may have introduced bias.

• Finally, the study was performed in South Korea, and the practice of performing a delayed thoracic CT following cardiac CT is not necessarily endorsed in the United States.

M. L. Rosado de Christenson, MD

Pulmonary Nodules

Perifissural Nodules Seen at CT Screening for Lung Cancer
Ahn MI, Gleeson TG, Chan IH, et al (Vancouver General Hosp, British Columbia, Canada; et al)
Radiology 254:949-956, 2010

Purpose.—To describe and characterize the potential for malignancy of noncalcified lung nodules adjacent to fissures that are often found in current or former heavy smokers who undergo computed tomography (CT) for lung cancer screening.

Materials and Methods.—Institutional review board approval and informed consent were obtained. Baseline and follow-up thin-section multidetector CT scans obtained in 146 consecutive subjects at high risk for lung cancer (age range, 50—75 years; >30 pack-year smoking history) were retrospectively reviewed. Noncalcified nodules (NCNs) were categorized according to location (parenchymal, perifissural), shape, septal connection, manually measured diameter, diameter change, and lung cancer outcome at 7½ years.

Results.—Retrospective review of images from 146 baseline and 311 follow-up CT examinations revealed 837 NCNs in 128 subjects. Of those 837 nodules, 234 (28%), in 98 subjects, were adjacent to a fissure and thus classified as perifissural nodules (PFNs). Multiple (range, 2—14) PFNs were seen in 47 subjects. Most PFNs were triangular (102/234, 44%) or oval (98/234, 42%), were located inferior to the carina (196/234, 84%), and had a septal connection (171/234, 73%). The mean maximal length was 3.2 mm (range, 1—13 mm). During 2-year follow-up in 71 subjects, seven of 159 PFNs increased in size on one scan but were then stable. The authors searched a lung cancer registry 7½ years after study entry and found 10 lung cancers in 139 of 146 study subjects who underwent complete follow-up; none of these cancers had originated from a PFN.

Conclusion.—PFNs are frequently seen on screening CT scans obtained in high-risk subjects. Although PFNs may show increased size at follow-up

CT, the authors in this study found none that had developed into lung cancer; this suggests that the malignancy potential of PFNs is low.

▶ Lung cancer is the most common fatal malignancy of US men and women. Improved survival may be associated with early diagnosis and complete surgical excision of the primary neoplasm. The earliest primary lung cancers may manifest as small pulmonary nodules, and such nodules are found in up to 50% of high-risk patients undergoing chest CT. However, the rate of lung cancer in resected small nodules varies from 0.3% to 2.7%, indicating that most indeterminate pulmonary nodules found on chest CT are benign. It has been reported that several CT features are seen in benign indeterminate nodules, including polygonal shape, long-to-short axis ratio of more than 1.78, peripheral location, absence of growth, and attachment to pulmonary vessels.

The authors identified a subset of pulmonary nodules found on thin section CT as part of a nonrandomized single-arm lung cancer screening trial in which the screened population was composed of current or former heavy smokers. The subset of nodules was characterized by their location adjacent to interlobar fissures. The authors postulated that these nodules might represent intrapulmonary lymphoid tissue and that they would demonstrate benign behavior. Patients with noncalcified nodules found on CT in this study underwent follow-up chest CT at 3- to 12-month intervals based on the largest dimension of the nodule. A cohort of the screening population was selected (146 consecutive patients imaged between September 29, 2001, and December 9, 2001) and was retrospectively evaluated. A subset of the nodules found was classified as perifissural if they were solid, well defined, smoothly marginated, and in contact with or within 5 mm of an interlobar or accessory fissure (Fig 3 in the original article). Clustered perifissural nodules were multiple and occurred within 10 mm of a fissure. Two-dimensional measurements (long axis and perpendicular short axis) and nodule shape were recorded as well as the location of the nodule with respect to the fissure, carina, and pulmonary segment.

In this study, 88% of the subjects had at least 1 noncalcified nodule. At the 7.5-year follow-up, there were 10 lung cancers diagnosed. The authors found no cancer originating in a perifissural nodule. The authors state that intrapulmonary lymph nodes are most frequent in subpleural locations and below the level of the carina. They quote studies that state that 70% of these lesions have a septal attachment, which was found in 73% of the perifissural nodules in this study. The authors postulate that the septal location may explain the triangular or rectangular shape exhibited by approximately 50% of perifissural nodules in their study. One of the perifissural nodules in this study exhibited growth, was excised, and was histologically proven to represent a lymph node. The authors postulate that growth in such nodules may represent a reaction to inhaled stimuli.

The authors acknowledge several limitations of their study:

- The nodules were not surgically proven to be benign; rather the authors used 2-year period of stability and 7.5 years of follow-up as evidence of benignity.
- The authors used linear electronic caliper measurements rather than volumetric analysis.
- The study design was that of a retrospective review.

It will be interesting to know whether the same findings are corroborated by larger prospective studies. The authors state that most radiologists have a tendency to ignore perifissural nodules or presume that they are benign. In my own practice, I usually describe such lesions as likely representing intrapulmonary lymphoid tissue and typically recommend no imaging follow-up, unless the nodules exceed 5 mm in size.

M. L. Rosado de Christenson, MD

Multiple Focal Pure Ground-Glass Opacities on High-Resolution CT Images: Clinical Significance in Patients With Lung Cancer

Tsutsui S, Ashizawa K, Minami K, et al (Nagasaki Univ Graduate School of Biomedical Sciences, Japan; Nagasaki Univ Hosp, Japan; Nagasaki Municipal Hosp, Japan)
AJR Am J Roentgenol 195:W131-W138, 2010

Objective.—The purpose of this study was to evaluate the clinical significance of multiple focal pure ground-glass opacities (GGOs) on high-resolution CT images of patients with lung cancer.

Materials and Methods.—The cases of 23 patients with proven lung cancer and associated multiple focal pure GGOs on high-resolution CT images were retrospectively reviewed. The number, size, distribution, and morphologic characteristics of focal pure GGOs were evaluated. Serial changes in focal pure GGOs that were not surgically resected were analyzed at follow-up high-resolution CT.

Results.—The number of focal pure GGOs was 196 in total. The size of the opacities ranged from 2 to 30 mm in largest diameter. Lung cancer and focal pure GGOs were seen in the same lobe and/or in the other lobes. One hundred seventy-one of the lesions (87%) had a well-defined border or round shape. Histologic findings were obtained for 15 lesions representing 74 focal pure GGOs that were surgically resected: 11 atypical adenomatous hyperplasia lesions, three bronchioloalveolar carcinomas, and one lesion of focal fibrosis. In 110 of the cases of focal pure GGOs, all of which were followed up with HRCT for a median duration of 1,351 days, the size of 105 lesions (95%) did not change, the size of one decreased, and four lesions disappeared.

Conclusion.—The size of most focal pure GGOs associated with lung cancer did not change during the follow-up period. Most of the small number of lesions histologically diagnosed were atypical adenomatous hyperplasia or bronchioloalveolar carcinoma. These data justify the therapeutic strategy of resecting the primary tumor without therapeutic intervention in the remaining focal pure GGOs (Fig 5).

▶ Much has been written about the varied imaging manifestations of adenocarcinoma and its premalignant precursor lesion, atypical adenomatous hyperplasia. It is well established that atypical adenomatous hyperplasia can be found

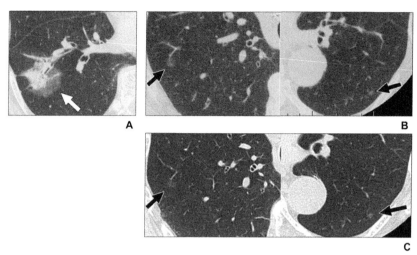

FIGURE 5.—74-year-old woman (patient 6) with adenocarcinoma of the lung and three focal pure ground-glass opacities (GGOs) (type 2). **A,** CT scan shows primary tumor (*arrow*) in right lower lobe that was resected by lobectomy. **B,** CT scan shows focal pure GGOs (*arrows*) in other lobes. **C,** CT scan shows focal pure GGOs (*arrows*) unchanged 2,093 days after **B.** (Reprinted with permission from the American Journal of Roentgenology, Tsutsui S, Ashizawa K, Minami K, et al. Multiple focal pure ground-glass opacities on high-resolution CT images: clinical significance in patients with lung cancer. *AJR Am J Roentgenol.* 2010;195:W131-W138, with permission from American Roentgen Ray Society.)

synchronously in pulmonary lobes resected for the treatment of lung cancer. In addition, atypical adenomatous hyperplasia may be indistinguishable from primary lung cancer, particularly well-differentiated noninvasive lesions. It should be noted that the finding of a nonsolid or ground-glass nodule is nonspecific, as it can be seen with alveolar collapse from various causes and nonneoplastic etiologies including fibrosis and inflammatory processes. Among neoplasms, adenocarcinoma, atypical adenomatous hyperplasia, and lymphoma can also produce this finding. Interim guidelines have been published for the management of subsolid nodules.[1] However, it is important to define the management of patients with lung cancer who have synchronous single or multifocal ground-glass or nonsolid nodules in the primary tumor lobe or in other lobes. One of the difficult areas regarding the new staging system of lung cancer has to do with the presence of multifocal lung malignancies, which may be classified as T3, T4, or M1a disease.

In this study, the authors investigated the occurrence of ground-glass nodules in patients with documented lung cancer. The study is a retrospective review of patients imaged and treated in 2 different institutions between January 2000 and December 2004 and yielded 23 eligible patients with a total of 30 tumors. The patients were studied with 2 different CT scanners (a single-detector and a 4-detector row multidetector CT). It appears that in all cases, the patients underwent additional high-resolution CT imaging, an unusual imaging strategy in the setting of lung cancer. The overwhelming majority of tumors (27) were histologically proven to be adenocarcinomas, including 4 cases of bronchioloalveolar carcinoma. (Since the publication of this article and the submission of this review, the term *bronchioalveolar carcinoma* is no longer in use, based on the February

2011 publication[2] of a new classification of lung adenocarcinoma.) The authors analyzed the number, size, location, and morphology of all the ground-glass opacity nodules associated with the adenocarcinomas. Four different scenarios were identified: single lung cancer with multifocal ground-glass opacity nodules in the same lobe, single lung cancer with multifocal ground-glass opacities in another lobe, single lung cancer with multifocal ground-glass opacities in the same lobe and in different lobes, and multifocal lung cancers with multifocal ground-glass opacities in various lobes. The most frequently encountered situation was single lung cancer with multifocal ground-glass nodules in the same lobe and in other lobes (Fig 5). A total of 196 ground-glass nodules were found ranging from 2 to 30 mm in size, with a range of 2 to 41 ground-glass nodules per patient. The majority (87%) of these lesions exhibited a round shape. Although 74 ground-glass nodules were excised, histologic proof only existed for 15 lesions as in some cases the lesions were too small to be found by the pathologist. Most of these lesions represented atypical adenomatous hyperplasia, and 10 of 11 were found in the lung cancer lobe.

The authors also found that the size of most of the focal nonsolid nodules (95%) did not change over a follow-up period ranging from 181 to 1382 days. The study has limitations that include the use of different protocols, absence of histologic proof for all ground-glass nodules, and the limited time of follow-up.

The authors conclude that their data support the resection of primary lung cancers in spite of the presence of ground-glass opacity nodules in the primary tumor lobe or in other lobes (Fig 5). However, because some of these lesions represent indolent malignancy, these patients may require long-term postoperative imaging follow-up.

M. L. Rosado de Christenson, MD

Reference

1. Godoy MCB, Naidich DP. Subsolid pulmonary nodules and the spectrum of peripheral adenocarcinomas of the lung: recommended interim guidelines for assessment and management. *Radiology.* 2009;253:606-622.
2. Travis WD, Brambilla E, Noguchi M, et al. International Association for the Study of Lung Cancer/American Thoracic Society/European Respiratory Society international multidisciplinary classification of lung adenocarcinoma. *J Thorac Oncol.* 2011;6:244-285.

Compliance with Fleischner Society guidelines for management of small lung nodules: a survey of 834 radiologists
Eisenberg RL, Bankier AA, Boiselle PM (Beth Israel Deaconess Med Ctr, Boston, MA)
Radiology 255:218-224, 2010

Purpose.—To determine the familiarity of radiologists with the Fleischner Society guidelines for management of small lung nodules and to assess whether their decisions for nodule management are consistent with these recommendations.

Materials and Methods.—Institutional review board exemption was granted for this electronic survey, which was sent to a sample of 7000 radiologists randomly selected from the Radiological Society of North America (RSNA) directory. Three clinical scenarios for nodule management were presented. Information about policies and guidelines for nodule management, awareness of published guidelines, and respondent demographics was obtained. Associations between these parameters and management recommendations were assessed by using a χ^2 test. Respondents were also asked about tube current settings for routine chest computed tomographic examinations and those performed solely for nodule follow-up.

Results.—Of 834 respondents (response rate, 11.9%), 649 (77.8%) were aware of the Fleischner Society guidelines and 490 (58.8%) worked in practices that employed them or similar guidelines. Management selections were consistent with the Fleischner guidelines in 34.7%-60.8% of responses for the three scenarios. A significantly higher rate of concordance was associated with awareness of the Fleischner guidelines, presence of written policies based on them, a teaching practice setting, practice in a group with at least one member having chest radiology fellowship training, and fewer than 5 years of experience practicing radiology ($P < .05$ for all associations). The spectrum of tube current settings used was similar between the subgroups of respondents who were aware and those who were unaware of the Fleischner guidelines.

Conclusion.—Among survey respondents, there was high awareness and adoption of the Fleischner guidelines, but radiologists showed varying degrees of conformance with these recommendations. Future efforts are necessary to bridge the gap between awareness and implementation of these evidence-based guidelines.

▶ Incidental indeterminate pulmonary nodules are a common finding on thoracic CT. In some cases, these nodules are identified in the lung bases on abdominal CT studies. The approach to the evaluation of such nodules has relied on follow-up imaging that typically spans a period of 2 years. In 2005, the "Guidelines for Management of Small Pulmonary Nodules Detected on CT Scans: A Statement From the Fleischner Society" was published in the journal *Radiology* and provided a method for evaluation of solid lung nodules based on the nodule size and the presence or absence of risk factors for lung cancer.[1] The authors performed an electronic survey of 7000 radiologists in the United States to evaluate their management strategies of incidentally discovered pulmonary nodules measuring 4 mm or smaller found during thoracic CT. The authors randomly selected survey recipients using the 2007 membership of the Radiological Society of North America and sent questionnaires to the electronic mail addresses listed in the directory. The survey included a variety of questions and asked whether the responders were familiar with the Fleischner Society and American College of Chest Physicians guidelines for management of pulmonary nodules. The questionnaire recipients were presented with 3 different scenarios regarding the evaluation of a small (≤4 mm) indeterminate nodule in 2 patients with low risk for lung cancer and 1 patient with high risk for lung cancer. The authors also included questions regarding demographic information of the responders, their practice types, and the manner in which they evaluated lung nodules on CT to determine whether they were using low-dose CT technique for the examinations performed for nodule follow-up.

Eight hundred thirty-four radiologists (11.9%) responded to the survey. Of these, 77.8% were aware of the Fleischner guidelines. However, responders in teaching hospitals, those with less than 5 years of practice experience and those with at least one member of the group having completed fellowship training in thoracic radiology demonstrated higher awareness of the guidelines. Fifty percent of responders work in practices that incorporated such guidelines into their written policies. However, there were variable degrees of conformance (34.7%-60.8%) with the recommendations when the responders were asked to select management options in various clinical scenarios related to the management of a small nodule.

The authors recognize several limitations to their study:

- Low response rate to the survey
- The clinical scenarios may lack nuances found in daily practice
- The responders were not provided copies of the guidelines
- A small number of respondents may be specialists in chest radiology

The article highlights the variability of practice in our country in spite of awareness of published guidelines and suggests that all practices might benefit from review and discussion of evidence-based guidelines in their practice meetings.

M. L. Rosado de Christenson, MD

Reference

1. MacMahon H, Austin JH, Gamsu G, et al. Guidelines for management of small pulmonary nodules detected on CT scans: a statement from the Fleischner Society. *Radiology.* 2005;237:395-400.

Malignant Neoplasia

Surveillance after surgical treatment of melanoma: Futility of routine chest radiography

Brown RE, Stromberg AJ, Hagendoorn LJ, et al (Univ of Louisville, KY; Univ of Kentucky, Lexington; Advertek Inc, Louisville, KY; et al)
Surgery 148:711-717, 2010

Background.—Current recommendations by the National Comprehensive Cancer Network and other groups suggest that follow-up of cutaneous melanoma may include chest radiography (CXR) at 6- to 12-month intervals. The aim of this study was to determine the clinical efficacy of routine CXR for recurrence surveillance in melanoma.

Methods.—Post hoc analysis was performed on data from a prospective, randomized, multi-institutional study on melanoma ≥1.0 mm in Breslow thickness. All patients underwent excision of the primary melanoma and sentinel node biopsy with completion lymphadenectomy for positive sentinel nodes. Yearly CXR and clinical assessments were obtained during follow-up. Results of routine CXR were compared with clinical disease states over the course of the study.

Results.—A total of 1,235 patients were included in the analysis over a median follow-up of 74 months (range, 12–138). Overall, 210 patients (17.0%) had a recurrence, most commonly local or in-transit. Review of CXR results showed that 4,218 CXR were obtained in 1,235 patients either before, or in the absence of, initial recurrence. To date, 88% ($n = 3,722$) CXR are associated with no evidence of recurrence. Of CXR associated with recurrence, only 7.7% ($n = 38$) of surveillance CXR were read as "abnormal." Overall, 99% ($n = 4,180$) of CXR were read as either "normal" or found to be falsely positive (read as "abnormal," but without evidence of recurrence on investigation). Only 0.9% ($n = 38$) of all CXR obtained were true positives ("abnormal" CXR, with confirmed first known recurrence). Among these 38 patients with true positive CXR, 35 revealed widely disseminated disease (multiorgan or bilateral pulmonary metastases); only 3 (0.2%) had isolated pulmonary metastases amenable to resection. Sensitivity and specificity for surveillance CXR in detecting initial recurrence were 7.7% and 96.5%, respectively.

Conclusion.—The routine use of surveillance CXR provides no clinically useful information in the follow-up of patients with melanoma. CXR does not detect recurrence at levels sufficient to justify its routine use and, therefore, cannot be recommended as part of the standard surveillance regimen for these patients.

▶ The authors state that the incidence of cutaneous melanoma is on the increase, with an estimated 68,720 new cases in the United States and 8650 deaths each year. They add that stage IV melanoma carries a very poor prognosis with a median survival of 8 months. They state that current recommendations from the National Comprehensive Cancer Network advocate follow-up of stage IIB and higher melanomas with chest radiography at 6- to 12-month intervals. The authors undertook this study to determine the utility of routine radiography for surveillance of these patients with the hypothesis that the use of such a follow-up scheme was not justified.

The authors performed a post hoc analysis of data from the Sunbelt Melanoma Trial, a multicenter prospective randomized study. The patient population included individuals between 18 and 71 years of age with invasive cutaneous melanoma > 1.0 mm in Breslow thickness without clinical evidence of metastatic disease. All patients underwent surgical excision of the melanoma and sentinel node biopsy. All patients were followed up with annual chest radiography. Patients with follow-up chest radiographs at less than 1 year and those without radiographic follow-up were excluded.

Most patients with recurrent disease had local recurrences followed by distant (nonpulmonary) metastases. Metastases to the lung only were present in 13.3% of recurrences. Radiographs were grouped as normal or abnormal based on the radiologist's report. It should be noted that the most common causes of false-positive results were nonmalignant incidental findings, including emphysema, granulomatous disease, and interstitial lung disease.

The authors characterize ideal screening tests as having high sensitivity, high specificity, easy availability, and low cost, as well as being noninvasive and able to detect the disease at an early stage. Based on their results, the authors conclude that chest radiography neither altered clinical course nor improved outcomes for the patients enrolled. They quote work by Mooney et al that estimates the cost of a 20-year chest radiography screening program in patients diagnosed with melanoma in 1996 between 27 and 32 million dollars.

In their study, only 3 of 1235 patients undergoing radiographic screening ultimately underwent therapeutic metastasectomy, and the authors extrapolate that 1406 chest radiographs would have to be performed to identify a single case of potentially resectable pulmonary metastasis. They also quote work by Tsao et al who found no survival benefit for patients with melanoma with early-detected asymptomatic pulmonary metastases.

The authors recognize several limitations to their study, including the fact that it is a post hoc analysis of data that were prospectively collected to evaluate other features of melanoma. As patients were randomized to various therapies, these could potentially alter the patterns of recurrence of the patients enrolled. Nevertheless they advocate that the current recommendations for routine radiographic screening of patients with melanoma be reevaluated. They suggest that cross-sectional and radionuclide imaging among others may be alternate methods for identifying regional disease.

M. L. Rosado de Christenson, MD

CT Findings in Patients with Pericardial Effusion: Differentiation of Malignant and Benign Disease

Sun JS, Park KJ, Kang DK (Ajou Univ School of Medicine, Yeongtong-gu, Suwon, Republic of Korea)
AJR Am J Roentgenol 194:W489-W494, 2010

Objective.—This study was designed to validate the usefulness of a CT finding of abnormal pericardial thickening and to investigate the value of associated thoracic changes in predicting the presence of malignant pericardial effusion.

Materials and Methods.—Seventy-four consecutively registered patients with pericardial effusion detected with transthoracic echocardiography were included in the study. The patients fulfilled the following criteria: undergoing pericardial fluid cytologic examination or pericardial tissue biopsy and undergoing chest CT examination less than 30 days after pericardial fluid or tissue examination. CT images were reviewed for the presence of pericardial thickening, the pattern of pericardial thickening, and the presence of pleural effusion and mediastinal lymph node enlargement.

Results.—Twenty-eight cases of malignant and 46 cases of benign pericardial effusion were identified. Mean pericardial thickening was greater in association with malignant disease (7.25 ± 2.91 mm) than with benign disease (4.11 ± 1.39 mm) ($p < 0.05$). Abnormal pericardial thickening ($p < 0.05$) and mediastinal lymph node enlargement ($p < 0.001$) were statistically significant findings of malignant pericardial effusion. The sensitivity of abnormal pericardial thickening was 42.9% and that of mediastinal lymph node enlargement was 60.7%.

Conclusion.—CT findings of irregular pericardial thickening and mediastinal lymphadenopathy have the potential to be reliably specific findings suggesting the presence of malignant pericardial effusion. It would be useful, however, to obtain pericardial fluid or tissue for cause-based management of pericardial effusion, especially in patients with malignant disease.

▶ Pericardial effusion may result from a variety of nonneoplastic and neoplastic disease processes, and the fluid may exhibit transudative or exudative characteristics, frank pus or blood, or a mixture of substances. According to the authors, large pericardial effusions are typically associated with malignant neoplasia, hypercholesterolemia, uremia, myxedema, and parasitic disease. Pericardial effusion is often managed by treating the underlying disease process, although emergent evacuation of the pericardial fluid may be required in patients with tamponade. Although echocardiography has been considered the imaging study of choice for evaluation of pericardial effusion, it is limited by its narrow field of view and the fact that it is an operator-dependent procedure. CT provides exquisite visualization of the normal and abnormal pericardium and has the added advantage of visualizing the entirety of the pericardium and associated abnormalities in adjacent thoracic and abdominal organs and locations.

The diagnosis of malignant pericardial effusion is important in the staging and management of patients with malignant neoplasms. The authors list the following entities as causes of pericardial effusion in the setting of malignancy: malignant involvement of the pericardium, radiation-induced pericarditis, drug-induced pericarditis, and idiopathic pericarditis. In fact, metastatic disease is the most common neoplasm affecting the pericardium and effusion is its most frequent manifestation. In addition, the authors cite literature stating that nonmalignant pericardial effusion is found on autopsy in up to 6% of patients with cancer. Thus, the authors performed this study to validate the usefulness of CT findings of abnormal pericardial thickening in differentiating malignant and benign pericardial diseases.

The authors performed a retrospective review of consecutive patients with pericardial effusion imaged at a 1100-bed tertiary referral university hospital between May 2003 and May 2007. The patients included in the study underwent echocardiography that showed pericardial effusion, cytologic evaluation of pericardial fluid, or pericardial tissue sampling and had a chest CT less than 30 days after evaluation of the pericardial fluid or tissue. The patients did not have a bulky pericardial soft tissue mass. Benign pericardial effusion was diagnosed by finding normal tissue or cytology at initial examination and no recurrence of effusion for at least 1 year of clinical and radiologic follow-up. Tuberculous pericardial effusion was diagnosed by the finding of tubercle bacilli in stains or cultures or the finding of tubercle bacilli or caseating granulomas at histological evaluation. The study population consisted of 78 patients examined with either a 16-row multidetector CT or a single-detector CT scanner. All CT studies were performed after the administration of intravenous contrast. The images were analyzed by 2 thoracic radiologists, and decisions were reached by consensus. The images were examined for pericardial thickening (> 3 mm pericardial thickness), pattern of thickening (irregular or smooth), and presence of pleural effusion or mediastinal lymphadenopathy. The majority of patients (42) had underlying malignancy, and most (23) had lung cancer, followed by breast cancer and lymphoma. There were 46 cases of benign effusion and 28 cases of malignant effusion. The etiologies of the benign effusions were mostly unknown (23) but also included tuberculosis (9 patients), pneumonia (6), radiation induced (4), systemic lupus erythematosus (2), and myocardial infarction and polymyositis (1 each).

The authors found that irregular pericardial thickening and mediastinal lymph node enlargement were significant CT findings of malignant pericardial effusion but have low sensitivities of 37.9% and 62.1%, respectively. They cite pericardioscopy-guided biopsy as having sensitivities of 93.3% to 97% for the diagnosis of malignancy. The authors found 9 cases of tuberculous pericarditis in their study that likely reflect the endemic nature of tuberculosis in their country, Republic of Korea.

The authors list several limitations of their study: the small number of cases, the different scanners used, and the use of cytologic or pathologic evaluation as the standard for benign pericardial effusion. It may be that the greatest limitation is that the CT studies followed an invasive procedure of the pericardium, which could have altered the morphologic features and as a result the CT appearance.

M. L. Rosado de Christenson, MD

Technique

Abandoning Daily Routine Chest Radiography in the Intensive Care Unit: Meta-Analysis
Oba Y, Zaza T (Univ of Missouri-Columbia)
Radiology 255:386-395, 2010

Purpose.—To systematically examine whether abandoning daily routine chest radiography would adversely affect outcomes, such as mortality and length of stay (LOS), and identify a subgroup in which daily routine chest radiography might be beneficial.

Materials and Methods.—This was a meta-analysis of clinical trials that examined the effect of abandoning daily routine chest radiography in adults in intensive care units (ICUs). Studies were identified through searches of MEDLINE, Cochrane Database, Database of Abstracts of

Reviews of Effects, Biological Abstracts, and CINAHL. The results were expressed as odds ratios (ORs) or weighted mean difference (WMD) along with their 95% confidence intervals (CIs).

Results.—Eight studies with a total of 7078 patients were identified. A pooled analysis revealed that the elimination of daily routine chest radiography did not affect either hospital or ICU mortality (OR, 1.02; [95% CI: 0.89, 1.17; $P =.78$ and OR, 0.92; 95% CI: 0.76, 1.11; $P =.4$, respectively). There was no significant difference in ICU LOS (WMD = 0.19 days; 95% CI: -0.13, 0.51; $P =.25$), hospital LOS (WMD = -0.29 days; 95% CI: -0.71, 0.13; $P =.18$), and ventilator days (WMD = 0.33 days; 95% CI: -0.12, 0.78; $P =.15$) between the on-demand and daily routine groups. Regression analyses failed to identify any subgroup in which performing daily routine chest radiography was beneficial.

Conclusion.—Systematic but unselective daily routine chest radiography can likely be eliminated without increasing adverse outcomes in adult patients in ICUs. Further studies are necessary to identify the specific patient population that would benefit from daily routine chest radiographs (Table 1).

▶ The daily bedside chest radiograph is a common imaging study for the assessment of patients in intensive care units (ICUs), particularly those requiring mechanical ventilation, and radiologists in the United States are quite familiar with interpreting the morning portables each day. This practice is supported by the American College of Radiology's (ACR's) Appropriateness Criteria for the performance of routine chest radiographs, which rates it as usually appropriate with the highest possible rating of 9 for patients with respiratory failure who are receiving mechanical ventilation. The same document also gives a rating of 9—usually appropriate to performing portable chest radiographs on this patient population based on clinical indications only and states that "...routine daily radiographs are indicated for patients with acute cardiopulmonary problems. In stable patients admitted for cardiac monitoring, or in stable patients admitted for extrathoracic disease only, an initial admission radiograph is recommended, with follow-up radiographs obtained only for specific clinical indications."[1] The ACR Appropriateness Criteria for routine chest radiograph were last reviewed in 2008.

The purpose of the authors' investigation was to determine whether abandoning routine daily radiography would adversely affect ICU patients (based on mortality and length of hospital stay) and to identify a group of patients in whom routine daily radiography would be beneficial. To this end, the authors searched for and identified relevant clinical trials (published between January 1, 1950 and December 31, 2008) that examined the impact of daily bedside radiography as compared with that of radiography for specific clinical indications. They selected randomized controlled or observational studies that compared outcome efficacy of routine versus clinically indicated radiography in adult patients admitted to medical or surgical ICUs. To be selected, the studies had to have hospital or ICU mortality, length of mechanical ventilation, hospital stay or adverse event rates as a primary outcome variable, and at least

TABLE 1.—Characteristics of Clinical Trials

Study	Study Design	No. of Patients	Duration (mo)	Type of Patients	Ventilated Patients (%)	Expected Mortality (%)*	Observed Mortality (%)	Quality Score†
Brivet et al (30)	Observational before-after	1529	36	97% medical, 3% surgical	43	23	16	5
Clec'h et al (3)	Randomized controlled trial	165	6	75% medical, 25% surgical	100	60	33	15
Hendrikse et al (9)	Observational before-after	736	18	48% medical, 52% surgical	62	16	16	10
Krinsley et al (31)	Observational before-after	2564	35	69% medical, 31% surgical	36	26	20	8
Kripoval et al (2)	Randomized controlled trial	94	10	Medical	100	Not available	24	12
Kroner et al (27)	Observational before-after	1490	11	26% medical, 74% surgical	100	21	18	11
Leong et al (32)	Observational before-after	300	7	Surgical	100	Not available	3	9
Rao et al (33)	Observational	200	Not available	Surgical	100	Not available	Not available	7

Editor's Note: Please refer to original journal article for full references.
*Based on Simplified Acute Physiology Score II or Acute Physiology and Chronic Health Evaluation Score II.
†Range, 0–22; 22 indicates the highest quality (10,11).

30% of patients in the study had to be mechanically ventilated. From an initial selection of 23 studies, a total of 8 were ultimately included in the published meta-analysis. See Table 1.

Of the 7078 ICU patients included, 3429 underwent daily routine chest radiography and 3649 underwent portable radiography for a clinical indication (on demand) with mean numbers of chest radiographs per patient ranging from 2.4 to 10.5 and 0.4 to 4.4, respectively. The mean patient age was 62.8 years, 59% were nonsurgical patients and 61% were mechanically ventilated. The mean mortality was 17%. The analysis showed that none of the patient subgroups had significant differences on any outcome when comparing the daily radiography to the on-demand radiography groups.

The authors conclude that the practice of daily radiography for ICU patients may not be necessary. They state that literature advocating daily radiography was mainly based on observational studies without a comparison group and without reporting objective data. They add that the performance of daily bedside radiography for a specific clinical indication rather than on a daily basis has benefits that include decreased workload, decreased radiation exposure to patients and medical personnel, and decreased health care costs. The authors highlight some of the limitations of their study including the following: 8 selected studies included both randomized control and observational studies, patient demographics were not similar in the 3 observational studies, the study may not be applicable to patient populations with higher mortality rates (than those included in the studies), and 1 included study had substantially more patients than the others. They conclude that daily routine radiography may be safely eliminated in most ICU patients and add that further studies are needed to identify specific populations that may benefit from the practice of routine radiography. It should be noted that the ability to discontinue the practice of obtaining routine portable radiographs on mechanically ventilated ICU patients will ultimately depend on how comfortable clinicians feel in forgoing radiography for the continued assessment and monitoring of their patients.

This article generated 2 letters to the editor published in the September 2010 issue of *Radiology*.[2,3] Milne points out the large variations between the ICUs and the patients in the selected studies and questions the effects of abandoning daily radiographs in such divergent patient groups. He also states that based on Fig 2 in the original article, in 7 of 8 ICUs, the resultant reduction of chest radiographs would only amount to 1.4 radiographs per patient.[2] Hejblum et al present data from their multicenter study published in 2009 in *Lancet*, which included 21 ICUs that were randomly assigned to the use of either routine radiography or on-demand radiography during 2 separate treatment periods. They report a mean decrease of 32% in the number of chest radiographs obtained and no significant difference between the groups of patients with respect to the following outcomes: diagnostic procedures or therapeutic interventions, length of ICU stay, and mortality while in the ICU.[3] They further state that their study supports the conclusions of the report by Oba et al.[4]

M. L. Rosado de Christenson, MD

References

1. American College of Radiology. ACR Appropriateness Criteria. Routine Chest Radiograph, http://www.acr.org/SecondaryMainMenuCategories/quality_safety/app_criteria/pdf/ExpertPanelonThoracicImaging/RoutineChestRadiographDoc7.aspx. Accessed August 26, 2010.
2. Milne EN. Imaging expertise in critical care units. *Radiology.* 2010;256:1013.
3. Hejblum G, Guidet B. Evidence-based data for abandoning unselective daily chest radiographs in Intensive Care Units. *Radiology.* 2010;256:1013-1014.
4. Hejblum G, Chalumeau-Lemoine L, Ioos V, et al. Comparison of routine and on-demand prescription of chest radiographs in mechanically ventilated adults: a multi-centre, cluster-randomised, two-period crossover study. *Lancet.* 2009;374:1687-1693.

Differentiation of Pleural Effusions From Parenchymal Opacities: Accuracy of Bedside Chest Radiography

Kitazono MT, Lau CT, Parada AN, et al (Hosp of the Univ of Pennsylvania, Philadelphia)
AJR Am J Roentgenol 194:407-412, 2010

Objective.—The purpose of this study was to determine, with CT as the reference standard, the ability of radiologists to detect pleural effusions on bedside chest radiographs.

Materials and Methods.—Images of 200 hemithoraces in 100 ICU patients undergoing chest radiography and CT within 24 hours were reviewed. Four readers with varying levels of experience reviewed the chest radiographs and predicted the likelihood of the presence of an effusion or parenchymal opacity on independent 5-point scales. The results were compared with the CT findings.

Results.—All readers regardless of experience had similar accuracy in detecting pleural effusions. Among 117 pleural effusions, 66% were detected on chest radiographs (53%, 71%, and 92% of small, moderate, and large effusions) with 89% specificity. Similarly, 65% of all parenchymal opacities were detected on chest radiographs, also with 89% specificity. Most (93%) of the misdiagnosed pulmonary opacities were simply not seen. Meniscus, apical cap, lateral band, and subpulmonic opacity were highly specific findings but had low individual sensitivity for effusions. The finding of homogeneous opacity, including both layering and gradient opacities, was the most sensitive sign of effusion. Atelectasis can occasionally mimic the pleural veil sign of effusion, accounting for most false-positive findings.

Conclusion.—Radiologists interpreting bedside chest radiographs of ICU patients detect large pleural effusions 92% of the time and can exclude large effusions with high confidence. However, small and medium effusions often are misdiagnosed as parenchymal opacities (45%) or are not seen (55%). Pulmonary opacities often are missed (34%) but are rarely misdiagnosed as pleural effusions (7%).

▶ The authors studied the ability of radiologists to detect pleural effusions on portable radiographs using chest CT as the gold standard for evaluation of the pleura. It is recognized that basilar airspace disease may mimic pleural fluid, particularly on portable radiographs performed without the benefit of lateral chest radiography. The authors retrospectively analyzed the radiographs of 100 patients in the surgical intensive care unit who had undergone chest CT less than 24 hours after the radiographs.

The authors list the following radiographic findings of pleural effusion on bedside radiography:

- Extrapulmonary opacities situated between the lung and chest wall or between the lung and diaphragm, including the meniscus sign, apical cap, lateral band, and subpulmonic opacity
- Homogeneous opacities overlying the hemithorax without obscuration of pulmonary markings, including layering and gradient opacities
- Analysis of the location of the mediastinum in cases of opaque hemithorax with mediastinal shift contralateral to the opaque hemithorax

The authors found an overall sensitivity of 66% for the diagnosis of pleural effusion on portable radiography and a specificity of 89%. Ninety-two percent of the large pleural effusions, 71% of the moderate pleural effusions, and 53% of the small pleural effusions were correctly diagnosed. However, 34% of the pleural effusions were missed on portable radiographs, and most of these were small. Almost half of the missed effusions were interpreted as parenchymal disease. In addition, 11% of the suspected effusions were false-positive findings in which airspace disease mimicked pleural fluid.

The meniscus, apical cap, lateral band, subpulmonic opacity, layering opacity, and gradient opacity were all highly specific but not sensitive signs of pleural effusion. Homogeneous opacity was the most sensitive sign of pleural effusion. Most false-positive findings were because of atelectasis. These findings should be taken into consideration when evaluating bedside radiographs of critically ill patients and when suggesting the presence of a pleural effusion.

M. L. Rosado de Christenson, MD

Extracardiac Findings on Coronary CT Angiograms: Limited Versus Complete Image Review
Johnson KM, Dennis JM, Dowe DA (Yale Univ School of Medicine, New Haven, CT; Univ of Utah School of Medicine, Salt Lake City; Atlantic Med Imaging, Galloway, NJ)
AJR Am J Roentgenol 195:143-148, 2010

Objective.—Cardiac CT often reveals findings outside the heart and great vessels. A few cardiologists have suggested that the field of interpretation be restricted to avoid false-positive diagnoses. Radiologists generally favor a comprehensive review to avoid false-negative findings. The purpose of this study was to examine this tradeoff by comparing broad and focused approaches with viewing coronary CT angiograms.

Materials and Methods.—Outpatient coronary CT angiography was performed on consecutively registered patients. In the broad approach to review, both the large field-of-view and small field-of-view image sets, including lung windows, were evaluated. In the focused approach, attention was centered on the heart, great vessels, and immediately adjacent structures and did not include lung windows. Each finding was classified as necessitating immediate therapy, timely additional workup, longer-term follow-up, or no action.

Results.—Among 6,920 patients, 1,642 (23.7%) had one or more extracardiac findings for a total of 1,901 findings in the broad viewing scheme. Of the 6,920 patients, 16.2% had a finding necessitating therapy, workup, or follow-up. In the focused viewing scheme, 90.9% of the findings necessitating therapy, 64.1% necessitating workup, and 51.2% necessitating follow-up were missed. Use of the focused approach resulted in fewer false-positive diagnoses, but five malignant tumors of the breast, 88 lung infiltrates, 43 cases of adenopathy, two cases of polycystic kidney disease, one breast abscess, and one case of splenic flexure diverticulitis were missed.

Conclusion.—Almost one fourth of all patients who underwent diagnostic coronary CT angiography in this study had extracardiac findings. Several serious diagnoses were missed with the limited viewing approach, but use of the broad viewing approach led to more workup and follow-up imaging.

▶ Several dedicated CT studies, including cardiac CT, yield information regarding organs outside the area of imaging interest. In the case of cardiac CT, there is the potential to evaluate a large portion of the lungs and mediastinum, chest wall, chest wall soft tissues, and parts of the upper abdomen. Cardiologists perform a large number of cardiac CT studies in the United States. Some of these specialists have suggested that evaluation of extracardiac structures should be limited to the subset of images used to diagnose cardiac disease, stating that a more comprehensive evaluation will lead to too many false-positive findings.

The authors undertook their study to compare the comprehensive and focused viewing approaches of consecutive coronary CT angiographic studies performed in an outpatient imaging center from March 2004 through November 2008. The studies were performed with 2 multidetector CT scanners: 64- and 16-detector rows. They defined extracardiac finding as any finding outside the pericardium and included aortic and pulmonary artery abnormalities. The sequelae of surgery or intervention were not included. Normal anatomic variants, artifacts, and insignificant abnormalities (bone islands, osteophytes, and healed rib fractures) were not recorded. Two data sets were reviewed: one with a small field of view (FOV) to encompass the heart and one with a large FOV to include the entire width of the chest. Extracardiac abnormalities were classified as those needing immediate therapy, timely further workup, longer-term follow-up, or no further action. Of 6920 patients in the study, 1642 had one or more extracardiac findings. Findings felt to require treatment, evaluation, or follow-up were present in 1119 patients (16.2% of the total). The most common finding was hiatus hernia, followed by pulmonary nodules (in 431 patients). Neoplastic disease was newly diagnosed in 5 patients.

The authors state that with the focused viewing approach, 90.9% of findings necessitating therapy, 64.1% of those necessitating workup, and 51.2% of those necessitating follow-up were missed. Among missed cases, the authors listed 88 infiltrates, 1 unsuspected metastatic renal cell carcinoma, 5 breast masses and 1 breast abscess, 3 malignant lung tumors, 2 cases of polycystic kidney disease, and 1 acute colonic diverticulitis. The authors stated that 33.9% of all extracardiac findings in the study were minor and could be dismissed at the time of image interpretation. The evaluation of the incidental findings resulted in additional costs of $83 035, with $39 597 spent on a single patient who had complications following lung biopsy. The average cost per patient was $86.00.

The authors acknowledge a series of limitations to their study:

- Lack of double reading of the images
- Subjective categorization of the findings with regard to the need for follow-up or work-up
- Lack of documentation of patient outcomes
- Lack of cost-benefit analysis

The authors recommend that any limited viewing should include evaluation of lung window images and advise evaluation of the vascular structures for exclusion of pulmonary emboli. They further state that because minor findings by far outnumber major findings, the ability to differentiate between the 2 will be the crucial factor in determining the cost-benefit ratio for the evaluation of such incidental abnormalities.

M. L. Rosado de Christenson, MD

A Prospective Evaluation of Dose Reduction and Image Quality in Chest CT Using Adaptive Statistical Iterative Reconstruction
Leipsic J, Nguyen G, Brown J, et al (Univ of British Columbia, Vancouver, Canada)
AJR Am J Roentgenol 195:1095-1099, 2010

Objective.—The purpose of this study was to compare the subjective image quality, image noise, and radiation dose of chest CT images reconstructed with a 30% blend of iterative reconstruction and 70% conventional filtered back projection (FBP) with those of images generated with 100% FBP.

Subjects and Methods.—Clinically indicated chest CT examinations of 292 consecutively registered patients were prospectively alternately assigned to two scanners on which different reconstruction techniques were used: adaptive statistical iterative reconstruction (ASIR) blended with FBP and 100% FBP. Both acquisitions were performed with dose modulation (noise index, 25 for ASIR and 21 for FBP). Patient demographics and habitus were recorded. Two radiologists blinded to the reconstruction algorithm independently scored subjective image quality on a 3-point Likert scale and measured image noise and radiation dose.

Results.—Compared with FBP images, ASIR images had significantly lower subjective image quality ($p = 0.01$), less image noise ($p = 0.02$), and less radiation dose ($p < 0.0001$). The CT dose index of the ASIR cohort (11.3 ± 51) was significantly lower than that of the 100% FBP cohort (15.4 ± 6.3) ($p < 0.0001$). Interobserver agreement on subjective image quality was excellent for both ASIR and FBP (Cronbach α, 0.92, $p < 0.0001$; Cronbach α, 0.85, $p < 0.0001$).

Conclusion.—In clinically indicated chest CT examinations, ASIR images had better image quality and less image noise at a lower radiation dose than images acquired with a conventional FBP reconstruction algorithm.

▶ The authors comment on the marked increase in the number of CT examinations in the United States ranging from 3 million studies in the early 1980s to 67 million studies in the year 2006 and the resultant increased radiation dose to the patient population, estimated as a 100- to 600-fold increase over the dose provided by conventional radiography. The association between ionizing radiation and malignant neoplasia raises real concerns about the effects of medical imaging on the health of the population, with estimates of approximately 2% of all incident cancers in the United States potentially related to the use of diagnostic CT. Because of these concerns, efforts are being made toward dose reduction with various techniques that include reduced tube voltage, automated tube current modulation, and decreased scan length. Many dose reduction techniques result in increased image noise. A recently introduced dose reduction technique, adaptive statistically iterative reconstruction (ASIR), is a complex method of image reconstruction with the object of reducing image noise that uses mathematic and statistical modeling to identify and reduce noise. This method is different from standard filtered back projection (FBP) CT reconstruction algorithms. Iterative reconstruction as a noise and dose reduction tool has been previously validated in abdominal CT and CT coronary angiography.

The authors studied and compared subjective image quality, image noise, and radiation dose of thoracic CT images reconstructed with a blend of 30% ASIR and 70% FBP with those of images reconstructed with 100% FBP. They prospectively scanned 292 consecutively registered patients referred from May 1, 2009, to October 14, 2009, for noncardiac-gated chest CT. Patients undergoing low-dose chest CT for nodule follow-up were excluded from the study. The scans were obtained in two 64-detector row CT scanners of the same manufacturer with similar scanning parameters that included tube voltage of 120 kV(p) for patients with body mass index (BMI) of more than 30 and 100 kV(p) for all others. Two radiologists blinded to the technique used evaluated the images for noise, image quality, and low contrast resolution. In addition, noise measurements were obtained from the picture archiving and communication systems images using the mid–descending aorta, and the CT noise index was recorded in all cases. ASIR was used in 130 cases and FBP in 162 cases without significant differences with respect to patient age, BMI, or tube voltage. Patients scanned with ASIR had a shorter scan length.

The authors found that ASIR was associated with a 25% dose reduction, with the most important risk factor associated with radiation dose being a high BMI. Patients scanned with ASIR had significantly lower CT dose indexes, lower measured image noise, and higher signal-to-noise ratios. Image quality was also superior in the images of patients scanned with ASIR.

The authors conclude that the use of ASIR allows the use of a higher noise index with a resultant reduction in tube current and radiation dose. They state that the resulting images have significantly reduced noise and increased subjective image quality. In addition, reconstruction times using ASIR were less than 5 minutes.

The authors list the following limitations to their study:

- The ASIR scanner was more advanced than the control scanner, which may have had an impact on differences in image quality.

- Iterative reconstruction techniques are not available across all platforms, but the authors state that several vendors are developing various forms of CT iterative reconstruction. Thus, the published results apply only to equipment available from 1 vendor.

- The use of ASIR on low-dose pulmonary nodule follow-up scans is not known as these studies were excluded.

Lastly, the authors do disclose that the first author of this article is on the speaker's bureau and advisory board for the company that manufactures the ASIR CT scanner.

M. L. Rosado de Christenson, MD

Diffuse Disease

Cryptogenic Organizing Pneumonia: Serial High-Resolution CT Findings in 22 Patients
Lee JW, Lee KS, Lee HY, et al (Sungkyunkwan Univ School of Medicine, Seoul, Republic of Korea)
AJR Am J Roentgenol 195:916-922, 2010

Objective.—We conducted a review of serial high-resolution CT (HRCT) findings of cryptogenic organizing pneumonia (COP).

Materials and Methods.—Over the course of 14 years, we saw 32 patients with biopsy-confirmed COP. Serial HRCT scans were available for only 22 patients (seven men and 15 women; mean age, 52 years; median follow-up period, 8 months; range, 5–135 months). Serial CT scans were evaluated by two chest radiologists who reached a conclusion by consensus. Overall changes in disease extent were classified as cured, improved (i.e., $\geq$ 10% decrease in extent), not changed, or progressed (i.e., $\geq$ 10%

increase in extent). When there were remaining abnormalities, the final follow-up CT images were analyzed to express observers' ideas regarding what type of interstitial lung disease the images most likely suggested.

Results.—The two most common patterns of lung abnormality on initial scans were ground-glass opacification (86% of patients [19/22]) and consolidation (77% of patients [17/22]), distributed along the bronchovascular bundles or subpleural lungs in 13 patients (59%). In six patients (27%), the disease disappeared completely; in 15 patients (68%), the disease was decreased in extent; and in one patient (5%), no change in extent was detected on follow-up CT. When lesions remained, the final follow-up CT findings were reminiscent of fibrotic nonspecific interstitial pneumonia in 10 of 16 patients (63%).

Conclusion.—Although COP is a disease with a generally good prognosis, most patients (73%) with COP have some remaining disease seen on follow-up CT scans, and, in such cases, the lesions generally resemble a fibrotic nonspecific interstitial pneumonia pattern (Fig 2).

▶ The authors present data on CT imaging follow-up of patients with biopsy-proven idiopathic cryptogenic organizing pneumonia (COP). They define COP as a lung disease characterized by plugs of granulation tissue that occupy small airways, alveolar ducts, and alveoli with associated chronic inflammatory cells in the airway walls. Affected patients often present with a subacute illness, symptoms of dyspnea and fever, and constitutional complaints including malaise and weight loss. Imaging findings of COP are characterized by bilateral patchy consolidations in the subpleural aspects of the lower lobes. High-resolution CT (HRCT) of COP is characterized by consolidations or pulmonary nodules that may be distributed along the bronchovascular bundles or

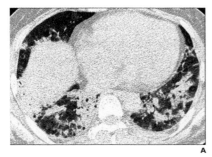 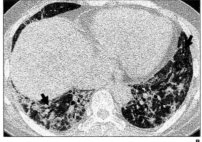

A   B

FIGURE 2.—56-year-old woman with cryptogenic organizing pneumonia showing improvement but remaining disease. **A,** Transverse thin-section (1.0-mm section thickness) CT scan obtained at level of liver dome shows bilateral patchy areas of consolidation and nodules distributed along bronchovascular bundles in lower lung zones. Total extent of parenchymal abnormalities on CT scans was 50% (consolidation, 40%; nodule, 10%). **B,** Nine-month follow-up CT scan obtained at similar level to panel A shows decreased extent of parenchymal lesions. Total extent of remaining lung lesions was 30% (ground-glass opacification, 20%; reticulation, 10%). Note associated traction bronchiectasis (*arrows*) in both lower lobes. Remaining abnormalities are suggestive of fibrotic nonspecific interstitial pneumonia. (Reprinted from Lee JW, Lee KS, Lee HY, et al. Cryptogenic organizing pneumonia: serial high-resolution CT findings in 22 patients. *AJR Am J Roentgenol.* 2010;195:916-922, with permission from the American Journal of Roentgenology.)

subpleural lung parenchyma. Patients with COP usually respond to corticosteroids and have a good prognosis, although disease progression is reported.

This study is a review of data gathered from patients with documented COP in a single tertiary care hospital identified through the retrospective review of all surgical biopsy files from January 1995 to May 2008 with a histologic diagnosis of organizing pneumonia. Seventy-two patients were found, but 40 were excluded, as they had associated collagen vascular disease, concurrent pulmonary infection, or drug-related lung disease. The 32 remaining patients were presumed to have a diagnosis of (idiopathic) COP. Ten of these patients had either no follow-up HRCT or a follow-up HRCT within a month of the original study, and none died of their disease. The remaining 22 patients had follow-up chest CT, with the shortest follow-up period being 2 months. Given the span of the data collection, images were acquired on a variety of CT scanners with variable technical parameters. Two chest radiologists reviewed the patterns and distribution of CT abnormalities at the initial and final CT studies, and conclusions were reached by consensus. Findings were categorized as completely resolved, improved (≥10% decrease in extent of involvement), stable, and progressed (≥10% increase in extent of involvement). All patients presented with dyspnea, cough, or fever. Pulmonary function studies (available for 19 patients) were recorded.

On initial HRCT, the most common abnormality was ground glass opacity (86%), followed by consolidation (77%). Disease was distributed along the bronchovascular bundles or subpleural lungs in 59%. The authors add that all initial scans showed involvement of the lower lobes, with lower lobe predominance in 55% of the cases.

On follow-up CT there was complete resolution of disease in 27% of patients and improvement in 68%. One patient showed no change, and no patients showed interval disease progression. The authors also note that 63% of patients with residual disease on follow-up HRCT had a pattern of involvement similar to that of fibrotic nonspecific pneumonia (NSIP) with basilar subpleural ground glass opacity and reticulation and traction bronchiectasis in 2 of these 10 patients (Fig 2). Other patterns of pulmonary disease in the remaining patients with residual lung disease were reminiscent of hypersensitivity pneumonitis, usual interstitial pneumonia (with honeycomb lung), and cellular NSIP.

Nine percent of patients had clinical recurrence of COP. The authors state that when reticular opacities are part of the initial imaging manifestations of COP, affected patients are less likely to respond to corticosteroids and may progress to pulmonary fibrosis. In their study, 4 patients exhibited initial reticulation and all 4 had residual abnormalities on follow-up HRCT. In addition, the authors state that approximately half of NSIP biopsy specimens exhibit areas of organizing pneumonia. Thus, they admit the possibility that some of the cases diagnosed as COP may have actually represented NSIP.

The authors acknowledge several limitations in their study:

- Retrospective review
- Small sample size
- Exclusion of the 10 patients who did not have follow-up HRCT
- Variability of follow-up intervals

They conclude that COP has a good prognosis in most patients and warn that residual CT abnormalities may mimic fibrotic NSIP.

M. L. Rosado de Christenson, MD

Interstitial Lung Disease

Biopsy-proved Idiopathic Pulmonary Fibrosis: Spectrum of Nondiagnostic Thin-Section CT Diagnoses

Sverzellati N, Wells AU, Tomassetti S, et al (Univ of Parma Padiglione Barbieri, Italy; Royal Brompton Hosp, London, England; Giovanni Battista Morgagni Hosp, Forlì, Italy; et al)
Radiology 254:957-964, 2010

Purpose.—To document the spectrum of misleading thin-section computed tomographic (CT) diagnoses in patients with biopsy-proved idiopathic pulmonary fibrosis (IPF).

Materials and Methods.—This study had institutional review board approval, and patient consent was not required. Three observers, blinded to any clinical information and the purpose of the study, recorded thin-section CT differential diagnoses and assigned a percentage likelihood to each for a group of 123 patients (79 men, 44 women; age range, 27–82 years) with various chronic interstitial lung diseases, including a core group of 55 biopsy-proved cases of IPF. Patients with IPF in the core group, in whom IPF was diagnosed as low-grade probability (<30%) by at least two observers, were considered to have atypical IPF cases, and the alternative diagnoses were analyzed further.

Results.—Thirty-four (62%) of 55 biopsy-proved IPF cases were regarded as alternative diagnoses. In these atypical IPF cases, the first-choice diagnoses, expressed with high degree of probability, were nonspecific interstitial pneumonia (NSIP; 18 [53%] of 34), chronic hypersensitivity pneumonitis (HP; four [12%] of 34), sarcoidosis (three [9%] of 34), and organizing pneumonia (one [3%] of 34); in eight (23%) of 34 cases, no single diagnosis was favored by more than one observer. Frequent differential diagnoses, although not always the first-choice diagnosis, were NSIP ($n = 29$), chronic HP ($n = 23$), and sarcoidosis ($n = 9$).

Conclusion.—In the correct clinical setting, a diagnosis of IPF is not excluded by thin-section CT appearances more suggestive of NSIP, chronic HP, or sarcoidosis (Fig 2).

▶ Idiopathic pulmonary fibrosis (IPF) is the clinical term used to describe patients with a histological diagnosis of usual interstitial pneumonia (UIP) characterized by temporal heterogeneity of the microscopic findings with admixed areas of fibrosis in various stages, inflammation, and scattered interspersed near-normal findings. It is important for the clinician to establish the diagnosis of IPF since it carries a worse prognosis than the other idiopathic interstitial pneumonias and a much worse prognosis than many malignancies. Radiologists play an important role in the diagnosis of this entity characterized

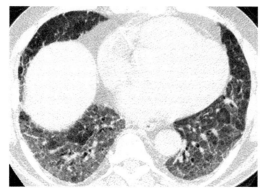

FIGURE 2.—Biopsy-proved IPF in 47-year-old man that was interpreted as high-probability (≥70%) NSIP by all three observers. Transverse thin-section CT scan obtained through the lower lungs shows a basilar peripheral predominant reticular pattern with ground-glass opacity and traction bronchiectasis. (Reprinted from Sverzellati N, Wells AU, Tomassetti S, et al. Biopsy-proved idiopathic pulmonary fibrosis: spectrum of nondiagnostic thin-section CT diagnoses. *Radiology.* 2010;254:957-964. Copyright by the Radiological Society of North America.)

by basilar predominant subpleural honeycomb lung on thin-section CT. However, it should be noted that other interstitial lung diseases can produce honeycomb lung and that the characteristic CT features of UIP are absent in up to 30% of patients according to the published literature.

The authors set out to identify the spectrum of CT differential diagnoses in patients with biopsy proven IPF. To this end, they retrospectively reviewed the interstitial lung disease databases of 3 different teaching hospitals in 2 different European countries (England and Italy) between January 1, 2003, and December 31, 2006. They identified a core group of consecutive patients with IPF consisting of 55 patients in the age group 44 to 74 years (mean age, 59 ± 6.2 years), comprising 39 men and 16 women. The diagnosis of UIP was confirmed by 2 pathologists applying current criteria. In addition, the authors randomly selected 2 other groups of patients with chronic interstitial lung disease and mixed them with the core study group. Patients with pulmonary infection, heart failure, and acute disease exacerbation at the time of CT were excluded. The patients were scanned with 3 different CT scanners (one 16-detector row multidetector scanner, one 64-detector row scanner, and one electron beam scanner). The vast majority of the images for 116 patients was transferred to CD-ROM and evaluated in 3 personal computers, and in 7 patients, hard-copy images were reviewed. The images were reviewed independently by 3 thoracic radiologists who listed their differential diagnoses and assigned a likelihood ratio to each diagnosis to the nearest 5%, totaling 100%. The authors separately assessed the clinical progression of disease by recording pulmonary functions 1 year later and defined functional deterioration as a decrease in the diffusing capacity of carbon monoxide of over 15%.

The observers interpreted the CT imaging findings as having high probability for IPF in 36%, 23% and 16% of the 55 patients. The first choice diagnosis most frequently recorded in the low probability for IPF cases was nonspecific interstitial pneumonia (Fig 2), followed by chronic hypersensitivity pneumonitis, sarcoidosis, and organizing pneumonia. The authors characterize these patients as having atypical CT findings of IPF. However, these patients appeared to have similar functional deterioration when compared with patients with typical IPF CT findings. Thus, the authors advice consideration of the diagnosis of IPF in patients with atypical CT findings who exhibit similar clinical deterioration as patients with IPF.

The authors acknowledge several limitations of their study. This study does not define the overall frequency of atypical CT appearances of IPF, as it was not a population-based study. The fact that the patient population was selected from centers specializing in pulmonary disease may have resulted in a bias toward complex or atypical cases. In addition, as the diagnosis of IPF may not require a biopsy in patients with typical CT findings, these patients with biopsy proven disease may have had a tendency for atypical CT manifestations. Finally, the radiologists who analyzed the images are experienced in pulmonary disease and may be more likely than other radiologists to consider alternate diagnoses.

M. L. Rosado de Christenson, MD

Pulmonary Thromboembolic Disease

Success of a Safe and Simple Algorithm to Reduce Use of CT Pulmonary Angiography in the Emergency Department

Stein EG, Haramati LB, Chamarthy M, et al (Albert Einstein College of Medicine, Bronx, NY)
AJR Am J Roentgenol 194:392-397, 2010

Objective.—The purpose of our study was to determine whether the radiation exposure to patients with suspected pulmonary embolism (PE) could be decreased by safely increasing the use of ventilation–perfusion (V/Q) scanning and decreasing the use of CT pulmonary angiography (CTPA) through an educational intervention.

Materials and Methods.—Collaborative educational seminars were held among the radiology, nuclear medicine, and emergency medicine departments in December 2006 and January 2007 regarding the radiation dose and accuracies of V/Q scanning and CTPA for diagnosing PE. To reduce radiation exposure, an imaging algorithm was introduced in which emergency department patients with a clinical suspicion of PE underwent chest radiography. If the chest radiograph was normal, V/Q scanning was recommended, otherwise CTPA was recommended. We retrospectively tallied the number and results of CTPA and V/Q scanning and calculated mean radiation effective dose before and after the intervention. False-negative findings were defined as subsequent thromboembolism within 90 days.

Results.—The number of CTPA examinations performed decreased from 1,234 in 2006 to 920 in 2007, and the number of V/Q scans increased from 745 in 2006 to 1,216 in 2007. The mean effective dose was reduced by 20%, from 8.0 mSv in 2006 to 6.4 mSv in 2007 ($p < 0.0001$). The patients who underwent CTPA and V/Q scanning in

2006 were of similar age. In 2007, the patients who underwent V/Q scanning were significantly younger. There was no significant difference in the false-negative rate (range, 0.8—1.2%) between CTPA and V/Q scanning in 2006 and 2007.

Conclusion.—The practice patterns of physicians changed in response to an educational intervention, resulting in a reduction in radiation exposure to emergency department patients with suspected PE without compromising patient safety (Fig 1).

▶ The increased utilization of diagnostic computed tomography (CT) in the United States and the resultant increasing dose of ionizing radiation to the population have received great attention in the media and the scientific literature. Over the past few decades, CT pulmonary angiography (CTPA) has almost supplanted ventilation-perfusion (V/Q) scintigraphy in the diagnosis of pulmonary thromboembolic disease. The authors state that the total effective radiation dose from CTPA is approximately 5 times larger than the total effective radiation dose from V/Q scintigraphy and that CTPA delivers a dose to the female breast approximately 20 to 40 times larger than V/Q scintigraphy. In addition, according to the Prospective Investigation of Pulmonary Embolism Diagnosis II trial, CTPA and V/Q scintigraphy have similar positive predictive values of 86% for CTPA and >85% for high-probability V/Q scintigrams. The purpose of their study was to determine whether a reduction in radiation dose to emergency department patients with suspected pulmonary thromboembolic disease could be achieved by increasing the use of V/Q scanning while reducing the use of CTPA.

The authors implemented an intervention designed to educate their physician colleagues in the emergency department with the hope of instituting the imaging algorithm shown on Figure 1 and described in the abstract. The authors retrospectively evaluated the result of their intervention by tallying the number and results of CTPAs and V/Q scintigrams performed quarterly the year before and the year after the educational intervention. They also calculated the mean effective dose for each patient in the study population with specific attention

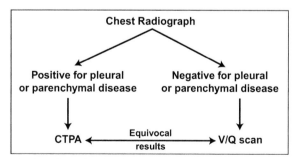

FIGURE 1.—Flowchart shows algorithm for suspected pulmonary embolism. CTPA = CT pulmonary angiography, V/Q scan = ventilation—perfusion scanning. (Reprinted from Stein EG, Haramati LB, Chamarthy M, et al. Success of a safe and simple algorithm to reduce use of CT pulmonary angiography in the emergency department. *AJR Am J Roentgenol.* 2010;194:392-397, with permission from American Journal of Roentgenology.)

to patients younger than 40 years. They assigned a dose of 2.2 mSv to each V/Q scan and a dose of 10 mSv to each CTPA according to the published work of Mettler et al.[1]

The authors found that 60% of their emergency department patients with suspected pulmonary thromboembolic disease were imaged with CTPA prior to the intervention, while approximately 60% were imaged with V/Q scintigraphy following the intervention. In addition, the population of patients evaluated with V/Q scanning subsequent to intervention was significantly younger than those evaluated with CTPA, and a significantly higher proportion of women were imaged with V/Q scanning before and after the intervention. They report a 20% reduction in mean effective dose for all patients after the intervention, a 32% reduction for women younger than 40 years, and a 34% reduction for all patients younger than 40 years.

The authors disclose the following limitations of their study: the retrospective nature of the study and the fact that objective clinical assessment of patients and D-dimer evaluations were not required prior to imaging. Uniform use of these additional criteria prior to imaging could potentially reduce the number of imaging studies performed for evaluation of patients with suspected pulmonary emboli. Based on the results of the study, it appears that an educational intervention can impact the way that our clinical colleagues practice and the kinds of imaging studies they order. If nothing else, such interventions would serve to educate clinicians in the area of radiation safety.

M. L. Rosado de Christenson, MD

Reference

1. Mettler FA Jr, Huda W, Yoshizumi TT, Mahesh M. Effective doses in radiology and diagnostic nuclear medicine: a catalog. *Radiology.* 2008;248:254-263.

Pulmonary Embolism in Pregnancy: CT Pulmonary Angiography Versus Perfusion Scanning
Shahir K, Goodman LR, Tali A, et al (Med College of Wisconsin, Milwaukee; et al)
AJR Am J Roentgenol 195:W214-W220, 2010

Objective.—The purpose of this study was to evaluate the equivalence of CT pulmonary angiography and perfusion scanning in terms of diagnostic quality and negative predictive value in the imaging of pulmonary embolism (PE) in pregnancy.

Materials and Methods.—Between 2000 and 2007 at a university hospital and a large private hospital, 199 pregnant patients underwent 106 CT pulmonary angiographic examinations and 99 perfusion scans. Image quality was evaluated, and the findings were reread by radiologists and compared with the original clinical readings. Three-month follow-up findings of PE and deep venous thrombosis were recorded.

Results.—PE was found in four of the 106 patients (3.7%) who underwent CT pulmonary angiography. The overall image quality was poor in 5.6% of cases, acceptable in 17.9%, and good in 76.4%. Fourteen CT and nine radiographic studies showed other clinically significant abnormalities. Six patients had indeterminate CT pulmonary angiographic findings, three had normal perfusion scans, and none underwent anticoagulation. All perfusion scan findings were normal. There was one incomplete study, and follow-up CT pulmonary angiography performed the same day showed PE. Two of 99 studies (2.02%) showed intermediate probability of the presence of PE; PE was not found at CT pulmonary angiography, but pneumonia was found. PE was found in one postpartum patient 9 weeks after she had undergone CT pulmonary angiography and ultrasound with normal findings. None of the patients died.

Conclusion.—CT pulmonary angiography and perfusion scanning have equivalent clinical negative predictive value (99% for CT pulmonary angiography; 100% for perfusion scanning) and image quality in the care of pregnant patients. Therefore, the choice of study should be based on other considerations, such as radiation concern, radiographic results, alternative diagnosis, and equipment availability. Reducing the amount of radiation to the maternal breast favors use of perfusion scanning when the radiographic findings are normal and there is no clinical suspicion of an alternative diagnosis.

▶ The evaluation of pulmonary embolism in pregnancy is a much discussed and controversial issue. Various clinical and radiological societies are in the process of drafting guidelines for the evaluation of these patients. The authors preface their findings by stating that women who are pregnant or in the postpartum period are 2 to 4 times as likely as nonpregnant subjects to develop venous thromboembolism. Ultrasound of the deep venous systems of the lower extremities is often performed because the study does not involve exposure to ionizing radiation. However, exclusion of deep venous thrombosis does not exclude the diagnosis of pulmonary thromboembolism (PTE). Currently, this diagnosis requires the use of ionizing radiation.

The authors state that a low-dose perfusion scintigraphic scan delivers a dose of 0.1 to 0.37 mGy (0.1-0.37 mSv) for a 1.5 mCi dose of technetium Tc 99m—labeled macroaggregated albumin to the embryo compared with 0.1 to 0.66 mGy with CT pulmonary angiography (CTPA). However, CTPA delivers a minimum radiation dose of 20 mGy per breast to an average-sized woman (compared with 3 mGy for standard mammography), whereas perfusion scanning delivers a much smaller dose of 0.11 to 0.31 mGy. CTPA also may expose the fetus to the theoretic risk of iodine-induced hypothyroidism. As these studies are consistently used for the diagnosis of PTE, the authors set out to determine which of the 2 had a better image quality and what was the likelihood of subsequent PTE after a negative diagnosis of PTE. They retrospectively analyzed image quality and the negative predictive value of CTPA in a sample of pregnant women evaluated for pulmonary embolus during the years 2000 to 2007.

One hundred patients underwent only CTPA, 93 only perfusion scanning, and 6 both. One hundred six patients were imaged at a university hospital and 93 at a private hospital. Acute PTE was diagnosed by finding a filling defect within a pulmonary artery or absence of opacification of a pulmonary artery. Chronic PTE was diagnosed when there was complete occlusion of a vessel smaller than the pulmonary arteries of the same order of branching, a peripheral eccentric filling defect along the vessel wall, and a band or web in a contrast-filled artery and/or smaller thick-walled contrast-filled arteries.

Objective criteria for image quality were based on the mean attenuation in the left lower lobe pulmonary artery at the beginning of its vertical course in an oval region of interest greater than two-thirds the width of the vessel; 169 Hounsfield unit (HU) or less was considered poor enhancement; 170 to 209 HU, acceptable enhancement; and 210 HU or more, good enhancement.

Perfusion scanning was performed by administering 1.0 to 1.5 mCi of technetium Tc 99m—labeled macroaggregated albumin, which is one half the radiopharmaceutical dose used in patients who are not pregnant. The patients were encouraged to empty their bladders frequently to minimize fetal dose. A positive result was one of high probability when there were ≥1.5 segmental perfusion defects. A negative result corresponded to normal perfusion; very low probability for PTE (nonsegmental or small subsegmental defects) or low probability for PTE (≤1 moderate size subsegmental perfusion defect). Intermediate probability and incomplete studies were considered indeterminate.

The authors report a very low incidence of PTE among their pregnant patients (2%). They found both scintigraphy and CT to have equal image quality. The percentage of nondiagnostic CTPA (6%) was not statistically different from the indeterminate perfusion scans (3%). Fourteen CTPAs showed additional findings.

The authors state that the risk of radiation to the fetus from perfusion scanning may be lower than that afforded by natural background radiation. The authors called for the formulation of specific clinical criteria for defining a high-risk group for PTE in pregnancy, given the low incidence of pulmonary embolism. The authors believe that perfusion scanning is preferable for patients with normal chest radiographs and low likelihood of having another disease to account for their symptoms.

M. L. Rosado de Christenson, MD

Pulmonary Embolism at CT Angiography: Implications for Appropriateness, Cost, and Radiation Exposure in 2003 Patients
Mamlouk MD, vanSonnenberg E, Gosalia R, et al (Univ of California, Irvine, Orange; St Joseph's Hosp and Med Ctr, Phoenix, AZ; et al)
Radiology 256:625-632, 2010

Purpose.—To determine whether thromboembolic risk factor assessment could accurately indicate the pretest probability for pulmonary embolism (PE), and if so, computed tomographic (CT) angiography might be targeted more appropriately than in current usage, resulting in decreased costs and radiation exposure.

Materials and Methods.—Institutional review board approval was obtained. Electronic medical records of 2003 patients who underwent CT angiography for possible PE during 1½ years (July 2004 to February 2006) were reviewed retrospectively for thromboembolic risk factors. Risk factors that were assessed included immobilization, malignancy, hypercoagulable state, excess estrogen state, a history of venous thromboembolism, age, and sex. Logistic regressions were conducted to test the significance of each risk factor.

Results.—Overall, CT angiograms were negative for PE in 1806 (90.16%) of 2003 patients. CT angiograms were positive for PE in 197 (9.84%) of 2003 patients; 6.36% were Emergency Department patients, and 13.46% were inpatients. Of the 197 patients with CT angiograms positive for PE, 192 (97.46%) had one or more risk factors, of which age of 65 years or older (69.04%) was the most common. Of the 1806 patients with CT angiograms negative for PE, 520 (28.79%) had no risk factors. The sensitivity and negative predictive value of risk factor assessment in all patients were 97.46% and 99.05%, respectively. All risk factors, except sex, were significant in the multivariate logistic regression ($P < .031$).

Conclusion.—In the setting of no risk factors, it is extraordinarily unlikely (0.95% chance) to have a CT angiogram positive for PE. This selectivity and triage step should help reduce current costs and radiation exposure to patients.

▶ The authors state that pulmonary embolism is one of the most common causes of unexpected death requiring prompt diagnosis. The diagnosis is usually achieved with CT pulmonary angiography (CTPA), which has sensitivity and specificity of 90% and 95%, respectively. The Prospective Investigation of Pulmonary Embolism Diagnosis II study emphasizes the need for determining the pretest clinical probability for pulmonary embolism to decide whether or when to perform CTPA. CTPA is a common study in all of our practices. The authors provide estimates of nearly 600 000 such examinations performed in the United States in 2008 at costs ranging from $2000 to $3000 at 2 of the authors' institutions. Not the least of the costs relate to the radiation burden on the population with its inherent risk of radiation-induced malignancies.

The authors retrospectively reviewed the electronic medical records of 2003 patients suspected of having pulmonary embolism who underwent CTPA for diagnosis between July 20, 2004, and February 24, 2006, at their 700-bed teaching hospital in Phoenix, Arizona. The patient population included 847 men and 1156 women with a mean age of 51 years, including both inpatients and patients evaluated in the emergency department. Dimerized plasmin fragment D (D-dimer) test results were available in 99 patients. It should be noted that none of the patients who had a negative D-dimer test result had pulmonary embolism. Patients were imaged with either 16-detector row or

64-detector row multidetector CT scanners. The following risk factors were assessed from a review of the charts: immobilization (as recorded on the chart or as presumed from a history of pelvic or long bone fracture requiring admission, postoperative state, neurologic events, and prolonged travel), malignancy, hypercoagulable state (from hereditary or systemic conditions known to result in hypercoagulability), excess estrogen state (including pregnancy, peripartum state, oral contraceptive use, or hormone replacement therapy), and a history of deep venous thrombosis or pulmonary embolism. In addition, age and gender were also analyzed, and patients were stratified into younger or older than 65 years groups.

The authors conclude that in the absence of risk factors for pulmonary thromboembolic disease, it is extremely unlikely to have a positive CTPA result for pulmonary embolism (0.95% chance). They add that when there is a combination of absent risk factors and negative D-dimer test results, a positive CTPA result would be extraordinarily rare. The authors make the following observations from their data:

- All risk factors were significant with the exception of excess estrogen state in 7 bivariate logistic regressions.
- All risk factors except for sex were significant with multivariate logistic regression.
- Patients with a positive CTPA result for pulmonary embolism most commonly had 2 risk factors.
- For positive CTPA result, the most common risk factor was age of 65 years or older, followed by immobilization, male sex, malignancy, prior pulmonary embolism or deep venous thrombosis, and hypercoagulable state.
- Inpatients were twice as likely as emergency department patients to have a positive CTPA result.

The authors add that the mean measured effective dose in patients scanned with the 64-detector row scanner was 19.9 ± 1.38 mSv per study. They add that absorbed organ doses are highest in skin, breast, esophagus, heart, and liver. They cite an article that reports an increased relative risk of breast or lung cancer in patients undergoing 1 CTPA, particularly young women.[1]

The authors list several limitations to their study: the retrospective nature of the review, review of CTPA results rather than the studies themselves, low number of D-dimer studies, subjective analysis of immobilization, and the probability equation for pulmonary embolism being based in patients in whom a study was obtained rather than in those in whom it was not.

M. L. Rosado de Christenson, MD

Reference

1. Hurwitz LM, Reiman RE, Yoshizumi TT, et al. Radiation dose from contemporary cardiothoracic multidetector CT protocols with an anthropomorphic female phantom: implications for cancer induction. *Radiology.* 2007;245:742-750.

Infection

H1N1 Influenza: Initial Chest Radiographic Findings in Helping Predict Patient Outcome

Aviram G, Bar-Shai A, Sosna J, et al (Tel Aviv Univ, Israel; Hadassah Hebrew Univ Med Ctr, Jerusalem, Israel)

Radiology 255:252-259, 2010

Purpose.—To retrospectively evaluate whether findings on initial chest radiographs of influenza A (H1N1) patients can help predict clinical outcome.

Materials and Methods.—Institutional review board approval was obtained; informed consent was waived. All adult patients admitted to the emergency department (May to September 2009) with a confirmed diagnosis of H1N1 influenza who underwent frontal chest radiography within 24 hours were included. Radiologic findings were characterized by type and pattern of opacities and zonal distribution. Major adverse outcome measures were mechanical ventilation and death.

Results.—Of 179 H1N1 influenza patients, 97 (54%) underwent chest radiography at admission; 39 (40%) of these had abnormal radiologic findings likely related to influenza infection and five (13%) of these 39 had adverse outcomes. Fifty-eight (60%) of 97 patients had normal radiographs; two (3%) of these had adverse outcomes ($P = .113$). Characteristic imaging findings included the following: groundglass (69%), consolidation (59%), frequently patchy (41%), and nodular (28%) opacities. Bilateral opacities were common (62%), with involvement of multiple lung zones (72%). Findings in four or more zones and bilateral peripheral distribution occurred with significantly higher frequency in patients with adverse outcomes compared with patients with good outcomes (multizonal opacities: 60% vs 6%, $P = .01$; bilateral peripheral opacities: 60% vs 15%, $P = .049$).

Conclusion.—Extensive involvement of both lungs, evidenced by the presence of multizonal and bilateral peripheral opacities, is associated with adverse prognosis. Initial chest radiography may have significance in helping predict clinical outcome but normal initial radiographs cannot exclude adverse outcome.

▶ The authors set out to retrospectively evaluate whether findings on initial chest radiography obtained in patients with influenza A (H1N1) can help predict clinical outcomes. To this end, they collected data from all consecutive patients admitted to the department of emergency medicine in their institution from May 1 to September 30, 2009, who fulfilled clinical criteria for the diagnosis of H1N1 infection, including body temperature of 100°F or higher, cough, sore throat, and real-time reverse transcriptase polymerase chain reaction assay positive for H1N1 virus. Patients with concurrent infections by other organisms were excluded.

Mechanical ventilation and death were established as main adverse outcome measures. All radiographs obtained within 24 hours of admission were included and were characterized as normal or abnormal. Abnormalities were characterized as ground glass opacity, consolidation, nodular opacities, patchy airspace disease, and confluent nodular opacities. The abnormalities were also characterized as central or peripheral and unilateral or bilateral, and their distribution was further assessed by describing whether the lesions affected the upper, middle, or lower lung zones.

The authors identified 179 adults with H1N1 during the study period, and 99 of these patients had frontal chest radiography within 24 hours of admission. Two patients were excluded because of concurrent pulmonary infection. Thus, the study population consisted of 97 patients with a mean age of 40.4 years and included 53 men and 44 women. Eighty-two percent of these patients were hospitalized, and the rest were discharged after initial evaluation. However, one of the discharged patients was subsequently admitted to a different hospital with progressive respiratory distress, received mechanical ventilation, and died 13 days later. Twenty-one percent of patients required admission to the intensive care unit, 9% required mechanical ventilation, and 5% died. These patients with adverse outcomes were significantly older.

Interestingly, only 40% of patients had chest radiographic findings on admission that were consistent with their influenza pulmonary infection. Sixty percent of patients had no imaging findings consistent with influenza, and 93% of these had normal chest radiographs. In addition, there was no significant difference in outcomes between patients with normal and abnormal chest radiographs.

The most frequent imaging abnormality was central ground glass opacity, followed by consolidation associated with ground glass opacity. Consolidations were patchy or nodular. The middle lung zones were most frequently involved, followed by the lower lung zones. Most patients had bilateral central involvement of multiple lung zones. Identification of bilateral peripheral involvement and involvement of 4 or more lung zones was helpful in predicting progression of disease to respiratory failure and adverse outcome.

Limitations of the study include: case interpretation by consensus and radiographic findings were not correlated with chest CT findings.

M. L. Rosado de Christenson, MD

Low Yield of Chest Radiography in a Large Tuberculosis Screening Program
Eisenberg RL, Pollock NR (Beth Israel Deaconess Med Ctr, Boston, MA)
Radiology 256:998-1004, 2010

Purpose.—To assess the frequency and spectrum of abnormalities on routine screening chest radiographs in the pre-employment evaluation of health care workers with positive tuberculin skin test (TST) results.

Materials and Methods.—The institutional review board approved this HIPAA-compliant retrospective study and waived the need for written informed patient consent. Chest radiographic reports of all 2586 asymptomatic individuals with positive TST results who underwent pre-employment evaluation between January 1, 2003, and December 31, 2007, were evaluated to determine the frequency of detection of evidence of active tuberculosis (TB) or latent TB infection (LTBI) and the spectrum of imaging findings. All chest radiographs interpreted as positive were reviewed by an experienced board-certified radiologist. If there was a discrepancy between the two readings, a second experienced radiologist served as an independent and final arbiter. Any follow-up chest radiographs or computed tomographic images that had been acquired by employee health services or by the employee's private physician as a result of a suspected abnormality detected at initial screening were also evaluated.

Results.—Of the 159 (6.1%) chest radiographic examinations that yielded abnormal results, there were no findings that were consistent with active TB. There were 92 cases of calcified granulomas, calcified lymph nodes, or both; 25 cases of apical pleural thickening; 16 cases of fibrous scarring; and 31 cases of noncalcified nodules. All cases of fibrous scarring involved an area smaller than 2 cm^2. All noncalcified nodules were 4 mm in diameter or smaller, with the exception of one primary lung malignancy and one necrotizing granuloma (negative for acid-fast bacilli) that grew *Mycobacterium kansasii* on culture.

Conclusion.—Universal chest radiography in a large pre-employment TB screening program was of low yield in the detection of active TB or increased LTBI reactivation risk, and it provided no assistance in deciding which individuals to prioritize for LTBI treatment.

▶ Most radiologists are familiar with the practice of obtaining chest radiographs in the setting of screening for pulmonary tuberculosis. This is particularly important in the evaluation of current and prospective hospital employees who may be exposed to tuberculosis and develop latent tuberculosis infection, as approximately 5% of them will develop active tuberculosis disease within the first 2 years, posing a risk to the very patients they care for. In the United States, most patients with latent tuberculosis infection are detected with the tuberculin skin test (TST). Based on the recommendations from the American Thoracic Society (ATS) and the Centers for Disease Control (CDC), such individuals are often screened with chest radiography to exclude the possibility of active tuberculosis infection.

The authors performed a retrospective study to evaluate the radiographic findings of individuals with positive TST results seeking employment at their hospital and included adults evaluated at their hospital and affiliated outpatient facilities between January 1, 2003, and December 31, 2007. Individuals with positive TST results underwent posteroanterior and lateral chest radiography. The authors defined the following imaging findings as consistent with active tuberculosis: cavitation, consolidation, and pleural effusion. Prior tuberculosis infection was inferred in the presence of focal pleural thickening, fibrous scarring, calcified pulmonary granulomas, calcified intrathoracic lymph nodes, and noncalcified lung nodules. As of 2006, all individuals with positive TST results demonstrating an induration of more than 10 mm underwent an in vitro diagnostic laboratory test for the diagnosis of latent tuberculosis infection.

The study population consisted of 2586 individuals with positive TST results, of whom 1422 were women. The subjects ranged in age between 18 and 65 years. Based on a prior smaller study, the authors estimated that approximately 95% of these individuals were foreign born and that approximately 93% had a history of vaccination with bacille Calmette-Guérin. They further estimated that approximately 70% of these individuals had risk factors for latent tuberculosis infection. They found 164 positive findings in 151 subjects (6.1% of the individuals in the study). Positive findings included calcified granulomas and/or lymph nodes (57.9%), apical pleural thickening (15.7%), fibrous scarring (10%), and small noncalcified nodules (19.5%).

The authors list 3 basic rationales for performing chest radiography on patients with positive TST results: (1) the exclusion of active tuberculosis; (2) the documentation of evidence of prior tuberculosis, which is associated with an increased risk for reactivation; (3) providing a baseline study to be used in the future as a comparative examination. The authors found no case of active tuberculosis in their study. They cite ATS and CDC statements regarding radiographic abnormalities in the setting of patients at risk for tuberculosis, which suggest that both nodules and fibrotic lesions pose an increased risk for reactivation of tuberculosis, whereas calcified nodules and pleural thickening suggest a lower risk of progression to active tuberculosis. One of the studies cited by the authors of the above guidelines suggest that fibrotic lung lesions larger than 2 cm^2 had an incidence of active tuberculosis almost twice as high as that of smaller lesions.

In this study, 94% of patients with positive TST results had negative chest radiographic findings. The rest had the findings listed above that are not suggestive of a significant risk of disease reactivation. In addition, patients with latent tuberculosis infection documented by positive in vitro test results were no more likely to have abnormal chest radiographic findings than those with negative test results, and no patient in either group exhibited large fibrotic lesions.

The authors conclude that screening chest radiography has an extremely low yield in this population. While they do not suggest that preemployment chest radiography be abandoned, they urge us to reflect on what it is that we learn from performing these studies and suggest that future large-scale studies be performed to clarify the reactivation risk associated with specific imaging abnormalities. They add that performing chest radiography in their study population did not help determine which individuals with latent tuberculosis infection should be prioritized for treatment.

M. L. Rosado de Christenson, MD

Trauma

Computed tomography in left-sided and right-sided blunt diaphragmatic rupture: experience with 43 patients

Chen H-W, Wong Y-C, Wang L-J, et al (Chang Gung Univ, Linkou, Taiwan)
Clin Radiol 65:206-212, 2010

Aim.—To investigate differences in the radiographic signs for left and right-sided blunt diaphragmatic rupture (BDR) in order to provide guidance to avoid missing these injuries.

Materials and Methods.—A retrospective review of the computed tomography (CT) examinations of 43 patients with BDR treated at our hospital between January 1995 and 2007 was undertaken. The presence of diaphragmatic discontinuity, diaphragmatic thickening, herniation of abdominal organs into the thoracic cavity, collar/hump sign, dependent viscera sign, abnormally elevated 4 cm or more above the dome of the other-sided hemi-diaphragm, and of associated injuries was recorded and their relationship to each other and to BDR diagnosis examined. A comparison between the use of axial and sagittal/coronal reconstruction images in diagnosis was also performed in 15 patients.

Results.—On axial imaging, left-sided diaphragmatic rupture occurred in 31 patients (72%) and right-sided in 12 (28%). Twenty-nine patients had associated injuries. More than 60% of the patients showed the "dependent viscera" sign, "abdominal organ herniation" sign, diaphragm thickening, or had a more than 4 cm elevation of one side of the diaphragm. "Diaphragmatic discontinuity" and "stomach herniation" were seen almost exclusively in left-sided rupture. Those with BDR and haemothorax had a significantly lower incidence of "diaphragm discontinuity" ($p = 0.034$) than those without haemothorax. Sagittal/coronal reconstruction slightly increased the number of band signs, diaphragmatic discontinuities and diaphragmatic thickenings seen.

Conclusions.—Of the CT signs examined in this study, when herniation of abdominal organs was used as a diagnostic marker, only a very small fraction of trauma patients identifiable by CT would be missed. Further, CT signs differ for left-sided and right-sided BDR, thus the possibility of BDR should be considered when any of the reported CT signs are present.

▶ Although diaphragmatic rupture is a rare consequence of blunt traumatic injury occurring in 3% to 8% of patients who undergo emergency laparotomy following trauma, up to 66% of such injuries are initially missed and may be later diagnosed at the time of surgery. Unfortunately, some of these injuries are not diagnosed during the patient's initial hospital admission and may manifest years later.

Diaphragmatic rupture in blunt traumatic injury is thought to result from a sudden increase in intra-abdominal pressure at the time of trauma. Diaphragmatic injury is reported to occur more frequently on the left side presumably because of the ability of the liver to dissipate the increased intra-abdominal pressure and a postulated greater strength of the right hemidiaphragm. However, some studies report relatively similar incidences of right and left diaphragmatic ruptures. Although this condition may be initially clinically silent, delayed diagnosis is associated with increased morbidity and mortality. The prospective diagnosis of such injuries requires a high index of suspicion on the part of the radiologist.

The authors undertook a retrospective review of 43 patients who had surgically proven diaphragmatic rupture after blunt injury to identify the CT differences between left and right diaphragmatic injuries and to determine the relationship between specific signs of diaphragmatic injury and CT evidence of chest injury. All the patients in the study were victims of motor vehicle collisions, and patients with diaphragmatic injury who had penetrating injury or who did not have CT examinations were excluded. Thirty-one patients had abdominal CT alone, and 12 patients had chest and abdominal CT, and all studies were performed with intravenous contrast and with a 4—detector row multidetector CT. All the patients had axial imaging, and 15 patients also had sagittal and coronal reformatted images (2.5 mm collimation and 1.25 reconstruction intervals). The authors acknowledge limitations to their study, including the retrospective nature of their review, the use of a 4-channel multidetector CT, and the fact that their study did not include cases in which the diagnosis of diaphragmatic injury was initially missed.

The following abnormalities were regarded as signs of diaphragmatic rupture:

- Diaphragmatic thickening, assessed by comparison to the contralateral side
- Herniation of abdominal organs into the thorax
- The collar sign, a waist-like appearance of herniated organs at the level of the diaphragm
- The hump sign, the presence of a rounded portion of the liver traversing the hemidiaphragm
- The band sign, a lucent band across the liver demarcating the torn diaphragm edge
- The dependent viscera sign, the absence of lung intervening between the posterior chest wall and the upper abdominal organs
- Abnormal diaphragmatic elevation of 4 cm or more above the apex of the contralateral hemidiaphragm

Liver injury was seen in 18.6% of patients but was found significantly more frequently in right diaphragmatic rupture. In addition, there was a significantly higher incidence of pulmonary injury in left diaphragmatic rupture. The authors advocate the use of modern multidetector CT for higher resolution and avoidance of motion or breathing artifacts and the use of multiplanar reformatted images for improved visualization of diaphragmatic abnormalities. It should be noted that associated hemothorax may obscure signs of diaphragmatic rupture. However, awareness of the various signs of diaphragmatic injury and a high index of suspicion in patients at risk should allow the prospective identification of these important injuries.

M. L. Rosado de Christenson, MD

Airway

Bronchial Collapsibility at Forced Expiration in Healthy Volunteers: Assessment with Multidetector CT

Litmanovich D, O'Donnell CR, Bankier AA, et al (Beth Israel Deaconess Med Ctr and Harvard Med School, Boston, MA)
Radiology 257:560-567, 2010

Purpose.—To assess forced-expiratory bronchial collapsibility in healthy volunteers by using multidetector computed tomography (CT) and to compare the results with the current diagnostic criterion for bronchomalacia.

Materials and Methods.—The institutional review board approved this HIPAA-compliant study. Following informed consent, 51 healthy volunteers with normal pulmonary function and no history of smoking were imaged by using a 64—detector row scanner with spirometric monitoring at total lung capacity and during forced exhalation. The total study population (in whom both main bronchi were imaged) included 25 men and 26 women (mean age, 50 years). Each scan was analyzed at a workstation by a fellowship-trained thoracic radiologist. Cross-sectional area measurements were obtained from end-inspiratory and forced-expiratory CT images for the right main bronchus (RMB), left main bronchus, (LMB), and bronchus intermedius (BI), and the mean percentage of expiratory collapse was calculated for each bronchus. The number of participants who exceeded the current diagnostic threshold level (>50% expiratory reduction in cross-sectional area) for bronchomalacia was calculated. Comparisons of airway dimensions and airway collapse according to bronchial segment and sex were made by using repeated-measures analysis of variance.

Results.—Mean percentage of expiratory collapse was 66.9% ± 19.0 (standard deviation) for the RMB and 61.4% ± 16.7 for the LMB. Thirty-seven (73%) of 51 participants exceeded the diagnostic threshold level for bronchomalacia. Significant differences were observed in mean percentage of expiratory collapse between the RMB (66.9% ± 19.0) and LMB (61.4% ± 16.7) ($P = .0005$). Among a subgroup of 37 participants in whom the BI was also imaged, the mean percentage of expiratory collapse was 61.8% ± 22.8, and 27 (73%) participants exceeded the diagnostic threshold level for bronchomalacia.

Conclusion.—Healthy volunteers demonstrate a wide range of forced-expiratory bronchial collapse, frequently exceeding the current diagnostic threshold level for bronchomalacia.

▶ Tracheobronchomalacia is increasingly recognized as an important central airways disease characterized by exaggerated expiratory collapsibility of the central airways. The diagnosis was traditionally established by bronchoscopic visualization of excessive tracheal and bronchial collapsibility. Recently, dynamic airway imaging has been presented as a diagnostic test for assessing the large airways. Traditionally, expiratory airway collapse in excess of 50% has been identified as a diagnostic criterion for tracheobronchomalacia. With this in mind, the authors set out to determine the validity of this diagnostic criterion by examining the forced expiratory collapsibility of the central bronchi in normal volunteers without lung disease or symptoms or risk factors for malacia.

The patient population in the study was originally investigated to determine the degree of tracheal collapsibility using multidetector CT in normal subjects. Healthy volunteers were enrolled from February to August 2008. Inclusion criteria included age from 25 to 75 years, absence of respiratory disease or symptoms, and no history of cigarette smoking. Pregnancy and risk factors for malacia (prior prolonged intubation, mediastinal radiation, and tracheal surgery) were exclusion criteria.

All patients underwent spirometry, and those with abnormal results were excluded. The study population was comprised by 51 individuals, 25 men, and 26 women with a mean age of 50 years. All patients were scanned in a 64-detector row scanner using a low-dose technique both during end inspiration and forced expiration. Postprocessing was performed to allow measurement of airway diameter and area perpendicular to the lumen of the bronchi. Seventy-three percent of the study population met current criteria for bronchomalacia. However, when the diagnostic criterion for malacia was increased to a collapsibility greater than 80%, only 21.6% of these normal subjects would have been diagnosed with bronchomalacia.

The authors recommend that the data available for normal subjects be compared to data from patients with proven malacia prior to proposing a definitive criterion for the CT diagnosis of the disease. However, they suggest that until such data is available, a threshold level of at least 70% expiratory collapse on dynamic expiratory CT be applied for considering the diagnosis. In addition, as normal subjects can exhibit such levels of airway collapsibility, a careful correlation with the presence or absence of clinical signs and symptoms of the disease is necessary.

Although the authors do not mention it, studies could be undertaken to determine the significance of severe airway collapsibility demonstrated on nondynamic CT in patients with expiratory imaging and dyspnea. It should be noted that this is a commonly encountered finding when performing chest CT of critically ill patients.

M. L. Rosado de Christenson, MD

2 Breast Imaging

Introduction

Have you ever been the new kid at school? I have been the new kid at school on several occasions. Each time I thought, "Everything is so different and new here. I'm not sure what to do or which way to go."

I am the new kid on the block as the YEAR BOOK breast imaging editor. For the first time I like being the new kid. I have received an outpouring of support. Dr Robyn Birdwell, who is quite a tough act to follow, graciously explained the responsibilities and offered her support. And Dr Anne Osborn ... I cannot say enough wonderful things about Dr Osborn! She is a GIANT of radiology and a role model for both female and male radiologists. The first time I met Dr Osborn was August 5, 1997, at the AFIP. She was a major source of encouragement to me then and to me now. I am so excited that she is the YEAR BOOK Editor-in-Chief. I must also thank Ruth Malwitz and Yonah Korngold, the Elsevier editors who patiently helped me navigate the editing process.

The articles I have chosen for this year's chapter are varied and reflect the broad range of issues that breast imagers encounter. I decided not to shy away from the controversial issues we faced this year. Our patients are knowledgeable and are aware of the controversy, so they will undoubtedly ask questions that we will need to answer.

I know I don't have all the answers, so I am thankful to my colleagues, Drs Le-Petross and Lane, for providing commentaries on two of the selections.

I sincerely hope our YEAR BOOK readers enjoy the breast imaging selections and find them useful in their daily practice.

Tanya W. Stephens, MD

Accuracy of ultrasonography and mammography in predicting pathologic response after neoadjuvant chemotherapy for breast cancer
Keune JD, Jeffe DB, Schootman M, et al (Washington Univ School of Medicine, St Louis, MO; et al)
Am J Surg 199:477-484, 2010

Background.—Neoadjuvant chemotherapy reduces tumor size before surgery in women with breast cancer. The aim of this study was to assess the ability of mammography and ultrasound to predict residual tumor size following neoadjuvant chemotherapy.

Methods.—In a retrospective review of consecutive breast cancer patients treated with neoadjuvant chemotherapy, residual tumor size estimated by diagnostic imaging was compared with residual tumor size determined by surgical pathology.

Results.—One hundred ninety-two patients with 196 primary breast cancers were studied. Of 104 tumors evaluated by both imaging modalities, ultrasound was able to size 91.3%, and mammography was able to size only 51.9% (χ^2 $P < .001$). Ultrasound also was more accurate than mammography in estimating residual tumor size (62 of 104 [59.6%] vs 33 of 104 [31.7%], $P < .001$). There was little difference in the ability of mammography and ultrasound to predict pathologic complete response (receiver operating characteristic, 0.741 vs 0.784).

Conclusions.—Breast ultrasound was more accurate than mammography in predicting residual tumor size following neoadjuvant chemotherapy. The likelihood of a complete pathologic response was 80% when both imaging modalities demonstrated no residual disease.

▶ Neoadjuvant chemotherapy can decrease tumor size in women with breast cancer, allowing these patients to undergo breast-conserving surgery. Monitoring treatment response allows for adjustments in therapy to provide the breast response and the opportunity for a more desirable surgical outcome.

Breast imaging plays a vital role in monitoring response to therapy. This article confirms the importance of breast imaging. The aim of the study was to assess the ability of mammography and ultrasound to predict residual tumor size following neoadjuvant chemotherapy.

Of the tumors evaluated, ultrasound was able to accurately estimate residual tumor size following neoadjuvant chemotherapy in approximately 90% of the tumors; mammography was able to accurately estimate residual tumor size in approximately half of the tumors.

For surgical decision making, the use of both modalities aids in the prediction of residual tumor size following neoadjuvant chemotherapy and complete pathologic response.[1]

T. W. Stephens, MD

Reference

1. Peintinger F, Kuerer HM, Anderson K, et al. Accuracy of the combination of mammography and sonography in predicting tumor response in breast cancer patients after neoadjuvant chemotherapy. *Ann Surg Oncol.* 2006;13:1443-1449.

ACR Appropriateness Criteria® on Nonpalpable Mammographic Findings (Excluding Calcifications)

Newell MS, Birdwell RL, D'Orsi CJ, et al (Emory Univ, Atlanta, GA; Brigham and Women's Hosp, Boston, MA; Emory Univ Hosp, Atlanta, GA; et al)
J Am Coll Radiol 7:920-930, 2010

Screening mammography can detect breast cancer before it becomes clinically apparent. However, the screening process identifies many false-positive findings for each cancer eventually confirmed. Additional tools are available to help differentiate spurious findings from real ones and to help determine when tissue sampling is required, when short-term follow-up will suffice, or whether the finding can be dismissed as benign. These tools include additional diagnostic mammographic views, breast ultrasound, breast MRI, and, when histologic evaluation is required, percutaneous biopsy. The imaging evaluation of a finding detected at screening mammography proceeds most efficiently, cost-effectively, and with minimization of radiation dose when approached in an evidence-based manner. The appropriateness of the above-referenced tools is presented here as they apply to a variety of findings often encountered on screening mammography; an algorithmic approach to workup of these potential scenarios is also included. The recommendations put forth represent a compilation of evidence-based data and expert opinion of the ACR Appropriateness Criteria® Expert Panel on Breast Imaging.

▶ No screening modality is perfect, and of course that includes screening mammography. Although screening mammograms detect breast cancers before they become clinically apparent, false-positive findings are also identified. There are tools available to the breast imager to help determine which findings truly represent malignancy. These tools include diagnostic mammography, breast ultrasound, breast MRI, and percutaneous biopsy.

This article discusses the appropriateness of the tools mentioned above as they apply to commonly encountered scenarios during the interpretation of screening mammograms and provides an algorithmic approach to the workup of the scenarios (Appendix A-D in the original article). This approach will be helpful in daily practice.[1]

T. W. Stephens, MD

Reference

1. Feig SA. Breast masses. Mammographic and sonographic evaluation. *Radiol Clin North Am.* 1992;30:67-92.

Barriers to Adherence to Screening Mammography Among Women With Disabilities

Yankaskas BC, Dickens P, Michael Bowling J, et al (Univ of North Carolina, Chapel Hill)
Am J Public Health 100:947-953, 2010

Objectives.—Given the lack of screening mammography studies specific to women with disabilities, we compared reasons offered by women with and without disabilities for not scheduling routine screening visits.

Methods.—We surveyed women in the Carolina Mammography Registry aged 40 to 79 years (n = 2970), who had been screened from 2001 through 2003 and did not return for at least 3 years, to determine reasons for noncompliance. In addition to women without disabilities, women with visual, hearing, physical, and multiple (any combination of visual, hearing, and physical) limitations were included in our analyses.

Results.—The most common reasons cited by women both with and without disabilities for not returning for screening were lack of a breast problem, pain and expense associated with a mammogram, and lack of a physician recommendation. Women with disabilities were less likely to receive a physician recommendation.

Conclusions.—Women with disabilities are less likely than those without disabilities to receive a physician recommendation for screening mammography, and this is particularly the case among older women and those with multiple disabilities. There is a need for equitable preventive health care in this population.

▶ There are approximately 45 million Americans living with disabilities. Although the Americans with Disabilities Act intends to level the playing field for disabled Americans, individuals with disabilities often have a very different health care experience than individuals without disabilities. While women with and without disabilities share many of the barriers to adherence to screening mammography, this study is welcome because it draws attention to the need for equitable preventive care for Americans with disabilities.

T. W. Stephens, MD

Breast Cancer Screening With Imaging: Recommendations From the Society of Breast Imaging and the ACR on the Use of Mammography, Breast MRI, Breast Ultrasound, and Other Technologies for the Detection of Clinically Occult Breast Cancer

Lee CH, Dershaw DD, Kopans D, et al (Memorial Sloan-Kettering Cancer Ctr, NY)
J Am Coll Radiol 7:18-27, 2010

Screening for breast cancer with mammography has been shown to decrease mortality from breast cancer, and mammography is the mainstay of screening for clinically occult disease. Mammography, however, has well-recognized limitations, and recently, other imaging including ultrasound and magnetic resonance imaging have been used as adjunctive screening tools, mainly for women who may be at increased risk for the development of breast cancer. The Society of Breast Imaging and the Breast Imaging Commission of the ACR are issuing these recommendations to provide guidance to patients and clinicians on the use of imaging to screen for breast cancer. Wherever possible, the recommendations are based on available evidence. Where evidence is lacking, the recommendations are based on consensus opinions of the fellows and executive committee of the Society of Breast Imaging and the members of the Breast Imaging Commission of the ACR.

▶ I cannot recall any of the previous US Preventive Services Task Force (USPSTF) recommendations receiving as much attention as the Task Force's 2009 recommendations on screening for breast cancer. As a breast imager, I must admit that I was quite pleased to see breast cancer screening in particular and screening mammography specifically as the main topic of discussion in face-to-face conversations and on the pages of Facebook.

Patients were asking questions. Nonimaging colleagues were asking questions. As breast imagers, we were called upon to answer everyone's questions. It is likely that the questions will continue and other imaging challenges and controversies will arise. Please know that we cannot answer questions if we are not informed.

I have included 2 articles with regard to breast cancer screening with imaging: the USPSTF recommendations[1] and the breast cancer screening with imaging recommendations from the Society of Breast Imaging and the American College of Radiology (SBI-ACR). Although the SBI-ACR recommendations were published after the USPSTF article, the SBI-ACR recommendations were not published as a response to the USPSTF publication.

T. W. Stephens, MD

Reference

1. US Preventive Services Task Force. Screening for breast cancer: U.S. preventive services task force recommendation statement. *Ann Intern Med.* 2009;151:716-726.

Can Computer-aided Detection Be Detrimental to Mammographic Interpretation?
Philpotts LE (Yale Univ School of Medicine, New Haven, CT)
Radiology 253:17-22, 2009

In conclusion, CAD has some potential advantages but also some important and potentially serious limitations. Awareness of the limitations discussed in this article is important for optimal use. A few suggestions to protect oneself from experiencing detrimental effects from the use of CAD in screening interpretation are as follows: (*a*) Never use CAD as a pre-screener. The present sensitivity of CAD is not sufficient, and many cancers will be missed with this approach. (*b*) Never use CAD as an initial step in mammogram interpretation. Again, for the same reasons, if one concentrates primarily on areas that CAD has marked, many important findings may be missed. (*c*) Interpret mammograms as usual, and only use CAD as a last step in a reading protocol. Do not decide not to recall a patient for a finding just because it is not marked by CAD. It might be worth considering that if one finds that CAD is consistently marking findings that the reader had not recognized initially and that appear important (ie, potentially worthy of recall) that the reader should maybe step away from reading for a rest until his or her acuity has resumed.

Understanding of the limitations of CAD is important for those interpreting mammograms; this cautious approach to the use of CAD should help optimize this presently imperfect system and minimize the possible detrimental effects.

▶ Interpreting mammograms is both rewarding and challenging. It is rewarding when cancers are detected and lives are saved and challenging, as the author of this article and others (references below)[1-3] have noted—approximately 20% of cancers are missed on mammography. Computer-aided detection (CAD) was developed to assist breast imagers with the challenging task of mammographic interpretation.

This article reviews the limitations of CAD and provides suggestions to protect the breast imager from the detrimental effects from the use of CAD in screening interpretation.

CAD is an important tool, and if we remember CAD's limitations, we can optimize its use.

T. W. Stephens, MD

References

1. Birdwell RL, Ikeda DM, O'Shaughnessy KF, Sickes EA. Mammographic characteristics of 115 missed cancers later detected with screening mammography and the potential utility of computer-aided detection. *Radiology.* 2001;219:192-202.
2. Fenton JJ, Taplin SH, Carney PA, et al. Influence of computer-aided detection on performance of screening mammography. *N Engl J Med.* 2007;356:1399-1409.
3. Majid AS, de Paredes ES, Doherty RD, Sharma NR, Salvador X. Missed breast carcinoma: pitfalls and pearls. *RadioGraphics.* 2003;23:881-895.

Cost-effectiveness of Breast MR Imaging and Screen-Film Mammography for Screening *BRCA1* Gene Mutation Carriers
Lee JM, McMahon PM, Kong CY, et al (Massachusetts General Hosp, Boston)
Radiology 254:793-800, 2010

Purpose.—To evaluate the clinical effectiveness and cost-effectiveness of screening strategies in which MR imaging and screen-film mammography were used, alone and in combination, in women with *BRCA1* mutations.

Materials and Methods.—Because this study did not involve primary data collection from individual patients, institutional review board approval was not needed. By using a simulation model, we compared three annual screening strategies for a cohort of 25-year-old *BRCA1* mutation carriers, as follows: *(a)* screen-film mammography, *(b)* MR imaging, and *(c)* combined MR imaging and screen-film mammography (combined screening). The model was used to estimate quality-adjusted life-years (QALYs) and lifetime costs. Incremental cost-effectiveness ratios were calculated. Input parameters were obtained from the medical literature, existing databases, and calibration. Costs (2007 U.S. dollars) and quality-of-life adjustments were derived from Medicare reimbursement rates and the medical literature. Sensitivity analysis was performed to evaluate the effect of uncertainty in parameter estimates on model results.

Results.—In the base-case analysis, annual combined screening was most effective (44.62 QALYs), and had the highest cost ($110973), followed by annual MR imaging alone (44.50 QALYs, $108641), and annual mammography alone (44.46 QALYs, $100336). Adding annual MR imaging to annual mammographic screening cost $69125 for each additional QALY gained. Sensitivity analysis indicated that, when the screening MR imaging cost increased to $960 (base case, $577), or breast cancer risk by age 70 years decreased below 58% (base case, 65%), or the sensitivity of combined screening decreased below 76% (base case, 94%), the cost of adding MR imaging to mammography exceeded $100000 per QALY.

Conclusion.—Annual combined screening provides the greatest life expectancy and is likely cost-effective when the value placed on gaining an additional QALY is in the range of $50000-$100000.

▶ It is well known that women with *BRCA1* gene mutations have a substantially increased lifetime risk of developing breast cancer.[1] Cancer detection in this group of patients is challenging because screening mammography detects less than one-half of prevalent and incident malignancies in these patients. Adjunct imaging with MRI for screening is recommended to assist in the detection of malignancies.

The authors of this article ask what is the best and most cost-effective screening strategy. The results of their analysis suggest that breast cancer screening outcomes for women with *BRCA1* gene mutations can be improved with annual combined screening with screen-film mammography and MRI.

T. W. Stephens, MD

Reference

1. Saslow D, Boetes C, Burke W, et al. American Cancer Society guidelines for breast screening with MRI as an adjunct to mammography. *CA Cancer J Clin.* 2007;57: 75-89.

Disclosing Harmful Mammography Errors to Patients

Gallagher TH, Cook AJ, Brenner RJ, et al (Univ of Washington, Seattle; Bay Imaging Consultants, Oakland, CA; et al)
Radiology 253:443-452, 2009

Purpose.—To assess radiologists' attitudes about disclosing errors to patients by using a survey with a vignette involving an error interpreting a patient's mammogram, leading to a delayed cancer diagnosis.

Materials and Methods.—We conducted an institutional review board–approved survey of 364 radiologists at seven geographically distinct Breast Cancer Surveillance Consortium sites that interpreted mammograms from 2005 to 2006. Radiologists received a vignette in which comparison screening mammograms were placed in the wrong order, leading a radiologist to conclude calcifications were decreasing in number when they were actually increasing, delaying a cancer diagnosis. Radiologists were asked (*a*) how likely they would be to disclose this error, (*b*) what information they would share, and (*c*) their malpractice attitudes and experiences.

Results.—Two hundred forty-three (67%) of 364 radiologists responded to the disclosure vignette questions. Radiologists' responses to whether they would disclose the error included "definitely not" (9%), "only if asked by the patient" (51%), "probably" (26%), and "definitely" (14%). Regarding information they would disclose, 24% would "not say anything further to the patient," 31% would tell the patient that "the calcifications are larger and are now suspicious for cancer," 30% would state "the calcifications may have increased on your last mammogram, but their appearance was not as worrisome as it is now," and 15% would tell the patient "an error occurred during the interpretation of your last mammogram, and the calcifications had actually increased in number, not decreased." Radiologists' malpractice experiences were not consistently associated with their disclosure responses.

Conclusion.—Many radiologists report reluctance to disclose a hypothetical mammography error that delayed a cancer diagnosis. Strategies should be developed to increase radiologists' comfort communicating with patients.

▶ As a breast imager at a large center, I have had several patients ask me whether their newly diagnosed breast cancer was missed on prior mammograms. While these can be difficult conversations, perhaps even more challenging is the specific situation described in the article. That is, when the patient does not ask about any possible error, but as radiologists, we are aware that one was made. This thought-provoking article made me reflect on what approach might be the best in these often-complicated encounters.

The literature suggesting that patients desire full disclosure of medical errors is often based on hypothetical situations or vignettes created for research purposes. Anecdotally, since reading this article, I asked a current breast cancer patient if she would want to be told of an error in the interpretation of her previous mammogram. She personally would not since her treatment and prognosis would be defined from the point of diagnosis and she would prefer that her focus was forward looking and optimistic. In her view, if she focused on a past error, she would be looking back and thinking "if only..." For her, there is no good in that. On the other hand, other patients might want to know every detail of any mistake. Patients are individuals and must be treated as such and not by invoking "blanket rules."

What do our patients truly want to know if a mistake has been made? Does it depend on their personality, educational level, or other variables? Does it vary depending on the stage of their cancer or whether it would have made a difference in their prognosis? And when do they want to know this information? At the time of their original diagnosis or later in the course of their treatment when the initial shock of their diagnosis has been absorbed? Further information about these issues may be gleaned by asking patients who have already begun their own cancer journey.

Concerning mammography, what constitutes an actionable medical error? Of course, there are blatant cancers that any reasonable radiologist would be expected to diagnose, but what about the more subtle cancers? Was last year's truly a false negative mammogram, or was the cancer visible at that time? Should it have been acted upon before now? As radiologists, these are all questions that we have to answer as we decide whether a mistake was indeed made. Often times, the errors that we do see might not necessarily be our own but rather those of our partners or perhaps another institution. How should we handle these situations? These are indeed difficult questions, and there is obviously need for further research and physician education on all of these issues.

Unfortunately, physicians are human, and medical mistakes are inevitable. As physicians, we would benefit from even more discussion regarding how and when to communicate possible errors to patients. We need specific information on precisely how such disclosure might affect patient satisfaction and any possible litigation. As physicians, we need to do what is right, letting our moral compass lead us, and we need to have open and honest conversations with our patients. This article is clearly a good step in identifying and defining these problems.

D. L. Lane, MD

FDG PET-CT in the management of primary breast lymphoma
Santra A, Kumar R, Reddy R, et al (All India Inst of Med Sciences, New Delhi)
Clin Nucl Med 34:848-853, 2009

Objective.—Primary breast lymphoma (PBL) is a rare disease and its management differs from other breast cancers. The purpose of this study is to evaluate the role of FDG PET-CT in the management of PBL. We carried out 16 PET-CT scans and reviewed the literature.

Materials and Methods.—A total of 16 FDG PET-CT scans were done in 8 female patients with PBL with a median age of 49 years (range: 27-68). Of the 16 PET-CT scans, 1 scan was done for primary diagnosis and staging (1 patient), 2 for staging (2 patients), 7 for evaluation of treatment response (6 patients), and 6 for detecting recurrence (4 patients). PET-CT image interpretation and analysis were performed qualitatively (visually) and semiquantitatively using standardized uptake value (SUV). Absence of uptake in the postchemotherapy follow-up PET-CT scan was considered as a complete response, and a fall of more than 50% of baseline SUV was considered as a significant response.

Results.—One patient was successfully diagnosed to have PBL and staged using PET-CT. Two patients were correctly staged with the help of FDG PET-CT. Complete response was noted in all 6 patients (3 had a positive baseline scan and showed complete resolution of FDG uptake, the other 3 who did not have baseline PET-CT and lesions were detected on CT, and also showed complete resolution). Of the 4 patients evaluated for recurrence, 1 patient was positive and 3 patients were negative for recurrence in follow-up PET-CT scans done after 18, 22, and 24 months, respectively.

Conclusion.—FDG PET-CT has a definitive role in every step of management (diagnosis, staging, treatment response evaluation, and detection of recurrence) in patients with primary breast lymphoma.

▶ Comprising 0.04% to 0.53% of breast cancers, primary breast lymphoma (PBL) is a rare entity. Although rare, the clinical and imaging features of PBL do not differ significantly from other more common types of breast cancer. The overlap of the clinical and imaging features may be problematic, for the treatment of PBL differs radically; therefore, it is vital to differentiate PBL from other breast malignancies.

The staging, treatment response monitoring, and restaging of lymphoma with fluorodeoxyglucose positron emission tomography-CT (PET-CT) is well known.

In this article, the authors evaluate a small series of patients with PBL and the literature for evaluating the role of PET-CT in the management of PBL (Figs 1-3 in the original article).

Although this series is small, it validates the role of PET/PET-CT in the initial staging, treatment response, and restaging in patients with PBL.

T. W. Stephens, MD

Identifying Minimally Acceptable Interpretive Performance Criteria for Screening Mammography
Carney PA, Sickles EA, Monsees BS, et al (Oregon Health & Science Univ, Portland; Univ of California, San Francisco; Univ School of Medicine, St Louis, MO; et al)
Radiology 255:354-361, 2010

Purpose.—To develop criteria to identify thresholds for minimally acceptable physician performance in interpreting screening mammography studies and to profile the impact that implementing these criteria may have on the practice of radiology in the United States.

Materials and Methods.—In an institutional review board—approved, HIPAA-compliant study, an Angoff approach was used in two phases to set criteria for identifying minimally acceptable interpretive performance at screening mammography as measured by sensitivity, specificity, recall rate, positive predictive value (PPV) of recall (PPV$_1$) and of biopsy recommendation (PPV$_2$), and cancer detection rate. Performance measures were considered separately. In phase I, a group of 10 expert radiologists considered a hypothetical pool of 100 interpreting physicians and conveyed their cut points of minimally acceptable performance. The experts were informed that a physician's performance falling outside the cut points would result in a recommendation to consider additional training. During each round of scoring, all expert radiologists' cut points were summarized into a mean, median, mode, and range; these were presented back to the group. In phase II, normative data on performance were shown to illustrate the potential impact cut points would have on radiology practice. Rescoring was done until consensus among experts was achieved. Simulation methods were used to estimate the potential impact of performance that improved to acceptable levels if effective additional training was provided.

Results.—Final cut points to identify low performance were as follows: sensitivity less than 75%, specificity less than 88% or greater than 95%, recall rate less than 5% or greater than 12%, PPV$_1$ less than 3% or greater than 8%, PPV$_2$ less than 20% or greater than 40%, and cancer detection rate less than 2.5 per 1000 interpretations. The selected cut points for performance measures would likely result in 18%—28% of interpreting physicians being considered for additional training on the basis of sensitivity and cancer detection rate, while the cut points for specificity, recall, and PPV$_1$ and PPV$_2$ would likely affect 34%—49% of practicing interpreters. If underperforming physicians moved into the acceptable range, detection of an additional 14 cancers per 100 000 women screened and a reduction in the number of false-positive examinations by 880 per 100 000 women screened would be expected.

Conclusion.—This study identified minimally acceptable performance levels for interpreters of screening mammography studies. Interpreting physicians whose performance falls outside the identified cut points should be reviewed in the context of their specific practice settings and be considered for additional training.

▶ The clinical usefulness of screening mammography continues to be challenged. As breast imagers, it is important that we interpret mammograms at an acceptable level.

The authors of this article identified criteria for minimally acceptable interpretive performance at screening mammography as measured by sensitivity (<75%), specificity (<88%), recall rate (<5% or >12%), positive predictive value (PPV) of recall (PPV1) (<3% or >8%) and of biopsy recommendation

(PPV2) (20% or >40%), and cancer detection rate (<2.5 per 1000 interpretations).

If the performance cut points for sensitivity and cancer detection are taken into account, 18% to 28% of interpreting physicians would be considered for additional training and if specificity, recall, and PPV1 and PPV2 considered, 34% to 49% of practicing interpreters would be considered for additional training.

Of course, values when evaluating performance-specific practice settings must be considered. If underperforming interpreters move into an acceptable range, it is expected that an additional 14 cancers per 100 000 women screened will be detected, and the number of false-positive examinations will be decreased by 880 per 100 000 women screened.

T. W. Stephens, MD

Incidental breast lesions detected on CT: what is their significance?
Moyle P, Sonoda L, Britton P, et al (Cambridge Univ Hosp NHS Trust, UK)
Br J Radiol 83:233-240, 2010

An increasing number of breast lesions are being detected incidentally on CT. The aim of this study was to investigate the rate of referrals to the breast unit for assessment of lesions identified on CT and the resulting yield of previously undiagnosed breast malignancies from this pathway. A retrospective review was undertaken of CT examinations conducted over a period of 14 years. All patients (with no previous history of breast cancer) whose report contained the keyword "breast" and who were referred to a specialist breast unit for assessment were reviewed. CT lesion morphology and enhancement pattern were identified and compared with the final diagnostic outcome. 70 patients were identified by retrospective analysis, yielding 78 incidental breast lesions, of which 22 (28.2%) were malignant (category B5). This gave a positive predictive value (PPV) for malignancy of 28.2%. The best morphological predictor of malignancy was spiculation (PPV, 76%) and irregularity (PPV, 58%), whereas calcification patterns (PPV, 36%) were diagnostically unhelpful. Malignant lesions were likely to be larger (mean, 28.5 mm) than benign lesions (mean, 20.2 mm; p<0.05). In conclusion, 30% of incidental breast lesions in this large series of patients proved to be unsuspected breast cancers, particularly irregular spiculated masses. Referral for formal triple assessment of CT-diagnosed breast lesions is worthwhile, and careful examination of the breast should be a routine part of CT examinations.

▶ At my institution I am fortunate to work with individuals who embrace a multidisciplinary and a multi-imaging speciality approach to health care. As imagers we may develop tunnel vision and focus our attention on the anatomy of interest for speciality and pay lesser attention to the surrounding anatomy.

This article reminds us that the approach to imaging diagnosis with the detection of incidental breast lesions on CT is important. Nearly 30% of the lesions in this large series proved to be unsuspected breast cancers. The careful examination of the breasts should be a routine part of CT examinations.[1−3]

T. W. Stephens, MD

References

1. Meller M, Cox J, Callanan K. Incidental detection of breast lesions with computer tomography. *Clinical Breast Cancer*. 2007;7:634-637.
2. Harish MG, Konda SD, MacMahon H, Newstaed GM. Breast lesions incidentially detected with CT: what the general radiologist needs to know. *RadioGraphics*. 2007;27:S37-S51.
3. Yi JG, Kim SJ, Marom EM, Park JH, Jung SI, Lee MW. Chest CT of incidental breast lesions. *J Thorac Imaging*. 2008;23:148-155.

Missed Breast Cancers at US-guided Core Needle Biopsy: How to Reduce Them

Youk JH, Kim E-K, Kim MJ, et al (Yonsei Univ College of Medicine, Seodaemun-ku, Seoul, South Korea)

Radiographics 27:79-94, 2007

Ultrasonographically (US) guided core needle biopsy is currently recognized as a reliable alternative to surgical biopsy for the histopathologic diagnosis of breast lesions. However, despite advances in biopsy devices and techniques, false-negative diagnoses are unavoidable and may delay the diagnosis and treatment of breast cancer. The most common reasons for false-negative diagnosis are *(a)* technical or sampling errors, *(b)* failure to recognize or act on radiologic-histologic discordance, and *(c)* lack of imaging follow-up after a benign biopsy result. Technical difficulties (eg, poor lesion or needle visualization, deeply located lesions, dense fibrotic tissue) cause inaccurate sampling but can be reduced by using modified standard techniques. Radiologic-histologic correlation is also of critical importance in US-guided core needle biopsy. Radiologic-histologic discordance occurs when the histologic results do not provide a sufficient explanation for the imaging features and indicates that the lesion may not have been sampled adequately, so that repeat biopsy is warranted. Appropriate follow-up imaging is invaluable; even patients with concordant benign findings after US-guided core needle biopsy are directed to undergo follow-up imaging because there may be delays in the recognition of false-negative findings. Optimization of technique, radiologic-histologic correlation, and postbiopsy follow-up protocols are recommended to reduce the occurrence of false-negative diagnosis at US-guided core needle biopsy performed by radiologists.

▶ Ultrasound (US)-guided biopsies are relatively easy and quick to perform.[1] Most patients would choose a US-guided biopsy over a stereotactic biopsy or an MRI-guided biopsy. US-guided core needle biopsies have a high sensitivity for the detection of breast cancer. Unfortunately every breast imager has experienced a false-negative diagnosis and should be prepared to perform a repeat biopsy or suggest surgical excision if a false-negative diagnosis is encountered. In the vast majority of cases, a repeat biopsy will definitively confirm the diagnosis of malignancy.

Although not recent, this is an important article. The authors list common causes of false-negative results with US-guided core needle biopsy, describe technical pitfalls of US-guided biopsies and discuss solutions to the pitfalls, and discuss ways to reduce missed breast cancers in US-guided core needle biopsies.

T. W. Stephens, MD

Reference

1. Schueller G, Schueller-Weidekamm C, Helbich TH. Accuracy of ultrasound-guided, large-core needle breast biopsy. *Eur Radiol.* 2008;18:1761-1763.

MR-Directed ("Second-Look") Ultrasound Examination for Breast Lesions Detected Initially on MRI: MR and Sonographic Findings
Abe H, Schmidt RA, Shah RN, et al (Univ of Chicago, IL)
AJR Am J Roentgenol 194:370-377, 2010

Objective.—The objective of our study was to assess the clinical utility of MR-directed ("second-look") ultrasound examination to search for breast lesions detected initially on MRI.

Materials and Methods.—A retrospective review was performed of the records of 158 consecutive patients (202 lesions) with breast abnormalities initially detected on MRI between July 2003 and May 2006. All lesions were detected as enhancing findings on a dynamic contrast MR study and were subsequently evaluated with ultrasound. Ultrasound was performed using MR images as a guide to lesion location, size, and morphology. Pathology findings were confirmed by subsequent percutaneous biopsy or lesion excision. Imaging follow-up was used for probably benign lesions, which were not biopsied.

Results.—Of the 202 MRI-detected lesions, ultrasound correlation was made in 115 (57%) including 33 malignant lesions and 82 benign lesions. The remaining 87 lesions were not sonographically correlated and included 11 malignant lesions and 76 nonmalignant lesions. Mass lesions identified on MRI were more likely to have a sonographic correlate than nonmasslike lesions (65% vs 12%, respectively); malignant mass lesions were more likely to show an ultrasound correlation (85%). The malignant lesions with successful sonographic correlation tended to present with subtle sonographic findings.

Conclusion.—MR-directed ultrasound of MRI-detected lesions was useful for decision making as part of the diagnostic workup. Malignant lesions were likely to have an ultrasound correlate, especially when they presented as masses on MRI. However, the sonographic findings of these lesions were often subtle, and careful scanning technique was needed for successful MRI—ultrasound correlation.

▶ The increased use of breast magnetic resonance imaging (MRI) for detecting additional ipsilateral and contralateral breast cancers that are mammographically occult in patients with newly diagnosed breast cancer has resulted in an increasing need for targeted or second ultrasound examination performed after MRI to evaluate the additional MRI-detected findings. This practice has been adapted because many centers do not have MRI-guided biopsy capabilities. However, that limitation is changing. At least one-third to half of all MRI-detected lesions has been reported to be sonographically occult, and therefore, MRI-guided biopsy is still required. Even though most of the sonographically occult lesions were benign, 13% to 28% of the MRI-detected lesions were malignant. This paper nicely summarizes the characteristics of lesions that are more likely to have an ultrasound correlation. The ability to determine which lesions should be evaluated by ultrasound and which should proceed directly to an MRI-guided biopsy would reduce the time from the initial preoperative MRI assessment to the start of definitive treatment. In addition, Abe and colleagues nicely confirmed the findings of other trials[1-4] showing that MRI-detected lesions with sonographic correlates were more likely to be malignant than lesions without sonographic correlates. More specifically, mass-like enhancing MRI-detected lesions have a higher sonographic detection rate than non—mass-like enhancing lesions. If the MRI-detected lesion is non—mass-like and has a suspicious ductal or segmental distribution with clumped internal enhancement, it is less likely to have a sonographic correlate. With such lesions, proceeding directly to an MRI-guided core biopsy without a second-look ultrasound examination would reduce the time from initial cancer diagnosis to the start of definitive therapy. In conclusion, MRI-detected mass-like lesions are more likely to be visible on second-look ultrasound and can be biopsied under ultrasound guidance regardless of the lesion size. MRI-detected nonmass lesions larger than 2 cm, with suspicious segmental distribution and clumped enhancement, warrant an MRI-guided biopsy, as a small percentage of sonographically occult MRI-detected lesions are malignant.

H. Le-Petross, MD

References

1. Destounis S, Arieno A, Somerville PA, et al. Community-based practice experience of unsuspected breast magnetic resonance imaging abnormalities evaluated with second-look sonography. *J Ultrasound Med.* 2009;28:1337-1346.
2. Meissnitzer M, Dershaw DD, Lee CH, Morris EA. Targeted ultrasound of the breast in women with abnormal MRI findings for whom biopsy has been recommended. *AJR Am J Roentgenol.* 2009;193:1025-1029.
3. Linda A, Zuiani C, Londero V, Bazzocchi M. Outcome of initially only magnetic resonance mammography-detected findings with and without correlate at second-look sonography: distribution according to patient history of breast cancer and lesion size. *Breast.* 2008;17:51-57.
4. LaTrenta LR, Menell JH, Morris EA, Abramson AF, Dershaw DD, Liberman L. Breast lesions detected with MR imaging: utility and histopathologic importance of identification with US. *Radiology.* 2003;227:856-861.

Palpable Presentation of Breast Cancer Persists in the Era of Screening Mammography

Mathis KL, Hoskin TL, Boughey JC, et al (Mayo Clinic and Mayo Foundation, Rochester, MN)

J Am Coll Surg 210:314-318, 2010

Background.—The aim was to describe cancer detection method and frequency of screening mammography in women undergoing breast cancer surgery in 2000.

Study Design.—Patients undergoing breast cancer surgery were identified through an institutional database. Charts were reviewed to determine presentation at time of diagnosis. Presentation was coded "palpable" if the woman presented with a breast complaint or if a new mass was detected on examination versus "screening" if detected on screening mammogram.

Results.—Five hundred ninety-two breast cancers were identified: 57% presenting by screening and 43% palpable. Cancer was more likely to present as palpable in patients with no previous screening mammography compared with those with previous mammography (67% versus 39%; p = 0.0002). Patients with palpable presentation were younger than those with screen-detected cancer (mean age 57 versus 62 years; p < 0.0001).

Conclusions.—Despite the frequent use of screening mammography, 43% of breast cancers presented as a palpable mass or otherwise symptomatic presentation.

▶ The aim of this study was to determine the method of breast cancer presentation and the frequency of participation in screening mammography in patients undergoing breast cancer surgery at a single institution.

In their series, these authors showed that breast cancer is more likely to present as a palpable finding in patients with no previous screening mammogram. In this series, patients were younger than those patients with screening-detected malignancies, were less likely to have had prior screening mammograms, and presented with larger tumors at more advanced stage at diagnosis.

Although the 2003 Cochrane Review concluded that women should not perform breast self-examination and the 2009 U.S. Preventive Services Task Force report found insufficient evidence for or against routine use of clinical breast examination, this study suggests that both breast self-examination and clinical breast examination still have a role in the detection of breast cancer.

T. W. Stephens, MD

Risk of Upgrade of Atypical Ductal Hyperplasia after Stereotactic Breast Biopsy: Effects of Number of Foci and Complete Removal of Calcifications
Kohr JR, Eby PR, Allison KH, et al (Univ of Washington Med Ctr, Seattle)
Radiology 255:723-730, 2010

Purpose.—To determine if patients with fewer than three foci of atypical ductal hyperplasia (ADH) who have all of their calcifications removed after stereotactic 9- or 11-gauge vacuum-assisted breast biopsy (VABB) have a rate of upgrade to malignancy that is sufficiently low to obviate surgical excision.

Materials and Methods.—An institutional review board—approved, HIPAA-compliant retrospective review of 991 cases of consecutive 9- or 11-gauge stereotactic VABB performed during a 65-month period revealed 147 cases of atypia. One pathologist performed a blinded review of the results of procedures performed to assess for calcifications and confirmed ADH in 101 cases with subsequent surgical excision. Each large duct or terminal duct—lobular unit containing ADH was considered a focus and counted. Postbiopsy mammograms were reviewed to determine whether all calcifications were removed. Upgrade to malignancy was determined from excisional biopsy pathology reports. Upgrade rates as a function of both number of foci and presence or absence of residual calcifications were calculated and compared by using χ^2 tests.

Results.—Upgrade to malignancy occurred in 20 (19.8%) of the 101 cases. The upgrade rate was significantly higher in cases of three or more foci of ADH (15 [28%] of 53 cases) than in cases of fewer than three foci (five [10%] of 48 cases) ($P=.02$). Upgrade rates were similar, regardless of whether all mammographic calcifications were removed (seven [17%] of 41 cases) or all were not removed (nine [20%] of 45 cases) ($P=.77$). Upgrade occurred in two (12%) of 17 cases in which there were fewer than three ADH foci and all calcifications were removed.

Conclusion.—The upgrade rate is significantly higher when ADH involves at least three foci. Surgical excision is recommended even when ADH involves fewer than three foci and all mammographic calcifications have been removed, because the upgrade rate is 12% (Table 3).

▶ The obviation of surgery excision after the diagnosis of atypical ductal hyperplasia (ADH) in patients with less than 3 foci and who have all of their calcifications removed after stereotactic 9- or 11-gauge vacuum-assisted biopsy is of particular importance and interest to me. The authors of this paper come to a different conclusion than authors at my institution (Sneige et al)[1] and Ely et al.[2] Sneige et al[1] and Ely et al[2] found no upgrade with less than 3 ADH foci (Table 3).

There is conflicting evidence as to whether subgroups of patients with ADH and complete lesion excision at percutaneous biopsy may avoid surgical excision. Variable upgrade rates in patients with ADH have been found. Some authors have found that upgrade to malignancy does not occur when fewer foci of ADH are identified at biopsy and/or when the lesion is completely

TABLE 3.—Published Data on ADH Upgrade versus Number of Foci

Study	Biopsy Method	Overall Upgrade Rate	Upgrade Rate with <3 ADH Foci	Upgrade Rate with ≥3 ADH Foci
Bonnett et al (9)*	11-Gauge VABB and 14-gauge CNB	30/73 (41)	16/49 (33)	14/24 (58)
Ely et al (37)†	11- and 14-Gauge	17/47 (36)	0/24 (0)	17/23 (74)
Forgeard et al (32)	11-Gauge VABB	29/116 (25)	5/44 (11)	24/72 (33)
Sneige et al (36)	11- and 14-Gauge VABB	3/42 (7.1)	0/28 (0)	3/14 (21)
Wagoner et al (33)	11-Gauge VABB and 14-gauge CNB	22/123 (17.9)	6/82 (7.3)	16/41 (39)
Current study	9- and 11-Gauge VABB	20/101 (19.8)	5/48 (10)	15/53 (28)

Note.—Except for the Study column, numbers in parentheses are percentages. CNB = core-needle biopsy.
Editor's Note: Please refer to original journal article for full references.
*This study included ADH, atypical lobular hyperplasia, and a heterogeneous group of non-ADH or atypical lobular hyperplasia.
†VABB or core-needle biopsy was not specified in this study.

removed percutaneously. Other authors have found lower upgrade rates in similar groups of patients but that upgrade rates are too high to avoid surgical excision.

These authors found that upgrade to ductal carcinoma in situ or invasive carcinoma was significantly less likely when ADH involved fewer than 3 foci than when it involved 3 or more foci; however, they found upgrade of ADH when there were fewer than 3 foci and all mammographic calcifications were removed. Also, the authors found no significant difference in upgrade rates based on whether calcifications were completely removed or not. Therefore, these authors recommend surgical excision for all patients with a diagnosis of ADH after stereotactic vacuum-assisted biopsy.

T. W. Stephens, MD

References

1. Sneige N, Lim SC, Whitman GJ, et al. Atypical ductal hyperplasia diagnosis by directional vacuum-assisted stereotactic biopsy of breast microcalcifications. Considerations for surgical excision. *Am J Clin Pathol.* 2003;119:248-253.
2. Ely KA, Carter BA, Jensen RA, Simpson JF, Page DL. Core biopsy of the breast with atypical ductal hyperplasia: a probabilistic approach to reporting. *Am J Surg Pathol.* 2001;25:1017-1021.

Screening for Breast Cancer: U.S. Preventive Services Task Force Recommendation Statement
U.S. Preventive Services Task Force (Agency for Healthcare Res and Quality, Rockville, MD)
Ann Intern Med 151:716-726, 2009

Description.—Update of the 2002 U.S. Preventive Services Task Force (USPSTF) recommendation statement on screening for breast cancer in the general population.

Methods.—The USPSTF examined the evidence on the efficacy of 5 screening modalities in reducing mortality from breast cancer: film mammography, clinical breast examination, breast self-examination, digital mammography, and magnetic resonance imaging in order to update the 2002 recommendation. To accomplish this update, the USPSTF commissioned 2 studies: 1) a targeted systematic evidence review of 6 selected questions relating to benefits and harms of screening, and 2) a decision analysis that used population modeling techniques to compare the expected health outcomes and resource requirements of starting and ending mammography screening at different ages and using annual versus biennial screening intervals.

Recommendations.—The USPSTF recommends against routine screening mammography in women aged 40 to 49 years. The decision to start regular, biennial screening mammography before the age of 50 years should be an individual one and take into account patient context, including the patient's values regarding specific benefits and harms. (Grade C recommendation).

The USPSTF recommends biennial screening mammography for women between the ages of 50 and 74 years. (Grade B recommendation).

The USPSTF concludes that the current evidence is insufficient to assess the additional benefits and harms of screening mammography in women 75 years or older. (I statement).

The USPSTF concludes that the current evidence is insufficient to assess the additional benefits and harms of clinical breast examination beyond screening mammography in women 40 years or older. (I statement).

The USPSTF recommends against clinicians teaching women how to perform breast self-examination. (Grade D recommendation).

The USPSTF concludes that the current evidence is insufficient to assess additional benefits and harms of either digital mammography or magnetic resonance imaging instead of film mammography as screening modalities for breast cancer. (I statement).

▶ I cannot recall any of the previous US Preventive Services Task Force (USPSTF) recommendations receiving as much attention as the Task Force's 2009 recommendations on screening for breast cancer. As a breast imager, I must admit that I was quite pleased to see breast cancer screening in particular and screening mammography specifically as the main topic of discussion from face-to-face conversations to the pages of Facebook.

Patients were asking questions. Nonimaging colleagues were asking questions. As breast imagers, we were called upon to answer everyone's questions. It is likely that the questions will continue and other imaging challenges and controversies will arise. Please know that we cannot answer questions if we are not informed.

I have included 2 articles with regard to breast cancer screening with imaging: the USPSTF recommendations and the breast cancer screening with imaging recommendations from the Society of Breast Imaging and the American College of Radiology (SBI-ACR).[1] Although the SBI-ACR recommendations were published after the USPSTF article, the SBI-ACR recommendations were not published as a response to the USPSTF publication.

T. W. Stephens, MD

Reference

1. Lee CH, Dershaw DD, Kopans D, et al. Breast cancer screening with imaging: recommendations from the Society of Breast Imaging and the ACR on the use of mammography, breast MRI, breast ultrasound, and other technologies for the detection of clinically occult breast cancer. *J Am Coll Radiol.* 2010;7:18-27.

Sonographic Confirmation of a Mammographically Detected Breast Lesion
Ellis RL (Gundersen Lutheran Health System, La Crosse, WI)
AJR Am J Roentgenol 196:225-226, 2011

Objective.—The purpose of this article is to describe a method for efficiently and effectively confirming mammographic—sonographic concordance before biopsy.

Conclusion.—With the increase in mammographic detection of smaller nonpalpable lesions, it is sometimes challenging to confirm that the lesion identified with subsequent sonography for additional lesion characterization is the same lesion. When additional confirmation is necessary, instillation of radiopaque contrast material under sonographic guidance followed by repeat mammography examination can help confirm lesion correlation.

▶ Breast imaging technology has markedly improved, making the detection of smaller and vague nonpalpable lesions on mammography commonplace. As noted by the author, nonspecific lesions are identified by sonography as well. So as breast imagers, our job has become more challenging and interesting as we attempt to determine mammographic-sonographic correlation.

The author provides a technique using the instillation of contrast that may be used for mammographic-sonographic correlation prior to biopsy. Other techniques to provide mammographic-sonographic correlation of masses include using a retractable localization needle such as a Homer needle or a biopsy marker clip.

When using contrast agents, the breast imager must be mindful of contrast allergies and must use injection precautions.

T. W. Stephens, MD

Stereotactic Vacuum-Assisted Breast Biopsy Is Not a Therapeutic Procedure Even When All Mammographically Found Calcifications Are Removed: Analysis of 4,086 Procedures

Penco S, Rizzo S, Bozzini AC, et al (European Inst of Oncology, Milan, Italy)
AJR Am J Roentgenol 195:1255-1260, 2010

Objective.—The purpose of our study was to assess whether in case of total removal of microcalcifications there is still residual tumor on the surgical specimen and, secondarily, to assess whether complete rather than partial excision of the imaging target with microcalcifications may result in increased diagnostic accuracy.

Materials and Methods.—We retrospectively reviewed 4,086 stereotactic vacuum-assisted breast biopsy (VABB) procedures for microcalcifications and histologic findings to determine the frequency of malignancy, histologic underestimation, and complete removal of cancer.

Results.—No residual microcalcifications on postbiopsy mammograms were seen in 1,594 of 4,047 (39.4%) procedures successfully completed: 351 of 1,594 lesions were malignant, 1,109 benign and 134 atypical. After partial removal of microcalcifications at VABB, the postsurgical specimen had infiltrating carcinoma in 130 of 566 cases (23%), whereas in case of total removal of microcalcifications, the underestimation occurred in 13 of 234 (5.5%) cases. The atypical ductal hyperplasia underestimation rate was 6.6% when the mammography target was completely removed and 38.7% when the target was only sampled. The percentage of lobular carcinoma in situ underestimation was the same for the two groups with partial and total removal of microcalcifications (21.2%). Among 1,016 VABB procedures with pathologic result of malignancy, 882 (86.6%) had residual cancer at surgery. In the group with complete removal of microcalcifications at VABB, residual cancer was found in 70% of cases.

Conclusion.—VABB may not be considered a therapeutic procedure, even in the case of complete removal of microcalcifications. However, a complete removal of microcalcifications may result in low rates of underestimation of malignancy and may consequently increase the diagnostic accuracy of the diagnostic procedure.

▶ When I perform percutaneous biopsies, many patients ask if additional surgery is required if the finding is completely removed at the time of the biopsy. This is a very logical question.

The authors of this article studied partial and complete removal of calcifications by stereotactic vacuum-assisted breast biopsies. They assessed whether residual tumor was present in the surgical specimen after complete removal of the calcifications and if complete versus partial removal of calcifications lead to increased diagnostic accuracy.

The conclusion of the study is that stereotactic vacuum-assisted breast biopsies, even with the complete removal of the calcifications, may not be considered therapeutic.[1−3] Please see references for further reading.

T. W. Stephens, MD

References

1. Kohr JR, Eby PR, Allison KH, et al. Risk of upgrade of atypical ductal hyperplasia after stereotactic breast biopsy: effects of number of foci and complete removal of calcifications. *Radiology.* 2010;255:723-730.
2. Ely KA, Carter BA, Jensen RA, Simpson JF, Page DL. Core biopsy of the breast with atypical ductal hyperplasia: a probabilistic approach to reporting. *Am J Surg Pathol.* 2001;25:1017-1021.
3. Nguyen CV, Albarracin CT, Whitman GJ, Lopez A, Sneige N. Atypical ductal hyperplasia in directional vacuum-assisted biopsy of breast microcalcifications: considerations for surgical excision. *Ann Surg Oncol.* 2011;18:752-761.

Targeted Ultrasound in Women Younger Than 30 Years With Focal Breast Signs or Symptoms: Outcomes Analyses and Management Implications
Loving VA, DeMartini WB, Eby PR, et al (Seattle Cancer Care Alliance, WA)
AJR Am J Roentgenol 195:1472-1477, 2010

Objective.—The purpose of this article is to assess the accuracy of targeted breast ultrasound in women younger than 30 years presenting with focal breast signs or symptoms.

Materials and Methods.—Retrospective review of the electronic medical records identified all ultrasound examinations from January 1, 2002, through August 30, 2006, performed for focal breast signs or symptoms in women younger than 30 years. BI-RADS assessments were recorded. Outcomes were determined by biopsy, 24 months of ultrasound surveillance, and linkage with the regional tumor registry. The overall cancer yield, sensitivity, specificity, negative predictive value (NPV), positive predictive value (PPV) 2, and PPV3 of ultrasound were calculated.

Results.—Among 830 study patients, lesions were assessed as BI-RADS category 1 or 2 in 526 (63.4%), BI-RADS category 3 in 140 (16.9%), BI-RADS category 4 in 163 (19.6%), and BI-RADS category 5 in one (0.1%) patient. Three malignancies were detected, for a cancer yield of 0.4%. No BI-RADS category 3 lesions, two BI-RADS category 4 lesions, and the single BI-RADS category 5 lesion were malignant. Ultrasound sensitivity was 100%, specificity was 80.5%, NPV was 100%, PPV2 was 1.8%, and PPV3 was 1.9%.

Conclusion.—Women younger than 30 years with focal breast signs or symptoms have a very low (0.4%) incidence of malignancy. The 100% sensitivity and NPV of targeted ultrasound in our study substantiates its use as an accurate primary imaging test in this clinical setting. We found no malignancies in BI-RADS category 3 lesions, supporting ultrasound surveillance over biopsy in this patient population.

▶ We don't usually perform mammograms on patients younger than 30 years. There is a very low prevalence of breast cancer in women younger than 30 years. Usually, this patient population has very dense breast tissue that decreases the sensitivity of mammography and because of the ionizing radiation associated with mammography.[1] The American College of Radiology (ACR) recommends sonography as the first imaging modality and recommends mammography for high-risk patients or for further evaluation of clinically or sonographically suspicious cases.[2]

The authors of this article assessed the accuracy of targeted sonography in women younger than 30 years presenting with focal breast signs or symptoms. This is important because many institutions recommend biopsy of all symptomatic solid breast masses, regardless of imaging appearance or patient age.

The authors' results support the ACR recommendation mentioned above. All cancer types in their study were identified by ultrasound. Their negative predictive value was 100%. The authors had no false-negative ultrasound for which the addition of a mammographic work-up would have added diagnostic value. The overall incidence of breast cancer in their study was 0.4%, which suggests that most young patients will have a benign cause for their focal breast concerns. No Breast Imaging Reporting and Data System 3 (BI-RADS 3) category masses were malignant in this study. All cancers were either BI-RADS category 4 or BI-RADS category 5 masses. Strict adherence to the use of BI-RADS criteria supports the safety of surveillance of probably benign masses over biopsy of these masses.

As with all studies, this one had limitations. One of which, the examinations were performed by radiologists specializing in breast imaging. Further studies are needed to determine whether the authors' results may be generalized to other practice settings.

T. W. Stephens, MD

References

1. Palmer ML, Tsangaris TN. Breast biopsy in women 30 years old or less. *Am J Surg.* 1993;165:708-712.
2. Graf O, Helbich TH, Hopf G, Graf C, Sickles EA. Probably benign breast masses at US: is follow-up an acceptable alternative to biopsy? *Radiology.* 2007;244: 87-93.

3 Musculoskeletal System

Introduction

The articles chosen this year include some that may be groundbreaking, some that may remind us of how to improve our value to our colleagues, and some that are simply beautiful reviews of difficult topics.

A review of new articles on musculoskeletal tumor imaging resulted in little new information. However, one very nice feasibility study of a unique application of proton MR spectroscopy is included to help our readers stay abreast of this possibility. The second tumor study chosen for review includes a discussion of the methodology used for histological evaluation of osteosarcoma; this directly affects clinical decision making and may be less closely related to the imaging of the tumor than one might expect. Any radiologist involved in bone sarcoma work should find this article to be of great interest.

Trauma articles held little new information this year. One study included in this chapter serves as a nice reminder that adult and childhood injuries may differ significantly despite having a common mechanism; the specific example here is of hyperextension of the knee resulting in anterior femoral physeal injury and posterior femoral periosteal disruption. Radiation dose from multidetector CT (MDCT) remains uppermost in our minds; one article discusses methodology for limiting dose in cervical spine MDCT, while another serves as a model retrospective research study establishing scenarios with 2 cohorts of trauma patients who deserve follow-up of a normal MDCT by MR.

There were several valuable articles discussing systemic diseases affecting the musculoskeletal system. With a nod to the ever-increasing number of patients with diabetes, one article describing diabetic myopathy is particularly valuable. Its description of MR features as well as its discussion of the hazards of biopsy in these patients is worth a review by all radiologists. Another growing patient population includes those with lung transplants; one of our articles describes the typical painful periostitis that can be associated with long-term use of voriconazole, used as prophylaxis and treatment of aspergillis in virtually all of these patients. This represents a new process to add to this author's differential diagnosis list of polyostotic periostitis. Another article revisited the criteria used to determine osteonecrosis in scaphoid fractures; the results may be surprising to some radiologists in that the most reliable method is actually one of the older rather than newer ones.

There were interesting offerings related to systemic metabolic disease. One of the most important relates fatty atrophy of the thigh muscles to vitamin D deficiency. While clinicians and especially those specializing in geriatrics are becoming aware of the prevalence of vitamin D deficiency in the elderly and its association with balance, falls, and broken bones, it would serve the public well if radiologists started paying attention to this as well. There was also an excellent study that shows a methodology for individualization of screening for bone mineral density. This article should become a landmark for cost/benefit discussions and is well worth reading. Finally, there is an excellent review that discusses innovations in imaging of both osteoporosis and osteoarthritis.

Arthritis is an important topic in our field, and newer research is expanding beyond the simple demonstration of arthritis by means of MR and ultrasound. One interesting report discusses the value of whole-body MR of joints in patients with unclassified arthritis. Another discusses the utility of power Doppler ultrasound in patients with very early inflammatory arthritis, relating cost of imaging to cost of treatment. This study may become important in developing cost-efficient diagnostic algorithms. Another article was particularly interesting in pointing out specific findings in MR of the hand that may differentiate psoriatic from rheumatoid arthritis. This specificity is valuable to clinicians, and radiologists should become aware of it.

Some very interesting articles were chosen that relate to sports and joint injury. One that may become controversial demonstrates that MR and MRA imaging of the shoulder is more accurately interpreted by subspecialty trained radiologists than general radiologists. This study might serve as a model as radiology groups enter into discussions of who should serve as the primary interpreters of musculoskeletal imaging. While it may not be a popular discussion, it is one that is needed in many community-based groups as well as perhaps at a national level as radiologists seek to demonstrate their value to the practice of medicine.

One nice review article discusses the shoulder rotator interval morphology and abnormalities. The discussion, graphics, and images are excellent, and this is an article I expect my fellows to master. Another shoulder article discusses abnormal translation of superior labral anterior-posterior (SLAP) lesions using the controversial abduction and external rotation (ABER) positioning.

Four hip articles were chosen. Two continue the discussion of proper imaging and interpretation of MR arthrography for femoral acetabular impingement (FAI), and one tackles the important issue of radiologists' failure to suggest FAI based on radiographic images. This article shows a tremendous preponderance of FAI in the young adult population presenting with hip pain and also demonstrates an embarrassing rate of under-diagnosis of the initial radiographs.

As was found with the discussion at the Society of Skeletal Radiology this year, many articles showed that we still have plenty to learn about the knee. Articles are included that discuss patellofemoral morphology, a new classification of discoid meniscus, and new observations regarding the association of meniscal tears and anterior cruciate injury.

The foot and ankle continue to confound many radiologists. Two articles were chosen that discuss the difficulties we seem to have with diagnoses as apparently simple as pes planus. Finally, I have included a review article discussing MR of ankle and hindfoot impingement; these eminent authors have contributed another outstanding article with beautiful illustrative images that will be appreciated by all radiologists concerned with foot and ankle imaging.

B. J. Manaster, MD, PhD

Tumor

A Feasibility Study of Quantitative Molecular Characterization of Musculoskeletal Lesions by Proton MR Spectroscopy at 3 T

Fayad LM, Wang X, Salibi N, et al (The Johns Hopkins Med Insts, Baltimore, MD; Siemens Healthcare USA, Earth City, MO; et al)
AJR Am J Roentgenol 195:W69-W75, 2010

Objective.—The purpose of this study is to establish the feasibility and potential value of measuring the concentration of choline-containing compounds by proton MR spectroscopy (MRS) in musculoskeletal lesions at 3 T.

Subjects and Methods.—Thirty-three subjects with 34 musculoskeletal lesions (four histologically proven malignant, 13 histologically proven benign or proven benign by follow-up analysis, and 17 posttreatment fibrosis with documented stability for 6–36 months) underwent single-voxel 3-T MRS studies. In each case, both water-suppressed and water-unsuppressed scans were obtained. The quality of the scans was recorded as excellent, adequate, or nondiagnostic, and the choline concentration was measured using water as the internal reference. The choline concentrations of benign and malignant lesions were compared using the Mann-Whitney test.

Results.—Spectral quality was excellent in 26 cases, adequate in four cases, and nondiagnostic in four cases. For malignant lesions (three sarcomas), the choline concentrations were 1.5, 2.9, and 3.8 mmol/kg, respectively. For five benign lesions (two neurofibromas, two schwannomas, and one enchondroma), the choline concentrations were 0.11, 0.28, 0.13, 0.8, and 1.2 mmol/kg, respectively. For seven benign lesions (two hematomas, two bone cysts, one lipoma, one giant cell tumor, and one pigmented villonodular synovitis), the spectra showed negligible choline content. For three posttreatment fibrosis cases, the choline concentration range was 0.2–0.4 mmol/kg. For the remaining 12 posttreatment fibrosis cases, the spectra showed negligible choline content. Average choline concentrations were different for malignant and benign lesions (2.7 vs 0.5 mmol/kg; $p = 0.01$).

Conclusion.—The measurement of choline concentration within musculoskeletal lesions by MRS is feasible using an internal water-referencing method at 3 T and has potential for characterizing lesions for malignancy.

▶ There has been a long search for a reliable methodology to differentiate benign from malignant musculoskeletal tumors. It is also acknowledged to be difficult to differentiate postoperative (and other posttherapeutic) change from local recurrence. Currently, most sarcoma services rely on imaging with contrast for both initial imaging and follow-up of musculoskeletal tumors, with the understanding that, while some lesions are reliably diagnosed, it is not always possible to differentiate benign from malignant or recurrence with this methodology.

There have been numerous attempts to develop different varieties of functional imaging to characterize musculoskeletal tumors and the results of their treatment. All have suffered from technical limitations, but we are seeing continual improvements in methodology. The most important limitation in this research seems to be the patient numbers because malignant musculoskeletal tumors are relatively rare. Thus, it is difficult for any single institution to collect a significant number of patients to study; it can be even more difficult to follow a reasonable number of these individuals, especially because they often return to home institutions for these follow-up examinations. Therefore, many reports in the literature suffer from fairly unconvincing statistics, though they are often cautiously encouraging.

Dr Fayad and her colleagues have been persistent in evaluating the utility of MR spectroscopy for musculoskeletal tumor imaging. This article is unique in seeking to establish the feasibility of proton MR spectroscopy for determining the choline concentration within musculoskeletal lesions using an internal water-referencing method. The patient numbers in this study are more impressive than in many others, and the results are definitely encouraging for differentiating benign from malignant lesions, though the follow-up portion of the study did not include enough recurrences to yield definitive recommendations. However, I would encourage radiologists to keep abreast of this avenue of research. Although we may still be several years from routine use of MR spectroscopy for evaluation of musculoskeletal tumors, it is worth reading articles that describe such well-crafted research, as is done by this group.

B. J. Manaster, MD, PhD

Tumor necrosis in osteosarcoma: inclusion of the point of greatest metabolic activity from F-18 FDG PET/CT in the histopathologic analysis
Costelloe CM, Raymond AK, Fitzgerald NE, et al (The Univ of Texas M. D. Anderson Cancer Ctr, Houston)
Skeletal Radiol 39:131-140, 2010

Objective.—To determine if the location of the point of maximum standardized uptake value (SUVmax) being included in or not included in the histopathologic slab section corresponded to tumor necrosis or survival.

Materials and Methods.—Twenty-nine osteosarcoma patients underwent post-chemotherapy [fluorine-18]-fluoro-2-deoxy-D-glucose (FDG) positron-emission tomography-computed tomography (PET/CT) prior to resection. PET/CT images were correlated with slab-section location as determined by photographs or knowledge of specimen processing. The location of the point of SUVmax was then assigned as being 'in' or 'out' of the slab section. Cox's proportional hazard regression was used to evaluate relationships between the location and value of SUVmax and survival. Logistic regression was employed to evaluate tumor necrosis.

Results.—No correlation was found between the SUVmax location and survival or tumor necrosis. High SUVmax correlated to poor survival.

Conclusion.—High SUVmax value correlated to poor survival. Minimal viable tumor (> 10%) following chemotherapy is a known indicator of poor survival. No correlation was found between the location of SUVmax and survival or tumor necrosis. Therefore, the SUVmax value either does not correspond to a sufficient number of tumor cells to influence tumor necrosis measurement or it was included in the out-of-slab samples that were directed to viableappearing areas of the gross specimen. Since high SUVmax has been previously found to correspond to poor tumor necrosis, and tumor necrosis is simply an estimate of the amount of viable tumor, SUVmax likely represents many viable tumor cells. Therefore, when not in the slab section, SUVmax was likely included in the tumor necrosis measurement through directed sampling, validating our current method of osteosarcoma specimen analysis.

▶ Patients with conventional osteosarcoma are treated with neoadjuvant chemotherapy, followed by wide surgical resection and then continued chemotherapy. Because of this treatment regimen, clinicians have the ability to evaluate the effectiveness of the neoadjuvant chemotherapy midway through the overall treatment process. This is done by histological evaluation of the resected tissue; if the tumor shows < 90% necrosis, the chemotherapy regimen is considered to have had suboptimal effect and strong consideration is given to changing the postoperative chemotherapy to a more aggressive regimen. Because there is a direct effect on clinical decision making and patient morbidity/mortality, it is clearly crucial that representative tissue be evaluated for determination of percent tumor necrosis.

Unlike the evaluation of prostate and other tumor specimens, histological evaluation of osteosarcoma specimens does not use the entire specimen. The specimens are usually large, and it is cost prohibitive to look at every cell. As indicated by the authors of this article, the usual procedure at oncologic institutions is to evaluate a single central slab of the bone, cut longitudinally, as well as evaluation of other regions that the pathologist and tumor surgeon believe may look like viable tumor in the gross specimen rather than tumor necrosis. It is important that imagers understand this process in that they may be able to influence the pathologist to evaluate regions that are suspicious on the restaging MR or positron emission tomography/CT.

This article is interesting in that the authors sought to evaluate whether the point of maximum standardized uptake value (SUV_{max}) was included in the central slab that was histologically evaluated and whether this correlated with patient survival (based on the known correlation between high SUV_{max} and poor patient survival in osteosarcoma). The results are of interest, along with the excellent discussion of methodology of histological evaluation and potential reasons for their results.

B. J. Manaster, MD, PhD

Trauma

Posterior Periosteal Disruption in Salter-Harris Type II Fractures of the Distal Femur: Evidence for a Hyperextension Mechanism

Kritsaneepaiboon S, Shah R, Murray MM, et al (Children's Hosp Boston and Harvard Med School, MA)
AJR Am J Roentgenol 193:W540-W545, 2009

Objective.—Patterns of periosteal disruption are important factors in assessing the mechanism of injury of radiologically evident Salter-Harris (SH) fractures. The purpose of this study is to assess the frequency of posterior periosteal disruption on MRI in radiographically occult or subtle SH type II fractures of the distal femur and to evaluate associated soft-tissue findings that support a hyperextension mechanism of injury.

Conclusion.—We found that all children in our experience with occult or subtle SH type II fractures of the distal femur have posterior periosteal disruption and other MRI findings to indicate a hyperextension mechanism of injury. Direct indicators of fracture may be inconspicuous, and the presence of posterior periosteal disruption is a clue that should prompt a search for other features of this serious pediatric injury, which may be followed by limb shortening or angular deformity.

▶ Radiologists who are not additionally trained in the subspecialty of pediatric radiology should maintain a healthy skepticism of their ability to diagnose subtle osseous injuries in children and adolescents. It is well worthwhile for the general radiologist to remember that while the mechanisms of injury in patients of this age group is often similar to that in adults, the resultant injury often is not. This is because of the differing relative strengths of bone, physes, and ligaments in children versus adults. Thus, an injury mechanism that leads to anterior cruciate rupture in adults may result in tibial spine avulsion relatively more frequently in children.

This article is a small retrospective study demonstrating that Salter Harris injuries of the distal femur often result in an anteromedial metaphyseal portion (Thurston Holland fracture fragment) that then extends through the remainder of the physis. The images serve to remind those of us who spend most of our time with adult imaging of just how subtle the radiographic findings can be in the absence of gross displacement of a fragment. Furthermore, by demonstrating that these fractures are usually a result of a hyperextension injury, the authors remind us to look for associated periosteal disruption along the posterior physis and even periosteal entrapment within the physis. Such periosteal entrapment, along with physeal widening should be part of the evaluation of every MR of a joint in an adolescent.

B. J. Manaster, MD, PhD

40-Slice Multidetector CT: Is MRI Still Necessary for Cervical Spine Clearance after Blunt Trauma?
Menaker J, Stein DM, Philp AS, et al (Univ of Maryland Med Ctr, Baltimore)
Am Surg 76:157-163, 2010

We have recently demonstrated that 16-slice multidetector CT (MDCT) is insufficient for cervical spine (CS) clearance in patients with unreliable examinations after blunt trauma. The purpose of this study was to determine if a negative CS CT using 40-sliceMDCT is sufficient for ruling out CS injury in unreliable blunt trauma patients or if MRI remains necessary for definitive clearance. In addition, we sought to elucidate the frequency by which MRI alters treatment in patients with a negative CS CT who have a reliable examination with persistent clinical symptoms. The trauma registry was used to identify all patients with blunt trauma who had a negative CS CT on admission using 40-slice MDCT and a subsequent CS MRI during their hospitalization from July 2006 to July 2007. Two hundred thirteen patients were identified. Overall, 24.4 per cent patients had abnormal MRIs. Fifteen required operative repair; 23 required extended cervical collar; and 14 had collars removed. A total of 8.3 per cent of patients with an unreliable examination and 25.6 per cent of reliable patients had management changed based on MRI findings. Overall, MRI changed clinical practice in 17.8 per cent of all patients. Despite newer 40-slice CT technology, MRI continues to be necessary for CS clearance in patients with unreliable examinations or persistent symptoms.

▶ The established practice in many high-volume trauma centers for clearing cervical spines by means of clinical exam and multidetector CT (MDCT) is more sophisticated and evidence based than the Advanced Trauma Life Support's recommendations of using radiographs. However, there is continued controversy regarding whether even the most sophisticated CT is reliable enough to obviate the use of MRI for evaluation of the integrity of the spinal cord and ligaments in 2 situations that occur relatively frequently: (1) the patient who has a normal CT but persistently unreliable clinical examination after blunt trauma and (2) the patient who has a negative MDCT with persistent pain on palpation, range of motion, or subtle neurological deficit, including paresthesias.

The literature is currently inconsistent regarding imaging recommendations in these 2 patient cohorts, with some claiming that CT is adequate and others claiming that MRI will demonstrate important abnormalities in a small number of patients. However, these studies uniformly suffer either from inadequate patient numbers or else imprecise definition of terms such as unreliable. The trauma and imaging communities are lucky that the University of Maryland's Shock Trauma Center had the foresight to establish an excellent trauma registry. These investigators thus have the means to study these issues both with sufficient numbers of patients and with a precision of terminology that is convincing. This article's conclusion that MRI should be performed in the 2 cohorts of patients discussed above is believable and should be strongly considered in such clinical situations.

B. J. Manaster, MD, PhD

Radiation Dose to the Thyroid Gland and Breast From Multidetector Computed Tomography of the Cervical Spine: Does Bismuth Shielding With and Without a Cervical Collar Reduce Dose?
Gunn ML, Kanal KM, Kolokythas O, et al (Univ of Washington, Seattle)
J Comput Assist Tomogr 33:987-990, 2009

Purpose.—This study aimed to assess the radiation dose reduction that could be achieved using an in-line bismuth shielding over the thyroid gland and breast and to determine the effect of a cervical spine collar on thyroid dose reduction and image noise when performing computed tomography of the cervical spine using automatic tube current modulation.

Materials and Methods.—An anthropomorphic phantom was scanned using a commercially available 64-channel computed tomographic scanner. A standardized trauma cervical spine protocol was used. Scans were obtained with and without a standard cervical spine immobilization collar and with and without bismuth-impregnated thyroid and breast shields. Thermoluminescent dosimeters were placed over the thyroid gland and breasts for each scan. A paired t test was used to determine whether the skin entry dose differed significantly between the shielded and unshielded thyroid and breast and to determine whether placing the thyroid shield over a cervical immobilization collar resulted in a significant dose reduction. Region of interest of pixel values was used to determine image noise.

Results.—The average measured skin entry dose for the unshielded thyroid gland was 21.9 mGy (95% confidence interval, 18.9–4.7). With a bismuth shield applied directly over the skin, the dose to the thyroid gland was reduced by 22.5% ($P < 0.05$). With the bismuth shield applied over the cervical spine collar, the dose reduction to the thyroid was 10.4%, which was not statistically significant ($P = 0.16$) compared with the dose reduction without the cervical collar. Skin entry dose over the breasts was significant, although they were outside the primary scan range. Without bismuth shielding, the skin entry dose was 1.5 mGy, and with bismuth shielding, the dose was significantly reduced by 36.6% ($P < 0.01$). Image noise increased most when shielding was used with an immobilization collar.

Conclusions.—There is a significant dose reduction to the thyroid gland and breasts when a bismuth shield is placed on the skin. The dose saving achieved by placing the shield on the cervical collar is approximately halved compared with placement on the skin, and this did not reach statistical significance, and this was accompanied by an increase on image noise. Bismuth shields should not be used in combination with cervical immobilization collars.

▶ Beyond producing diagnostic images and making correct diagnoses, it is the radiologist's job to protect the patient from excessive medical radiation. Numerous articles, both in the medical and lay literature, decry the exponential increase in use of CT over the past decades and the associated significant increase in radiation to the population. In addition to the increased diagnostic use of CT, the development of multidetector CT results in radiation exposure well beyond the region being scanned.

This article discusses the use of bismuth shielding during CT of the cervical spine, to protect the thyroid gland (directly in the field) as well as the breasts (which may be exposed to the primary radiation beam with 64-channel multidetector CT and steep pitches). Although the design of the experiment is somewhat limited (only 1 scanner type and a single tube current modulation technique were tested; a phantom was used, which does not account for different body habitus; and effects of shielding on diagnostic accuracy were not assessed), the study is an important step in consideration of patient radiation safety. It not only demonstrated significant savings in radiation dose to both the thyroid and breasts with cervical shielding with the shield placed directly on the patient's neck, but also showed that placement of the shield on the cervical collar is in fact detrimental because the radiation dose is not significantly decreased while the image noise is demonstrably increased. Thus, if it is an institutional policy to use bismuth shielding with cervical spine CTs, it is important that the shield not be used if a cervical collar is in place. Subtleties such as this are important in obtaining optimal diagnostic accuracy as well as patient protection, and it is important that the radiologist and radiation safety staff stay abreast of such developments.

B. J. Manaster, MD, PhD

Systemic

Diabetic Myopathy: MRI Patterns and Current Trends

Huang BK, Monu JUV, Doumanian J (Univ of Rochester Med Ctr, NY; Rush Copley Med Ctr, Aurora, IL)
Am J Roentgenol 195:198-204, 2010

Objective.—This study retrospectively evaluates diabetic myopathy in a large referral hospital population. It describes the MRI findings and the distribution of muscle involvement, including comparison with clinical parameters.

Materials and Methods.—MRI reports of the lower extremities from July 1999 through January 2006 were reviewed and compared with clinical parameters for patients with diabetic myopathy. Clinical parameters (e.g., type of diabetes, hemoglobin A_{1C} level, creatine kinase level, and erythrocyte sedimentation rate [ESR]) and the presence of complications, including nephropathy, neuropathy, and retinopathy, were noted. The distribution of muscle involvement and imaging features were reviewed.

Results.—Over a 79-month period, 21 extremities (11 thighs and 10 calves) of 16 patients were imaged. Fourteen (88%) patients had type 2 diabetes, and two (12%) had type 1 diabetes. Four patients (25%) had disease in more than one location. In the thigh, the anterior compartment was involved in all patients. The posterior compartment was affected in nine (90%) of 10 calves. Muscle infarction and necrosis was seen in eight (38%) extremities. The creatine kinase level, ESR, and hemoglobin A1C level were elevated in the majority of cases. Coexisting nephropathy (50%), neuropathy (50%), and retinopathy (38%) were present in these patients.

Conclusion.—Diabetic myopathy may occur more frequently in patients with type 2 diabetes than previously reported. In this population, T2-weighted and contrast-enhanced images have similar findings, and the increased coexistence of nephropathy makes administration of gadolinium-based contrast agents ill-advised. With a typical clinical presentation and MRI findings, a confident diagnosis can be made, and potentially harmful biopsy is avoided.

Diabetic myopathy encompasses a spectrum of diseases, including muscle inflammation, ischemia, hemorrhage, infarction, necrosis, fibrosis, and fatty atrophy. It is usually seen with long-standing, poorly controlled diabetes.

▶ With the exponentially increasing numbers of cases of diabetes in the developed world, radiologists must be prepared to evaluate these patients for diabetic myopathy. It is important to distinguish the magnetic resonance (MR) findings of diabetic myopathy from those indicating other muscle processes that may require surgical intervention, such as pyogenic myositis and, particularly, necrotizing myositis. There is a paucity of literature regarding the imaging findings of diabetic myopathy.

This article suffers from reporting on a relatively small number of cases. However, the observations made are useful. Perhaps of greatest importance is the observation that diabetic myopathy not infrequently develops in type 2 diabetic patients, whereas the prior literature suggested a strong predominance in type 1 diabetic patients. Many of this study's type 2 diabetic patients were insulin dependent, but the most common feature seems to be poor control of the disease. As with the type 1 diabetic patients noted in earlier studies, presence of myopathy in type 2 diabetic patients portends a poor disease prognosis.

This article confirms predominance of disease in the lower extremities, but shows that the calf may be affected nearly as frequently as the thigh, which differs from previous reports. The MR findings of subcutaneous edema, T2 hyperintensity, and enhancement of multicompartment muscles are nonspecific, as is the more advanced finding of hemorrhagic necrosis. However, the authors emphasize that the MR appearance, in conjunction with clinical findings, may allow conservative treatment without the necessity (and possible complications) of biopsy.

B. J. Manaster, MD, PhD

Medication-induced periostitis in lung transplant patients: periostitis deformans revisited
Chen L, Mulligan ME (UMMS, Baltimore)
Skeletal Radiol 2010 [Epub ahead of print]

We report five cases of diffuse periostitis resembling hypertrophic osteoarthropathy and perostitis deformans in lung transplantation patients on chronic voriconazole, a fluoride-containing compound. Although drug-related periostitis has long been known, the association of lung transplant medication with periostitis was only recently introduced in the literature. To our knowledge, imaging findings have not been fully characterized in the radiology literature. Imaging features along with clinical history help to distinguish this benign condition from other disease entities. In this article, we review the current literature and illustrate the variety of imaging characteristics of this entity so that interpreting radiologists can make accurate diagnoses and avoid unnecessary work up.

▶ Radiologists are well used to searching for periosteal reaction as an indicator of osseous abnormality. When periosteal reaction is discovered in multiple bones, and the patients' clinical symptoms are of joint pain (in the absence of radiographic joint abnormalities), radiologists raise the question of hypertrophic osteoarthropathy (HOA), either primary or secondary. The primary form of HOA is rare; the more common secondary form is most often associated with a pulmonary abnormality (most frequently lung cancer); other associations include medications (prostaglandins, hypervitamin A, and fluorosis).

This article demonstrates the findings of HOA in a newly described clinical presentation, that of lung transplant patients and relatively long-term and chronic use of the medication voriconazole. It is speculated that the reaction may relate to the fluoride component of voriconazole, but the pathogenesis is not known.

The number of patients with lung transplant is growing worldwide. Voriconazole is a widely used medication in lung transplantation patients for both prophylaxis and treatment of aspergillus infection. Therefore, it is worthwhile for radiologists to become familiar with this new association for diffuse periostitis and consider it when discussing such a case. Becoming familiar with its manifestations, as described in this article, should obviate a more extensive workup for the periostitis and associated pain in these lung transplant patients.

B. J. Manaster, MD, PhD

Assessment of Scaphoid Viability With MRI: A Reassessment of Findings on Unenhanced MR Images

Fox MG, Gaskin CM, Chhabra AB, et al (Univ of Virginia, Charlottesville)
AJR Am J Roentgenol 195:W281-W286, 2010

Objective.—The purpose of this article is to evaluate the accuracy of unenhanced T1-weighted MR images in predicting the vascular status of the proximal pole of the scaphoid in patients with chronic scaphoid fracture nonunions.

Materials and Methods.—A database search identified 29 patients with chronic scaphoid nonunions who underwent a preoperative MRI examination and intraoperative assessment of scaphoid viability from 2004 to 2009. T1-weighted MR images were evaluated by two musculoskeletal radiologists. If the proximal pole demonstrated diffusely decreased T1-weighted signal (less than or equal to that of skeletal muscle), the patient was placed in a moderate-to-high risk for avascular necrosis (AVN) category. Otherwise, the patient was placed in a viable-to-low risk for AVN category. Scaphoid viability or necrosis was diagnosed intraoperatively depending on whether punctate bleeding was present. After the patients were classified according to the T1-weighted appearance, the appearance on STIR images was recorded.

Results.—There were 29 patients (25 male) with a mean age of 21 years. When we compared the MRI results, using only the T1-weighted images, with the surgical findings, unenhanced MRI had a sensitivity, specificity, and accuracy of 55%, 94%, and 79%, respectively, for diagnosing AVN. Increased proximal pole STIR signal was noted with similar frequencies in patients with and without AVN.

Conclusion.—T1-weighted unenhanced MRI is an acceptable alternative to delayed contrast-enhanced MRI in the preoperative assessment of the vascular status of the proximal pole of the scaphoid in patients with chronic fracture nonunions. STIR images were not beneficial in determining proximal pole viability.

▶ MR imaging has long been thought to have great potential in diagnosing the vascular status and potential viability of regions of osteonecrosis. Since the early 1990s, investigators have offered various MR sequences as accurate depictions of the viability of bone. Surgeons may rely on these impressions, planning either vascularized or nonvascularized bone grafting based on them. There is a significant difference in surgical technical requirements, time, and cost in the vascularized versus nonvascularized surgical procedures; accurate preoperative assessment of the vascular status of the involved bone would be of great value.

The clinical investigations available thus far suffer from low patient numbers, arbitrary and not easily reproduced criteria, and often long periods of time between the MRI and surgery, the gold standard. The latter limitation is particularly problematic with osteonecrosis in the scaphoid, as it is known that scaphoid fractures may heal over a very long period of time, even when initially thought to be a nonunion.

The authors of this study seek a simpler solution to the use of delayed-contrast enhancement imaging. Their study is retrospective and has a reasonably large number of patients but suffers, as do all the previous studies, from substantial delay between MRI and surgery in several cases. However, the article is well worth reading in detail because it carefully describes apparent discrepancies among previous study results and reasonably speculates about their causes. It allows the reader to better understand the limitations of MR as it is currently practiced in the evaluation of osteonecrosis and viability of fragments in scaphoid fractures and may promote more caution in interpretation.

B. J. Manaster, MD, PhD

Relationship Between Fatty Degeneration of Thigh Muscles and Vitamin D Status in the Elderly: A Preliminary MRI Study

Tagliafico AS, Ameri P, Bovio M, et al (Univ of Genoa, Italy)
AJR Am J Roentgenol 194:728-734, 2010

Objective.—The purpose of this study was to study the relationship between fatty degeneration of thigh muscles and vitamin D status in elderly adults.

Subjects and Methods.—For six months, 121 patients 65 years old or older were evaluated. Myopathy, muscular impairment, and conditions influencing vitamin D status other than diet and sunlight were exclusion criteria. Twenty patients (10 men and 10 women; mean age, 77.6 years) underwent MRI. Thigh muscles were scanned from the hip to the knee with T1- and T2-weighted spin-echo sequences. Skeletal muscles were evaluated for fatty degeneration and atrophy from grade 0 to 3 (grade 0 = normal appearance, grade 3 = severe changes). The relationship between muscular fatty degeneration, 25-hydroxyvitamin D (25-OHD) levels, and scores on Tinetti scales for balance and gait were examined.

Results.—In the evaluation of the extensor muscles for fatty degeneration and atrophy, grade 0 was present in three patients (15%), grade 1 in 11 (55%), and grade 2 in six (30%). In the flexor muscles, grade 0 was found in one patient (5%), grade 1 in five (25%), and grade 2 in

14 (70%); grade 3 changes were not seen. Muscular fatty degeneration negatively correlated with 25-OHD levels ($r = -0.50$, $p < 0.01$) and the Tinetti scores (balance: $r = -0.40$, $p < 0.05$; gait: $r = -0.50$, $p < 0.05$). In 11 vitamin D−deficient patients (55%), there was selective complete atrophy of at least one thigh muscle. The gracilis and sartorius muscles were spared.

Conclusion.—In elderly adults, fatty degeneration of thigh muscles was associated with vitamin D deficiency and impaired balance and gait. Selective complete fatty degeneration of single muscles was observed.

▶ As the baby boomers start to head into their geriatric years, radiologists will see more and more imaging in this patient group. Clinicians and radiologists alike are becoming aware of the importance of diagnosing osteoporosis and the complications of therapy for osteoporosis such as bisphosphonate fractures. However, radiologists seem less aware than geriatricians are about the hazards of vitamin D deficiency in the elderly (defined as > 65 years of age). There in fact is a very high prevalence of this vitamin deficiency, especially in the elderly population. This deficiency is associated with loss of muscle strength, decreased muscle mass, myopathy, and increased risk of falling. This article nicely addresses the issue of vitamin D deficiency and is a good study examining the musculature of the thigh, relating atrophy to vitamin D deficiency as well as the Tinetti balance and gait scales. It is worth a review, with particular note of the findings of selective complete muscle atrophy and the relative sparing of the sartorius and gracilis. The study is admittedly small, with preliminary results, but represents a good start on an important topic.

B. J. Manaster, MD, PhD

Timing of Repeat BMD Measurements: Development of an Absolute Risk-Based Prognostic Model

Frost SA, Nguyen ND, Center JR, et al (St Vincent's Hosp, Sydney, New South Wales, Australia)

J Bone Miner Res 24:1800-1807, 2009

This study attempted to address the following questions: for an individual who is at present nonosteoporotic, given their current age and BMD level, what is the individual's risk of fracture and when is the ideal time to repeat a BMD measurement? Nonosteoporotic women ($n = 1008$) and men ($n = 750$) over the age of 60 in 1989 from the Dubbo Osteoporosis Epidemiology Study were monitored until one of the following outcomes occurred: (1) BMD reached "osteoporosis" level (i.e., T-scores ≤ -2.5) or (2) an incident fragility fracture. During the follow-up period (average, 7 yr), 346 women (34%) and 160 men (21%) developed osteoporosis or sustained a low-trauma fracture. The risk of osteoporosis or fracture increased with advancing age (women: RR/10 yr, 1.3; 95% CI, 1.1−1.6; men: RR/10 yr, 2.3; 95% CI, 1.7−2.9) and lower BMD levels (women: RR per -0.12 g/cm^2, 3.2; 95% CI, 2.6—4.1; RR per -0.12 g/cm^2, 2.6; 95% CI, 2.0—3.3). Using the predicted risk (of osteoporosis or fracture) of 10% as a cut-off level for repeating BMD measurement, the estimated time to reach the cut-off level varied from 1.5 (for an 80-yr-old woman with a T-score of -2.2) to 10.6 yr (for a 60-yr-old man with a T-score of 0). These results suggest that, based on an individual's current age and BMD T-score, it is possible to estimate the optimal time to repeat BMD testing for the individual. The prognostic model and approach presented in this study may help improve the individualization and management of osteoporosis.

▶ Patient screening for costly disease processes or their consequences is now recognized as being cost effective in many instances. Because of the prevalence of osteoporosis and associated insufficiency fractures in many patient populations, bone mineral density (BMD) screening is becoming accepted as an important tool. However, the technique is quite costly if applied indiscriminately to all individuals who may be theoretically at risk (eg, all those older than 60 years). Additionally, there is no established guideline to the optimal timing of repeat BMD measurements, except that repeat measurements more frequently than every 12 months are unlikely to be informative.

This article should be considered a landmark for helping to establish a prognostic model approach to individualization in the management of osteoporosis. The methods used in the study have resulted in the physician being able to estimate the optimal time to repeat BMD testing based on the individual's current age and BMD T-score. This should result in optimizing individual patient care while conserving resources, as opposed to widespread overuse of BMD testing. Individualized medical testing should represent an important advance in public health discussions.

B. J. Manaster, MD, PhD

The Founder's Lecture 2009: advances in imaging of osteoporosis and osteoarthritis
Link TM (Univ of California at San Francisco)
Skeletal Radiol 39:943-955, 2010

The objective of this review article is to provide an update on new developments in imaging of osteoporosis and osteoarthritis over the past three decades. A literature review is presented that summarizes the highlights in the development of bone mineral density measurements, bone structure imaging, and vertebral fracture assessment in osteoporosis as well as MR-based semiquantitative assessment of osteoarthritis and quantitative cartilage matrix imaging. This review focuses on techniques that have impacted patient management and therapeutic decision making or that potentially will affect patient care in the near future. Results of pertinent studies are presented and used for illustration. In summary, novel developments have significantly impacted imaging of osteoporosis and osteo-arthritis over the past three decades.

▶ Most radiologists find both osteoporosis and osteoarthritis to be as common as dirt. The diagnosis of each is made on a qualitative basis multiple times daily, without much additional thought. However, there is tremendous ongoing research that may soon change our approach to these diseases. Although it is not necessary or even possible at this point for every radiologist to keep abreast of each research effort, occasionally there is a review article that makes the task of keeping updated relatively easy. Such is the case of this article, which is based on a lecture of the same title given at the International Skeletal Society meeting in honor of Dr Harry K Genant, who pioneered the study of osteoporosis by imaging.

Dr Link's article nicely segues the study of bone mineral density by means of quantitative CT and, more recently, dual X-ray absorptiometry, to structural analysis of osseous (trabecular) quality with multidetector CT and high resolution MR imaging. Additionally, bone strength imaging is described using water content of cortical bone using ultrashort echo time techniques.

Cartilage matrix imaging techniques are also described, relating to osteoarthritis. I recommend this article as a comfortable resource in maintaining awareness of the current state of the art.

B. J. Manaster, MD, PhD

Arthritis

Contrast-Enhanced Whole-Body Joint MRI in Patients With Unclassified Arthritis Who Develop Early Rheumatoid Arthritis Within 2 Years: Feasibility Study and Correlation With MRI Findings of the Hands

Kamishima T, Fujieda Y, Atsumi T, et al (Hokkaido Univ Hosp, Sapporo City, Japan; et al)
AJR Am J Roentgenol 195:W287-W292, 2010

Objective.—The purpose of this article is to examine the feasibility of whole-body joint MRI for detecting systemic joint synovitis and for analyzing the relationship between the hands and systemic joint involvement in patients with unclassified arthritis who later develop early rheumatoid arthritis (RA).

Materials and Methods.—The study included 17 patients (five men and 12 women; median age, 65 years [range, 38−77 years]; median symptom duration, 3 months [range, 1−6 months]). MRI of the systemic joints was performed for patients with unclassified arthritis without radiographic evidence of RA and who were diagnosed as having RA according to 1987 revised classification criteria within 2 years.

Results.—The chosen 4-point scale for image quality was moderate to excellent. MRI findings of systemic joints were in accordance with joint swelling and tenderness (chi-square test, $p < 0.0001$). Sixty percent (45/75) of hand joints and 67% (12/18) of systemic joints other than hands showed MR synovitis without swelling. With regard to the correlation of MRI findings between hands and joints other than hands, there was a statistically significant positive correlation in the joint count ($r = 0.5514$ and $p = 0.0218$) and semiquantitative value of hand synovitis ($r = 0.5382$ and $p = 0.0258$).

Conclusion.—Whole-body joint MRI in early RA is feasible in terms of image quality and agreement with the results of clinical examination. MRI may be more sensitive for depicting synovitis-positive joints than clinical examination. Estimation of the systemic burden of synovitis detected by MRI may be possible via MRI of the hands.

▶ With the advent of new disease-modifying drug therapy, the prognosis of rheumatoid arthritis has altered significantly in recent years. Additionally, research has shown that MR and ultrasound may demonstrate joint involvement far earlier than traditional radiography, allowing earlier diagnosis of the disease. In recognition of the relative insensitivity of the criteria for diagnosis of rheumatoid arthritis established in 1987, the American College of Rheumatology has recently established new criteria[1]; one of the major changes includes quantification of the number of joints involved. Recognizing that evaluation of number of joints may be optimized by whole-body MRI, this study was instituted.

The study used patients who had undifferentiated arthritis, not yet meeting the criteria for rheumatoid arthritis, but for whom the diagnosis was established over the ensuing 2-year period. Whole-body MR, as performed in this study, proved to usually produce interpretable images (excluding the elbows). In several cases, synovitis was noted in joints that were clinically not noted to be swollen. Interestingly, joint pain did not always correlate well with synovitis. This article provides techniques and suggests that whole-body MR for evaluation of synovitis is both feasible and perhaps desirable. Because of the relatively small number of patients studied, it remains preliminary.

B. J. Manaster, MD, PhD

Reference

1. Aletaha D, Neogi T, Silman AJ, et al. 2010 Rheumatoid arthritis classification criteria: an American College of Rheumatology/European League Against Rheumatism collaborative initiative. *Arthritis Rheum.* 2010;62:2569-2581.

A diagnostic algorithm for persistence of very early inflammatory arthritis: the utility of power Doppler ultrasound when added to conventional assessment tools
Freeston JE, Wakefield RJ, Conaghan PG, et al (Univ of Leeds, UK)
Ann Rheum Dis 69:417-419, 2010

Objectives.—The aim of this study was to assess the value of power Doppler ultrasound (PDUS) in combination with routine management in a cohort of patients with very early inflammatory arthritis (IA).

Methods.—50 patients with ≤ 12 weeks of inflammatory symptoms with or without signs had clinical, laboratory and imaging assessments.

Diagnosis was recorded at 12 months. Assuming a 15% pre-test probability of IA, post-test probabilities for various assessments were calculated and used to develop a diagnostic algorithm.

Results.—All patients positive for rheumatoid factor (RF) and/or cyclic citrullinated peptide (CCP) developed persistent IA, so the added value of PDUS was assessed in the seronegative (RF and CCP negative) group. The probability of IA in a seronegative patient was 6%. The addition of clinical and radiographic features raised the probability of IA to 30% and, with certain ultrasound features, this rose to 94%.

Conclusions.—In seronegative patients with early IA, combining PDUS with routine assessment can have a major impact on the certainty of diagnosis.

▶ With the success of new drug treatments for inflammatory arthritis, clinicians and patients alike are eager to make the diagnosis of inflammatory arthritis as early as possible in the disease process so as to institute therapy and prevent irrevocable arthritic change. However, it has been found that the traditional American College of Rheumatology criteria are not useful in diagnosing rheumatoid arthritis earlier than at 12 weeks. In the interest of establishing cost-effective diagnostic criteria for early diagnosis, the authors evaluated the usefulness of power Doppler ultrasound in patients with very early inflammatory arthritis. This is the first study to address the diagnostic benefit of adding ultrasound to conventional clinical tools in this cohort of patients. The study shows that while power Doppler does not add particular value to those patients who have positive rheumatoid factor and cyclic citrullinated peptide, it is particularly valuable in diagnosing seronegative patients in whom 1 to 3 conventional features are positive; positive ultrasound features can raise the probability in these patients from 2%-30% to 50%-94%. This type of information is particularly valuable in developing cost-efficient diagnostic algorithms.

B. J. Manaster, MD, PhD

MRI Findings in Psoriatic Arthritis of the Hands
Spira D, Kötter I, Henes J, et al (Eberhard-Karls-Univ, Tübingen, Germany)
AJR Am J Roentgenol 195:1187-1193, 2010

Objective.—The purpose of this essay is to provide a practical review of the spectrum of morphologic and functional MRI findings in psoriatic arthritis of the hand joints.

Conclusion.—The MRI findings of psoriatic arthritis include enthesitis, bone marrow edema, and periostitis accompanying articular or flexor tendon sheath synovitis in the early stage accompanied by destructive and proliferative bony changes, subluxation, and ankylosis in the late stage (Figs 7A and 8A).

▶ Clinically evident psoriatic arthritis (PSA) has prevalence in persons with psoriasis estimated at 13.8%. However, these authors cite references that

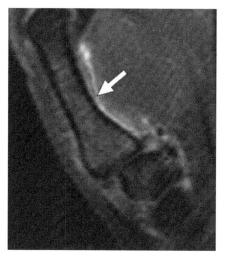

FIGURE 7.—69-year-old woman with psoriatic arthritis. **A,** Coronal oblique fat-saturated gadolinium-enhanced T1-weighted MR image shows periosteal thickening and hyperemia (*arrow*) in metacarpal bone of right first digit. (Reprinted with permission from the American Journal of Roentgenology. Spira D, Kötter I, Henes J, et al. MRI findings in psoriatic arthritis of the hands. *AJR Am J Roentgenol.* 2010;195:1187-1193, with permission from American Roentgen Ray Society.)

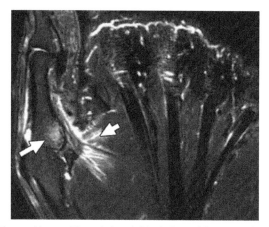

FIGURE 8.—52-year-old man with psoriatic arthritis. **A,** Coronal fat-saturated gadolinium-enhanced T1-weighted MR image shows bone marrow edema and hyperemia beginning at corner of proximal phalanx of thumb at insertion of thenar musculature and then spreading to involve adjacent bone (*arrow*). (Reprinted with permission from the American Journal of Roentgenology. Spira D, Kötter I, Henes J, et al. MRI findings in psoriatic arthritis of the hands. *AJR Am J Roentgenol.* 2010;195:1187-1193, with permission from American Roentgen Ray Society.)

suggest that PSA is underdiagnosed since many cases may have subclinical disease. Because the changes of PSA can be successfully treated with tumor necrosis factor α blockers, early diagnosis is considered optimal. MRI is gaining currency as the best modality for not only identifying the presence of disease but also adding specificity to the diagnosis.

This article nicely reviews the spectrum of MRI findings in PSA of the hands and helps to differentiate these findings from those of rheumatoid arthritis (RA). Unlike RA, PSA can be thought of as a synovioenthetic process. Thus, although the articular synovitis seen in PSA is not differentiated from that of RA by MRI, the early features of enthesitis in PSA may be a valuable feature. The review emphasizes that PSA tenosynovitis tends to be isolated to the flexor tendons of the hand. It also stresses that early disease may be seen as bone marrow edema at the corner of the phalanx at the insertion of the capsule (Fig 8A), then spreading to involve the entire bone with disease progression. Inflammation of the periosteum is another differentiating factor (Fig 7A), as is muscular fascial thickening/edema or pronounced soft tissue edema spreading to the subcutis.

A good radiologist will pursue subtle findings outlined in this article to differentiate early RA from PSA, proving their worth to their clinical colleague. It is no longer sufficient to simply note early synovitis or tenosynovitis with bone marrow edema and identify it as a nonspecific arthritis.

B. J. Manaster, MD, PhD

Prevalence, Distribution, and Morphology of Ossification of the Ligamentum Flavum: A Population Study of One Thousand Seven Hundred Thirty-Six Magnetic Resonance Imaging Scans
Guo JJ, Luk KDK, Karppinen J, et al (The First Affiliated Hosp of Soochow Univ, Suzhou, China; The Univ of Hong Kong, China; Univ of Oulu, Finland)
Spine 35:51-56, 2010

Study Design.—Large scale, cross-sectional imaging study of a general population.

Objective.—To evaluate the prevalence, morphology, and distribution of ossification of the ligamentum flavum (OLF) in a population, and synthesize the scientific literature on the prevalence of OLF and some factors associated with its occurrence.

Summary of Background Data.—OLF is a rare disease in which the pathogenesis has not been conclusively established. Little is known about its epidemiology. To date, there is no study that comprehensively assessed the distribution and prevalence of OLF in the whole spine using magnetic resonance imaging (MRI).

Methods.—A total of 1736 southern Chinese volunteers (1068 women; 668 men) between 8 and 88 years of age (mean, 38 years) were recruited by open invitation. MRI was administered to all the participants. T2-weighted, 5-mm spin-echo MRI sequences of the whole spine were obtained. Presence of OLF was identified as an area of low signal intensity in the T2 sagittal sequence located in the posterior part of the spinal canal, and subsequently confirmed by computed tomography scans showing areas of ossification within the ligamentum flavum. The distribution of OLF was classified into 3 types: the isolated type, continuous type, and noncontinuous type. While the morphology of the lesion was classified into triangular, round, and beak shapes based on the pattern of ossification on T2-weighted sagittal MRIs.

Results.—OLF was identified in a total of 66 subjects or 3.8% of the population (52 women and 14 men). In 45(68.2%) cases, OLF was present at a single-level (isolated type), whereas in 21 (31.8%) cases OLF was present at multiple levels. The isolated type was found in 45 (68.2%) cases, continuous type in 11 (16.7%), and noncontinuous type in 10 (15.2%). The most common site of involvement is the lower thoracic spine, but they can also occur in the upper thoracic spine. The majority of the segments had a round morphology (n = 75: 81.5%), while 17 (18.5%) segments were triangular in shape. A literature review of the past 26 years showed only 4 reports on the prevalence of OLF, all were in special patient groups.

Conclusion.—Case reports have described postoperative paraplegia from failure to identify and decompress all stenotic segments of OLF. This study demonstrated that OLF is not uncommon, and that some 15% of the lesions are noncontinuous, and therefore could be missed. The authors recommend that for patients undergoing surgical decompression for 1 level of OLF, the whole spine should be routinely screened for other stenotic segments. Failure to do so could result in paraplegia from the nondecompressed levels.

▶ Ossification of the ligamentum flavum (OLF), like ossification of the posterior longitudinal ligament, may be easily overlooked on routine MR examination of the spine, yet may represent a significant cause of spinal stenosis. Although multiple case reports have adequately described this lesion, there has thus far been no large population study describing the prevalence and distribution of OLF. This study provides a very large cross-sectional imaging study of a general population from Southern China. It shows that in this population the prevalence is relatively high (3.8%) and that, furthermore, lesions may be multiple (38%) and noncontiguous (15%). Although care must be taken with extrapolating data from the Chinese population to other populations, the author suspects that the prevalence in the general population likely approaches that shown in this article. This new, well-documented information should lead radiologists to conscientiously search for OLF; additionally, if a single OLF lesion is noted, evaluation of the entire spine should be strongly considered in order to avoid missing an even more significant lesion. This should be an important component of preoperative planning in patients with documented OLF.

B. J. Manaster, MD, PhD

Joints/Sports Injuries

Magnetic resonance imaging and magnetic resonance arthrography of the shoulder: dependence on the level of training of the performing radiologist for diagnostic accuracy
Theodoropoulos JS, Andreisek G, Harvey EJ, et al (Univ of Toronto, Ontario, Canada; McGill Univ, Montreal, Quebec, Canada; et al)
Skelet Radiol 39:661-667, 2010

Purpose.—Discrepancies were identified between magnetic resonance (MR) imaging and clinical findings in patients who had MR imaging examinations evaluated by community-based general radiologists. The purpose of this study was to evaluate the diagnostic performance of MR imaging examinations of the shoulder with regard to the training level of the performing radiologist.

Methods.—A review of patient charts identified 238 patients (male/female, 175/63; mean age, 40.4 years) in whom 250 arthroscopies were performed and who underwent MR imaging or direct MR arthrography in either a community-based or hospital-based institution prior to surgery. All MR imaging and surgical reports were reviewed and the diagnostic performance for the detection of labral, rotator cuff, biceps, and Hill—Sachs lesions was determined. Kappa and Student's t test analyses were performed in a subset of cases in which initial community-based MR images were re-evaluated by hospital-based musculoskeletal radiologists, to determine the interobserver agreement and any differences in image interpretation.

Results.—The diagnostic performance of community-based general radiologists was lower than that of hospital-based sub-specialized musculoskeletal radiologists. A sub-analysis of re-evaluated cases showed that musculoskeletal radiologists performed better. κ values were 0.208, 0.396, 0.376, and 0.788 for labral, rotator cuff, biceps, and Hill—Sachs lesions (t test statistics: $p=<0.001$, 0.004, 0.019, and 0.235).

Conclusions.—Our results indicate that the diagnostic performance of MR imaging and MR arthrography of the shoulder depends on the training level of the performing radiologist, with sub-specialized musculoskeletal radiologists having a better diagnostic performance than general radiologists.

▶ Orthopedic surgeons tend to hold general radiologists (as opposed to musculoskeletal subspecialty-trained radiologists with whom they work closely) in rather low esteem. I believe that this unfortunate situation relates to 2 factors: first, most orthopods are quite accurate in their evaluation of trauma radiographs (although that accuracy drops significantly when anything unusual is encountered such as infection or superimposed tumor) and second, most general radiologists have never mastered the correct terminology for orthopedic implants and do not understand complications of orthopedic procedures. This combination has led to orthopods often interpreting their own radiographs, feeling strongly that the radiologist does not add value in their interpretation.

Most orthopedic surgeons still rely on radiologists to interpret cross-sectional imaging. However, it is important for us to remember that an excellent physical examination may prove to be highly sensitive (up to 90%) and specific (up to 85%); if orthopods lose faith in MR interpretations, they may limit their preoperative evaluation to physical examination in many straightforward cases. However, some literature has shown that the therapeutic decision may be changed in up to 49% of cases that undergo MR examination, leading many orthopedic surgeons to order preoperative MR on nearly all their cases.

The authors of this article have undertaken a likely unpopular task: comparing diagnostic accuracy of general radiologists versus subspecialty-trained musculoskeletal radiologists. They find that the diagnostic performance of community-based general radiologists is lower than that of hospital-based subspecialized musculoskeletal radiologists with regard to their study of MR and magnetic resonance angiography of the shoulder. Similar observations have been made in other subspecialties of radiology. Perhaps it is time for radiology groups to reconsider policies of allowing all members to interpret musculoskeletal imaging. Although such a practice may seem cost-effective in the short run, it may in fact cost that group a great deal in terms of eventual loss of imaging numbers or contracts.

B. J. Manaster, MD, PhD

The Rotator Interval: A Review of Anatomy, Function, and Normal and Abnormal MRI Appearance

Petchprapa CN, Beltran LS, Jazrawi LM, et al (New York Univ Langone Med Ctr)
AJR Am J Roentgenol 95:567-576, 2010

Objective.—The purpose of this article is to review imaging of the rotator interval, an anatomically complex region in the shoulder that plays an important role in the normal function of the shoulder joint. The rotator interval can be difficult to evaluate by imaging, and it is not routinely evaluated arthroscopically unless the clinical examination or imaging findings suggest an abnormality of the rotator interval. Rotator interval pathology is implicated in glenohumeral instability, biceps instability and adhesive capsulitis—entities which remain a challenge to diagnose and treat.

Conclusion.—Imaging can play an important role in increasing suspicion for injury to the rotator interval so that this region can be evaluated and appropriate treatment can be initiated (Figs 5 and 7).

▶ The rotator interval of the shoulder is a complex anatomic region containing multiple structures that may be difficult to visualize on MRI, though they may be seen more confidently using MR arthrography. These structures contribute

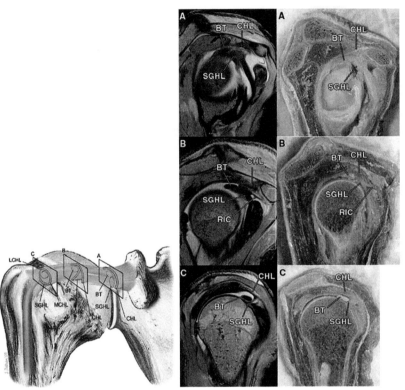

FIGURE 5.—Biceps pulley. A—C, Illustration (*left*) of biceps pulley with corresponding proton density—weighted saline MR arthrograms and bandsaw sagittal sections of cadaver specimen through medial (**A**), middle (**B**), and lateral (**C**) rotator interval. SGHL = superior glenohumeral ligament, BT = biceps tendon, CHL = coracohumeral ligament, MCHL = medial coracohumeral ligament, LCHL = lateral coracohumeral ligament, RIC = rotator interval capsule. (Reprinted with permission from the American Journal of Roentgenology, Petchprapa CN, Beltran LS, Jazrawi LM, et al. The rotator interval: a review of anatomy, function, and normal and abnormal MRI appearance. *AJR Am J Roentgenol.* 2010;95:567-576, with permission from American Roentgen Ray Society.)

importantly to the stability of the shoulder and specifically to the bicipital tendon as it extends through its intra-articular path to the bicipital tendon groove.

Though I have trained as an anatomist, this is one anatomical region that has always been difficult for me to confidently assess. However, this article beautifully demonstrates the anatomy, allowing a full understanding of the structures. Both graphic diagrams and cadaveric arthrographic images show them well, in all planes. Be aware that some of the cadaveric images are obtained in oblique planes designed to demonstrate the anatomy and will not be duplicated on routine MR exams. The drawings of the Bennett classification of biceps instability (Fig 7) are particularly helpful, as are the combined graphic images of the biceps pulley (Fig 5). This is an article that I keep bookmarked for reference and teaching.

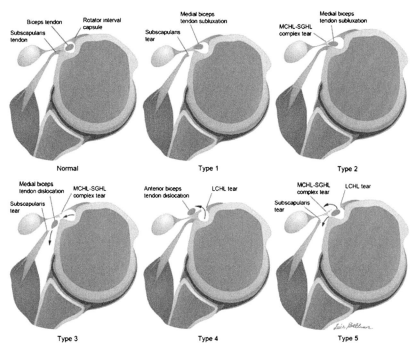

FIGURE 7.—Bennett classification of biceps instability. Illustration shows normal appearance and lesions involving biceps pulley in axial plane. Rotator interval capsule is composed of coracohumeral ligament, superior glenohumeral ligament (SGHL), and capsular fibers, which all blend together along insertions medial and lateral to bicipital groove, maintaining biceps tendon within groove. Medial aspect of coracohumeral ligament (MCHL) blends with SGHL forming medial sheath (or MCHL—SGHL complex), which along with superior fibers of subscapularis tendon form medial supporting structures of bicipital groove. Lateral aspect of coracohumeral ligament (LCHL) blends with most anterior fibers of supraspinatus tendon forming lateral supporting structures of bicipital groove. Type 1 lesions are isolated tears of superior fibers of subscapularis tendon. Type 2 represents tear of medial sheath (MCHL—SGHL complex), allowing medial subluxation of biceps tendon. Type 3 represents lesion of both medial sheath and subscapularis tendon, allowing medial dislocation of biceps tendon from bicipital groove. Type 4 involves LCHL and most-anterior fibers of supraspinatus tendon, allowing biceps tendon to dislocate anterior to subscapularis and coracohumeral ligament. Type 5 combines all structures (subscapularis tendon, medial sheath, LCHL, and supraspinatus tendon), which allows biceps tendon to dislocate either anteriorly or medially. (Reprinted with permission from the American Journal of Roentgenology, Petchprapa CN, Beltran LS, Jazrawi LM, et al. The rotator interval: a review of anatomy, function, and normal and abnormal MRI appearance. *AJR Am J Roentgenol.* 2010;95:567-576, with permission from American Roentgen Ray Society.)

Because the coracohumeral ligament and glenohumeral ligament are important structures in adhesive capsulitis, this entity is discussed as well, along with representative images.

B. J. Manaster, MD, PhD

Radiographic Prevalence of Femoroacetabular Impingement in a Young Population with Hip Complaints Is High

Ochoa LM, Dawson L, Patzkowski JC, et al (William Beaumont Army Med Ctr, El Paso, TX; Brooke Army Med Ctr, Fort Sam Houston, TX; et al)

Clin Orthop Relat Res 468:2710-2714, 2010

Background.—Femoroacetabular impingement (FAI) is reportedly a pre-arthritic condition in young adults that can progress to osteoarthritis. However, the prevalence of FAI is unknown in the young, active population presenting with hip complaints.

Questions/Purposes.—We sought to determine (1) the prevalence of radiographic findings of FAI in a young, active patient population with complaints localized to the region of the hip presenting to primary care and orthopaedic clinics; (2) the percentage of films with FAI with an official reading suggesting the diagnosis; and (3) whether the Tönnis grades of osteoarthritis corresponded to the findings of FAI.

Methods.—We performed a database review of pelvic and hip radiographs obtained from 157 young (mean age 32 years; range, 18−50 years) patients presenting with hip-related complaints to primary care and orthopaedic clinics. Radiographs were analyzed for signs of FAI (herniation pits, pistol grip deformity, center-edge angle, alpha angle, and crossover sign) and Tönnis grade. Radiology reports were reviewed for a diagnosis of FAI.

Results.—At least one finding of FAI was found in 135 of the 155 patients (87%). Four hundred thirteen of 487 radiographs (85%) had been read as normal and one read as showing FAI. Tönnis grades did not correlate with radiographic signs of FAI.

Conclusions.—Radiographic evidence of FAI is common in active patients with hip complaints. Increased awareness of FAI in primary care, radiology, and orthopaedic clinics and additional research into the long-term effects of management are warranted.

Level of Evidence.—Level II, diagnostic study. See the Guidelines for Authors for a complete description of levels of evidence.

▶ Femoral acetabular impingement (FAI) and the associated osseous morphologic abnormalities, with their predisposition to occur in patients developing early osteoarthritis, have been given tremendous attention over the past 6 years. Numerous investigations and research articles have made FAI almost a household word among musculoskeletal radiologists, hip orthopedic specialists, and sports medicine physicians. As we have come to understand the condition, many of us have discovered that we make the diagnosis from radiographs on almost a daily basis. At my institution, the residents even included the prevalence of the diagnosis in their end-of-year skit. That should make one wonder whether the process is being overdiagnosed, even within the setting of a sports medicine clinic.

The prevalence of FAI is estimated at 10% to 15% in the asymptomatic patient population. This article addresses the prevalence of radiographic morphologic abnormalities of the hip suggesting FAI in the active young adult (average age of 32 years) symptomatic population. It may be astounding to some to read that 87% of this symptomatic population had at least 1 radiographic finding of FAI. It is also bothersome that 85% of these cases were interpreted by the radiologists as normal (though the database covered the years 2001-2007, and many of the readings occurred before a good general understanding of FAI).

This study reassures me that the prevalence of our interpretations of FAI in the sports medicine setting is correct. It also suggests that when FAI is demonstrated in patients being seen in family medicine or general practice clinics, the radiologist should go to some effort to explain the process and likelihood of it as a prearthritic condition to these clinicians who are likely to be unfamiliar with FAI.

B. J. Manaster, MD, PhD

Acetabular Labral Tears and Cartilage Lesions of the Hip: Indirect MR Arthrographic Correlation With Arthroscopy—A Preliminary Study
Zlatkin MB, Pevsner D, Sanders TG, et al (Natl Musculoskeletal Imaging, Weston, FL; et al)
AJR Am J Roentgenol 194:709-714, 2010

Objective.—The purpose of this study was to assess the diagnostic correlation between indirect MR arthrography, conventional MRI, and arthroscopy in acetabular labral and cartilage lesions of the hip.

Materials and Methods.—Fourteen patients who underwent conventional and indirect MR arthrography with arthroscopic correlation were studied over the course of 18 months. MR studies were performed on a 1.5-T magnet. Sequences consisted of unilateral sagittal turbo spin-echo proton density fat-suppressed, axial turbo spin-echo T2 fat-saturated, and coronal turbo spin-echo proton density fat-saturated images. Whole-pelvis coronal T1 and STIR sequences were also performed. Patients received IV gadolinium contrast material and exercised for 15 minutes. Gadolinium-enhanced fat-saturated T1 sequences were obtained in three planes. Arthroscopy was performed by two orthopedic surgeons who specialize in treating hip disorders. Cases were then retrospectively reviewed by two experienced musculoskeletal radiologists who were blinded to the arthroscopic findings. Cases were examined for acetabular labral tears and chondral lesions. Extraarticular findings of femoral acetabular impingement were recorded. Unenhanced and gadolinium-enhanced images of the labrum were compared for differences and changes in diagnosis. Comparison was made between the arthroscopic and MR findings for analysis of the results.

Results.—Of the 13 labral tears found at arthroscopy, 85% were detected by conventional MRI, whereas 100% were identified via indirect MR arthrography. Seventy percent of the labral tears identified on conventional MRI were better delineated by indirect MR arthrography.

Identification of chondral abnormalities was not improved via indirect MR arthrography over conventional MRI.

Conclusion.—IV contrast-enhanced indirect MR arthrography appears to be an effective means of hip evaluation for labral tears. It does not appear to improve detection of cartilage abnormalities when compared with conventional MRI.

▶ The morphologies of femoral acetabular impingement and the various dysplasias of the hip are well recognized as contributing factors to early osteoarthritis. Once these morphologic abnormalities are noted, it is important to demonstrate labral tears and, even more importantly, cartilage thinning or defects to guide surgical treatment. As the authors of this article note, several articles show good correlation of the observed labral and cartilage defects seen via direct MR arthrography with the gold standard of arthroscopy. However, most radiologists who perform large numbers of hip MR arthrograms have observed that the procedure is not entirely benign. Although the likelihood of serious complications of the procedure is extremely low, many patients report significant and relatively long-lived hip pain that they relate to the arthrogram. Additionally, there is significant cost adding the procedure to the MR. Therefore, it would be useful to develop an alternative reliable method to determine both labral and cartilage abnormalities in this patient population.

The authors of this article were additionally concerned with situations where a radiologist was not available to perform the arthrographic portion of a direct MR arthrogram. This article discusses the accuracy of indirect MR arthrography of the hip, using arthroscopy as the gold standard. The results showing excellent accuracy of diagnosing labral injuries are said to be encouraging. However, these authors also believe that their results indicating poor accuracy in diagnosing cartilage defects are significant. Many surgeons will not accept an inadequate evaluation of cartilage defects, in terms of grade, location, and extent, since this information helps direct surgical decisions. Therefore, the radiologist who is contemplating switching from direct to indirect MR arthrography of the hip would do well to understand these implications and discuss the importance of accurate cartilage evaluation with his/her surgeon.

B. J. Manaster, MD, PhD

Degenerative changes in the ligamentum teres of the hip: cadaveric study with magnetic resonance arthrography, anatomical inspection, and histologic examination
Sampatchalit S, Barbosa D, Gentili A, et al (VA Med Ctr, San Diego, CA)
J Comput Assist Tomogr 33:927-933, 2009

Objective.—Review and classify the pathologic abnormalities of the ligamentum teres in degenerative hip joints.

Material and Methods.—Eleven cadaveric hip joints were examined with magnetic resonance arthrography and were then sectioned. The appearance of the ligamentum teres and its attachment seen by inspection of the anatomical sections was correlated with findings seen at magnetic resonance imaging. Histologic evaluation was done.

Results.—Magnetic resonance arthrographic and histologic findings showed a spectrum of ligamentum teres degeneration. The thickest ligamentum teres revealed mucoid and fibromatous degeneration with microscopic tear. Ligamentum teres with intermediate thickness revealed fatty replacement with and without fibromatous degeneration, fibromatous degeneration with and without mucoid degeneration, and eosinophilic change. The thinnest ligamentum teres was near-complete disruption of the ligament.

Conclusions.—The ligamentum teres revealed degenerative changes that were similar histologically to degenerative changes in tendons. Magnetic resonance arthrography provided a sensitive technique for demonstration of the ligamentum teres and various patterns of degeneration.

▶ One of the fairly hot topics in the world of sports medicine concerning the hip is acute tear of the ligamentum teres. Radiologists are beginning to make this diagnosis more frequently, indicating that they are including the ligamentum teres in their search pattern for abnormalities in hip MR. Interestingly, many of my colleagues admit that they are uncertain of the significance of the diagnosis and that their surgical colleagues are even more uncertain regarding treatment and prognosis.

Be that as it may, as with every new diagnostic entity, it is important to understand the normal appearance of the structure, including normal variation and normal degeneration expected with the aging process. This article is presented by Dr Resnick's team, armed with cadavers, bandsaw, and their usual careful observation and correlation with MR. This beautiful presentation of the expected appearance of a degenerative ligamentum teres represents a good start in our understanding of this structure. There is also an elegant presentation of the anatomy of the ligamentum teres as well as its likely mechanical functions.

B. J. Manaster, MD, PhD

Analysis of the Patellofemoral Region on MRI: Association of Abnormal Trochlear Morphology With Severe Cartilage Defects
Ali SA, Helmer R, Terk MR (Emory Univ, Atlanta, GA)
AJR Am J Roentgenol 194:721-727, 2010

Objective.—The objective of our study was to assess patellofemoral measurements on MRI and to correlate the measurements with different grades of cartilage defect.

Materials and Methods.—Axial and sagittal MR images of 100 patients with various pathologic knee conditions were analyzed. The patients were divided into two age groups: < 40 years and ≥ 40 years. Patellar measurements of facet asymmetry, the patella-to-patellar tendon ratio, and the amount of patellotrochlear cartilage overlap were obtained in each subject.

Similarly, trochlear measurements of the ventral trochlear prominence, trochlear depth, facet asymmetry, sulcus angle, and lateral inclination were obtained. Axial and sagittal MR images were reviewed to grade the severity of focal cartilage defects in the patellofemoral region on the basis of the depth of the lesion. Measurements in knees without a chondral defect were compared with knees with mild and severe chondral defects.

Results.—There was a statistically significant difference in the trochlear measurements of the ventral prominence ($p = 0.012$), trochlear depth ($p = 0.001$), sulcus angle ($p = 0.208$), and lateral inclination ($p = 0.154$) between normal knees and knees with severe cartilage defects in patients younger than 40 years. No significant difference was seen in the patellar measurements between normal knees and knees with severe cartilage defects.

Conclusion.—There is an association between abnormal trochlear morphology and severe patellofemoral cartilage defects in patients younger than 40 years.

▶ The patellofemoral joint is functionally complex; abnormal function of this joint results in chondromalacia and anterior joint pain. Radiographic measurements of the patella, femoral trochlea, and their relationship have long been used to predict patellar tracking disorders and associated chondromalacia. This article introduces MR measurements in the patellofemoral joint that they can demonstrate to correlate with chondromalacia. The methodology of the measurements is well shown with imaging and description, so that it can easily be followed in practice. Interestingly, the authors show that the trochlear morphology more closely relates to patellar chondromalacia than do patellar morphologic measurements. Although the conclusions are somewhat limited by numbers of patients, this is a well-reasoned and well-presented article and well worth a careful look. Radiologists who evaluate this article will be able to report on abnormal trochlear morphology more accurately, relating it to chondromalacia.

B. J. Manaster, MD, PhD

Increasing Incidence of Medial Meniscal Tears in Nonoperatively Treated Anterior Cruciate Ligament Insufficiency Patients Documented by Serial Magnetic Resonance Imaging Studies
Yoo JC, Ahn JH, Lee SH, et al (Sungkyunkwan Univ School of Medicine, Seoul, Korea; Armed Forces Capital Hosp, SeongNam-si, Korea)
Am J Sports Med 37:1478-1483, 2009

Background.—No consensus has been reached with regard to the ideal timing of anterior cruciate ligament reconstruction in terms of reducing secondary meniscal tears in anterior cruciate ligament-deficient knees.

Hypothesis.—Delay in anterior cruciate ligament reconstruction increases the incidence and severity of medial meniscal tears.

Study Design.—Case series; Level of evidence, 4.

Methods.—Thirty-one patients were evaluated with arthroscopic all-inside suturing of medial meniscal tears with concurrent anterior cruciate ligament reconstruction who had at least 2 preoperative magnetic resonance imaging studies. Patients were evaluated during the acute phase of injury, but anterior cruciate ligament reconstruction surgery was delayed at least 6 months. Mean interval between first and second imaging studies was 36.8 months. Subsequent medial meniscal tears were identified as longitudinal or bucket-handle types. Relationships between medial meniscal lesions and patient age, time interval between the date of initial injury and surgery, repetitive injury, and patient activity level were evaluated.

Results.—During the first preoperative magnetic resonance imaging studies, 14 knees had no medial meniscal tear, 15 a longitudinal tear, and 2 a bucket-handle-type tear; during the second preoperative imaging studies, 5 knees had no medial meniscal tear, 19 a longitudinal tear, and 7 a bucket-handle-type tear. The incidence of medial meniscal tears increased from 55% in first studies to 84% in second studies for chronic anterior cruciate ligament-insufficient knees ($P = .0054$). Eight knees without a tear during first studies had a longitudinal tear during second studies, 1 knee without a tear and 4 with a longitudinal tear in first studies had a bucket-handle-type tear in second studies. Thirteen knees (42%) had a worse meniscal status during the second studies.

Conclusion.—Delayed anterior cruciate ligament reconstruction increases the likelihood of a medial meniscal tear, suggesting that early anterior cruciate ligament reconstruction should reduce or prevent additional medial meniscal injury. The findings show that further medial meniscal damage is common if surgery is delayed by 6 months or more.

▶ The natural history of anterior cruciate ligament (ACL)-deficient knees remains controversial. This controversy influences individual decisions regarding ACL reconstruction. Some orthopedic surgeons and patients delay reconstruction for various reasons. Additionally, in the middle-aged patient population, some surgeons may counsel that it is reasonable to handle an ACL tear nonoperatively. Previous biomechanical studies demonstrated that the medial meniscus serves as a secondary stabilizing structure in the chronically ACL-deficient knee, limiting anterior tibial translation, and therefore is subject to additional stresses in these patients. These previous studies also showed the lateral meniscus to be less subject to new damage than the medial in knees with chronic ACL deficiency. This study confirms that delay in ACL reconstruction, even as little as 6 months, increases the likelihood of a significant medial meniscal tear. This is interesting information for radiologists, both from the point of view of discussions with orthopedic surgeons and patients and in suggesting that surveillance for these tears should be even more careful in these patients.

B. J. Manaster, MD, PhD

Inter- and Intraobserver Reliability in the Radiographic Evaluation of Adult Flatfoot Deformity

Sensiba PR, Coffey MJ, Williams NE II, et al (Miami Valley Hosp, Dayton, OH)
Foot Ankle Int 31:141-145, 2010

Background.—Adult acquired flatfoot is a complex deformity with numerous radiographic measurements described to define it. The purpose of this study was to evaluate the inter- and intraobserver reliability of six radiographic measurements using digital and conventional radiographs.

Materials and Methods.—Three digital weightbearing radiographs consisting of anteroposterior, lateral, and hindfoot alignment views were obtained at presentation for 20 consecutive patients. Six radiographic measurements were made for each patient: talus/second metatarsal angle, calcaneal pitch angle, talus/first metatarsal angle, medial cuneiform/fifth metatarsal distance, tibial/calcaneal displacement, and calcaneal angulation. Each radiograph was evaluated on multiple occasions by a senior orthopaedic surgery resident, a junior orthopaedic surgery resident, and a third-year medical student. Inter- and intraobserver reliability was determined using measurements made on digital radiographs.

Results.—Interobserver reliabilities were 0.830 for talus/second metatarsal angle, 0.948 for calcaneal pitch angle, 0.781 for talus/first metatarsal angle, 0.991 for medial cuneiform/fifth metatarsal distance, 0.870 for tibial/calcaneal displacement, and 0.834 for calcaneal angulation. Interobserver reliability was similar for digital and conventional radiographs, and intraobserver reliability increased with observer experience.

Conclusion.—Adult acquired flatfoot deformity is a complex condition that is difficult to quantify radiographically. The medial cuneiform/fifth metatarsal distance and the calcaneal pitch angle were found to have the highest inter-observer reliability. Intraobserver reliability increased with observer experience.

▶ Radiologists are often miserably inconsistent in their use of correct terminology and measurements of foot deformities. Adult flatfoot deformity can arise because of a multitude of abnormalities but most often is acquired because of posterior tibial tendon deficiency. Although the tendon abnormality is demonstrated on MRI, the resultant deformity is well seen on weight-bearing radiographs. There are standard measurements used on standard images (weight-bearing anteroposterior and lateral images of the foot as well as the hindfoot alignment radiograph); the radiologist should have a working knowledge of these. This article not only demonstrates those standard measurements but also shows the inter- and intraobserver variability of each. It is surprising that the most frequently advocated measurement (talus/first metatarsal angle on the lateral radiograph) had the greatest observer variability. Radiologists can profit from a brief review of this article, reviewing the methodology for correct measurement and gaining an appreciation for which observations are the most accurate.

B. J. Manaster, MD, PhD

New Radiographic Parameters Assessing Forefoot Abduction in the Adult Acquired Flatfoot Deformity

Ellis SJ, Yu JC, Williams BR, et al (The Hosp for Special Surgery, NY)
Foot Ankle Int 30:1168-1176, 2009

Background.—Stage II flatfoot secondary to posterior tibial tendon insufficiency may be subclassified into mild (IIa) and severe (IIb) deformity based on the degree of talonavicular abduction. Current assessment of this abduction is difficult. We hypothesized that two new anteroposterior radiographic parameters, the lateral talonavicular incongruency angle (IA) and incongruency distance (ID) would demonstrate good reliability, correlate with current abduction parameters, and differ in IIb deformity, IIa deformity, and controls.

Materials and Methods.—Preoperative radiographs for consecutive patients undergoing flatfoot reconstruction were reviewed and subdivided into those with a Stage IIb ($n = 32$) or Stage IIa ($n = 8$) deformity. A third group of patients without flatfoot served as control ($n = 30$). Radiographs were measured blindly by two investigators. Reliability was assessed with intraclass correlation coefficients (ICC), correlation with existing parameters with Pearson coefficients, and comparison between groups with analysis of variance.

Results.—The mean intrarater and interrater ICC's for the IA (0.88 and 0.81, respectively) were high. The IA correlated well with the coverage angle ($r = 0.86$) and uncoverage percent ($r = 0.76$). The IA was higher in the IIb versus IIa patients ($p = 0.007$) and in the IIb group versus control ($p < 0.001$). The ID demonstrated excellent reliability (ICC's of 0.83 and 0.83), but correlated poorly with the two other abduction parameters ($r = -0.59$ and -0.49) and failed to differentiate between the three groups ($p = 0.0528$).

Conclusion.—This data suggests that the IA is reliable and may help subclassify Stage II flatfoot deformity.

▶ Reading other radiologists' reports regarding foot and ankle deformities suggests to this author that there is generally a poor understanding of standard terminology and measurements of such. Similarly, corrective surgical procedures are often not recognized or correctly named and assessed. Although one might excuse this in a highly complex developmental deformity, the general radiologist should be able to accurately describe deformities and corrective procedures in the very common adult-acquired flatfoot deformity. The primary aim of this article is to suggest the use of a new measurement by which the surgeon might subclassify adult-acquired flatfoot deformity (related to posterior tibial tendon insufficiency), therefore suggesting specific surgical procedures in addition to the standard lateral column lengthening. This angular measurement appears to be internally consistent and useful. However, the article as a whole also nicely presents the current measurements and surgical considerations for adult-acquired flatfoot deformity and as such could be useful to any general radiologist who may be interested in improving the reporting of this disease process.

B. J. Manaster, MD, PhD

MRI of Ankle and Lateral Hindfoot Impingement Syndromes
Donovan A, Rosenberg ZS (Sunnybrook Health Sciences Centre, Toronto, Ontario, Canada; NYU Langone Med Ctr and NYU Hosp for Joint Diseases)
AJR Am J Roentgenol 195:595-604, 2010

Objective.—The objective of this article is to review the pathophysiology and clinical presentation of impingement syndromes at the ankle joint (anterolateral, anterior, anteromedial, posteromedial, and posterior) and the role of MRI in evaluating impingement at the ankle joint and at extraarticular locations, lateral to the ankle joint (talocalcaneal and calcaneofibular).

Conclusion.—MRI is valuable in assessing both osseous and soft-tissue abnormalities associated with impingement syndromes.

▶ Multiple sites of impingement about the ankle have been described. These are often associated with ankle sprains; most radiologists are used to seeking evidence of ankle impingement in the sports-injured patient group. However, it is important to remember that the older patient group with hindfoot valgus or patients with morphologic abnormalities leading to pes planus may have different sites of impingement, particularly at extra-articular lateral osseous sites (lateral talocalcaneal or calcaneofibular).

Clinical suspicion plays a large part in diagnosis of ankle impingement. MR examination may be confirmatory; it is important to know the signs and associations. There is a wide range of sensitivity and specificity in diagnosing impingement in nonarthrographic MR examination. This article, authored by world-authority Dr Rosenberg and her colleague Dr Donovan, beautifully explains the pathogenesis and MR appearance of the different types of ankle impingement. It also reminds us of the other ankle abnormalities that may coexist with impingement; it can be difficult to clinically differentiate between impingement and other structural abnormalities as a source of pain. All must be carefully evaluated on an MR examination. It is well worth spending some time studying this excellent review.

B. J. Manaster, MD, PhD

4　Pediatric Radiology

Introduction

Subspecialization, not to mention *subsubspecialization,* is now rife in pediatric radiology, especially in the biggest centers (AEO has been self-described as a pediatric conventional skeletal radiologist specializing in the proximal end of the left second metacarpal). For certain specific indications, one needs to seek out that individual with highly specific skills. Nonetheless, it behooves all pediatric radiologists, indeed all medical imagers, to be at least aware of most entities, either to give immediate advice or to guide the proper authorities. For example from this year's selections, the recognition of the bone changes suggesting the rare Stüve Wiedemann syndrome will alert all to the dangers of dysautonomia (including temperature instability) in an involved child. Many of our abstracts and commentaries can be faced in that spirit. Others are good old "Aunt Minnies"—such as the phalanges of Wolf-Hirschhorn syndrome. Still others require the radiologist to correctly identify the abnormalities, even if they cannot bundle them all into a single entity—PAGOD syndrome, for example.

Not only are radiologists subspecializing and *subsubspecializing,* advancements in image technology and new approaches to radiology research are being made. We have included some articles to reflect this: for example, the articles on handheld ultrasound devices and developing participatory research in pediatric radiology. For the technophiles among you, there isn't yet—but sometime soon, perhaps even as soon as next year—there may be an article on a new "app" and its impact on pediatric imaging.

Whether you are a general radiologist, a pediatric radiologist, or a pediatric radiologist with a subspecialist interest, we hope there is at least one article here for you. However, if you were hoping for an article dedicated to the left second metacarpal, you too may have to wait 'til next year (although prominent pseudoepiphysis of that site is mentioned in the Wolf-Hirschhorn article mentioned above).

Amaka C. Offiah, BSc, MBBS, MRCP, FRCR, PhD
Alan E. Oestreich, MD

Gastrointestinal

Severe gastric damage caused by button battery ingestion in a 3-month-old infant

Honda S, Shinkai M, Usui Y, et al (Kanagawa Children's Med Ctr, Yokohama, Japan)
J Pediatr Surg 45:E23-E26, 2010

Ingestion of a button battery has been considered a serious problem, causing necrosis and perforation, when impacted in the esophagus. However, such batteries in the stomach rarely cause any harm to the gastric wall, which is regarded as evidence supporting the use of conservative treatment. We present the rare case of a 3-month-old infant with severe gastric wall injury caused by a button battery lodged in the stomach. The present case suggests that button batteries located in the stomach should be removed as soon as possible, especially in infants.

▶ Every once in a while, an exception to conventional wisdom will lead to a new conventional wisdom (rather than being an exception that proves a rule). And here is an important example that should be brought to the attention of all radiologists, pediatricians, surgeons, and other pediatric health care providers. Formerly, it was believed that once an ingested button battery gets to the stomach, the child is safe. Not so! This 3-month infant had severe gastric antrum damage from a button battery, detected, and surgically treated, apparently 2 days after being fed it by a sibling. The supine abdominal radiograph showed the metallic object in the region of the pylorus and ultrasound imaging, Fig 1B, localized it specifically to the pylorus. The alerting authors strongly suggest that extreme vigilance is needed with a button battery in the stomach,

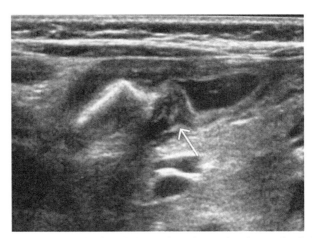

FIGURE 1.—B, Ultrasonography showed a hyperechoic object at the pylorus with a thickened gastric wall. (Reprinted from Honda S, Shinkai M, Usui Y, et al. Severe gastric damage caused by button battery ingestion in a 3-month-old infant. *J Pediatr Surg.* 2010;45:E23-E26, with permission from Elsevier.)

especially in the infant, with strong consideration to immediate removal absent rapid evidence of further passage; indeed, as you see in the abstract above, they advocate removal as soon as possible. What else can go wrong with button batteries even higher on the respiratory/gastrointestinal tract? A button battery can cause severe damage to the nasal septum when the battery lies in the nasal cavity.[1] Any first radiographs for foreign body ingestion, therefore, should still include a lateral view of the entire nasopharynx and nose. More than 1 toy (or jewelry) magnet in the nose can also cause severe necrosis.

A. E. Oestreich, MD

Reference

1. Guidera AK, Stegehuis HR. Button batteries: the worst case scenario in nasal foreign bodies. *N Z Med J.* 2010;123:68-73.

Assessment of retromesenteric position of the third portion of the duodenum: an US feasibility study in 33 newborns
Yousefzadeh DK, Kang L, Tessicini L (The Univ of Chicago, IL)
Pediatr Radiol 40:1476-1484, 2010

Background.—US can be used to assess bowel and does not require ionizing radiation or the administration of contrast material. Prior studies of the duodenum with US are limited.

Objective.—This study assesses the success rate of US demonstration of the third portion of the duodenum (D3) between the superior mesenteric artery (SMA) and the aorta in newborns to exclude malrotation based on embryologic and anatomic principles.

Material and Methods.—Thirty-three newborns underwent US studies. The structures between the SMA and the aorta, including D3, were evaluated in axial and longitudinal planes. The length of time to acquire diagnostic images was recorded.

Results.—In both the axial and longitudinal planes, D3 was seen between the SMA and the aorta in all 33 infants, including some with abundant bowel gas. The mean length of time to acquire diagnostic images was 34 s.

Conclusion.—Bedside US successfully illustrated the retromesenteric position of D3 in all 33 infants. Overlying gas-filled bowel was effectively effaced by graded compression. The short study duration indicates the practicality of the method. Further studies in broader patient populations and in correlation with other imaging and/or surgical findings is required to validate our technique.

▶ Once again, the inventive mind and thoughtful experience of Dr Yousefzadeh have led to a potentially major breakthrough in how children are imaged, and this time on a topic of great importance to the clinical care of infants. Although eyebrows have been raised as to "How could this be true if we never heard

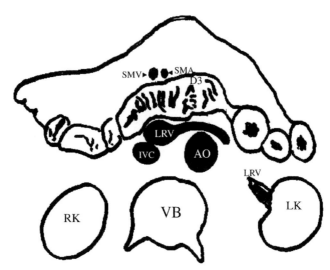

FIGURE 1.—Transverse anatomic sketch demonstrates the third portion of the duodenum (D3) between the SMA/SMV (*arrowheads*) and the aorta (*AO*). The left renal vein (*LRV*), inferior vena cava (*IVC*), left and right kidneys (*LK* and *RK*) and vertebral body (*VB*) are also shown. (With kind permission from Springer Science and Business Media: Yousefzadeh DK, Kang L, Tessicini L. Assessment of retromesenteric position of the third portion of the duodenum: an US feasibility study in 33 newborns. *Pediatr Radiol.* 2010;40:1476-1484.)

about it before?" the case for ultrasound rapid evaluation for duodenal position in the infant (and therefore in the vomiting infant as well) is strongly supported by the embryology and images presented. Fig 1 summarizes the position of the relevant structures on frontal coronal ultrasound, and Fig 2 of the original article summarizes the longitudinal findings. A large number of well-annotated ultrasound images follow, all of which support the thesis. Before this material was presented, the immediate first step to rule out volvulus in the newly vomiting infant has been a radiographic fluoroscopic upper gastrointestinal series. This ultrasound method does not use radiation, is available at the bedside, and may well save time before going to operation to save the vitality of the volvulused duodenum. More experience by many of us, now that we know the technique, will hopefully confirm that this new diagnostic pathway is a clear improvement.

A. E. Oestreich, MD

Congenital and acquired mesocolic hernias presenting with small bowel obstruction in childhood and adolescence
Villalona GA, Diefenbach KA, Touloukian RJ (Yale Univ School of Medicine, New Haven, CT)
J Pediatr Surg 45:438-442, 2010

Objective.—The objective was to present a case series of pediatric patients presenting with small bowel obstruction secondary to both congenital and acquired internal mesocolic hernias, and the use of imaging technology in the management of this condition.

Methods.—A retrospective review of patients treated at the Yale–New Haven Children's Hospital for small bowel obstruction from 1998 to 2008 (n = 6) who presented with acute small bowel obstruction secondary to internal mesocolic hernias was performed.

Results.—We present 6 patients with small bowel obstruction caused by congenital (n = 4) and acquired (n = 2) mesocolic hernias after previous surgery. The median age at presentation was 13 years. Small bowel obstruction with a mesocolic hernia was identified by preoperative abdominal computerized tomography in 3 patients (50%) and at operation in the others. The mean length of stay was 6 days, with no recurrent episodes in the follow-up period.

Conclusion.—Small bowel obstruction secondary to mesocolic hernias, although rare, may be considered in the differential diagnosis of patients with history of malrotation or abdominal wall defects owing to their association with congenital mesenteric anomalies. This condition requires special attention from the clinician because of its catastrophic consequences. Imaging studies are an important asset because of the difficulty in making an accurate clinical diagnosis and the rarity of internal hernias (Fig 2).

▶ Classically (ie, when I was younger), upper gastrointestinal and small bowel barium study was the principal means of establishing the diagnosis of internal hernia by imaging. One fine review of both the nature of internal hernias and of the fluoroscopic imaging was the little booklet of Ghahremani and Meyers.[1]

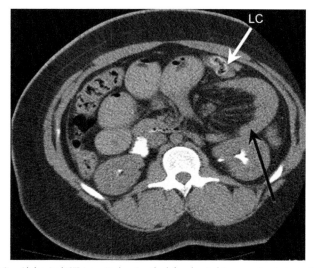

FIGURE 2.—Abdominal CT (case 2) showing the left colon (white arrow) anterior to the left mesocolic hernia (black arrow). (Reprinted from Villalona GA, Diefenbach KA, Touloukian RJ. Congenital and acquired mesocolic hernias presenting with small bowel obstruction in childhood and adolescence. *J Pediatr Surg.* 2010;45:438-442, with permission from Elsevier.)

This article extends the diagnostic capabilities to CT, as well as mentioning a role for ultrasound, and, indeed, conventional plain images. Fig 2 demonstrates nicely the basic CT findings to be sought. Interestingly, half of their patients had been born with omphalocele (1 case) or gastroschisis (2 cases). Because internal hernias are most often an asymptomatic abnormality, minus the small bowel obstruction, diagnosis is often elusive. In the imaging (CT or fluoroscopic) differential diagnosis, with or without small bowel obstruction, one should not forget abdominal cocoon, also known as sclerosing encapsulating peritonitis, in which a portion of the small bowel is enclosed in an encompassing membrane that, like internal hernia, causes a localized compartmentalized collection of small bowel obstruction.[2] In that latter condition, CT and sonography may be helpful as well,[2] not to mention classic barium small bowel study.

A. E. Oestreich, MD

References

1. Ghahremani GG. Internal abdominal hernias. *Surg Clin North Am.* 1984;64: 393-406.
2. Tombak MC, Apaydin FD, Colak T, et al. An unusual cause of intestinal obstruction: abdominal cocoon. *AJR Am J Roentgenol.* 2010;194:W176-W178.

Tuberculous abdominal cocoon: original article
Wani I, Ommid M, Waheed A, et al (SMHS Hosp, Srinagar, Kashmir, India; SKIMS, Srinagar, India)
Ulus Travma Acil Cerrahi Derg 16:508-510, 2010

Background.—Tuberculous abdominal cocoon is a rare disease, and diagnosis is seldom made preoperatively. The bowel is encased in a membrane in a cocoon-like fashion. Histopathology is confirmatory.

Methods.—This prospective case note review was a study of patients diagnosed with tuberculous abdominal cocoon from April 2005 - April 2008. There were 8 females and 3 males.

Results.—All patients had features of small bowel obstruction. All had laparotomy and the characteristic finding of absence of the greater omentum from the involved area and the absence of any stigmata of gut tuberculosis. Peeling of membrane is all that is required, and patients received anti-tubercular therapy postoperatively. In each case, evidence of tuberculosis on histopathology of membrane was present.

Conclusion.—Tuberculous abdominal cocoon is a rare entity. Females are commonly affected. Surgery is the preferred treatment.

▶ Every so often, the uncommon entity of abdominal cocoon belongs in the differential diagnosis of barium studies of the small bowel or cross-sectional imaging of the abdomen when small bowel loops seem isolated into an unnatural well-marginated compartment of the abdomen. The more common occurrence of internal hernia usually goes higher up in the list of differential diagnosis to explain the pattern. Although various disturbances in the abdomen may lead to the wrapping of an area of small bowel into the cocoon pattern, this article points to a specific infectious agent to be considered, tuberculosis, which has implications for infection safety during surgery as well as antituberculous treatment of the patient. At least in many areas of the world, finding a cocoon pattern preoperatively should lead to a skin test or other testing for tuberculosis. Surgery for abdominal cocoon may be done by laparoscope, as recently reported.[1] The catalog of possible medical/surgical manifestations of tuberculosis continues to expand.

A. E. Oestreich, MD

Reference

1. Qasaimeh GR, Amarin Z, Rawshdeh BN, El-Radaideh KM. Laparoscopic diagnosis and management of an abdominal cocoon: a case report and literature review. *Surg Laparosc Endosc Percutan Tech.* 2010;20:e169-e171.

Case report: actinomycosis of the appendix—an unusual cause of acute appendicitis in children
Liu V, Val S, Kang K, et al (Long Island College Hosp, Brooklyn, NY)
J Pediatr Surg 45:2050-2052, 2010

Abdominal actinomycosis in children is a rare disease, which is occasionally found on histologic examination after an operation for acute appendicitis. Because of its nonspecific clinical and radiological signs and symptoms and low prevalence, the diagnosis is hardly ever made before the patient undergoes an operation and tissue is available for pathologic evaluation. When the diagnosis is made, the patient should be treated with the appropriate long-term antibiotics. With antibiotic therapy, the prognosis is favorable.

We describe a 13-year-old girl who presented with acute appendicitis and was found to have abdominal actinomycosis after undergoing open appendectomy, which was treated successfully with penicillin and piperacillin-tazobactam.

▶ Actinomycosis is not common in most medical circles, but it is a well-known infectious agent that tends to disregard borders between compartments and anatomic structures (actinomycetes without borders). In contrast, ordinary appendicitis is common. The preoperative diagnosis of actinomycosis of the appendix is rarely made, so perhaps this case can teach us something. For example, the child had a 3-week history of intermittent periumbilical pain; on CT, shown in Fig 1, the initial observers found several calcific bodies in the 2.2-cm diameter appendix, and interoperatively, a large phlegmon was found involving cecum, rectosigmoid, bladder, and ileum with dense, almost woody, adhesions. Antibiotic treatment, such as with penicillin, is advised. The authors state that most abdominal actinomycoses have been associated with appendicitis

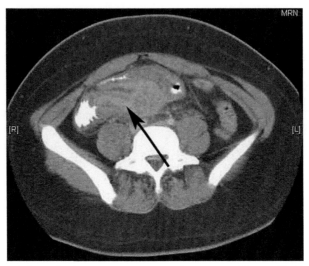

FIGURE 1.—Abdominal and pelvic CT scan with PO and IV contrast of 13-year-old girl presenting with right lower quadrant pain for 3 weeks showing tubular mass in right lower quadrant (arrow). (Reprinted from Liu V, Val S, Kang K, et al. Case report: actinomycosis of the appendix—an unusual cause of acute appendicitis in children. *J Pediatr Surg.* 2010;45:2050-2052, with permission from Elsevier.)

but that symptoms are often indolent. I wonder if a careful study of this case, and similar ones, including one in a cat,[1] might lead to preoperative diagnosis insofar as adjoining structures are involved and symptoms are subacute. MRI might reveal the transgression on borders and perhaps ultrasound as well in some cases.

A. E. Oestreich, MD

Reference

1. Sharman MJ, Goh CS, Kuipers von Lande RG, Hodgson JL. Intra-abdominal actinomycetoma in a cat. *J Feline Med Surg.* 2009;11:701-705.

Role of plain abdominal radiographs in predicting type of congenital pouch colon

Mathur P, Saxena AK, Bajaj M, et al (SMS Med College, Jaipur, Rajasthan, India; Univ of Oxford, UK; GBH American Hosp, Udaipur, Rajasthan, India; et al)
Pediatr Radiol 40:1603-1608, 2010

Background.—Congenital pouch colon (CPC) is a rare form of high ano-rectal malformation (ARM) in which part of or the entire colon is replaced by a pouch with a fistula to the genito-urinary tract. According to the Saxena-Mathur classification CPC is divided into five types. Although plain abdominal radiographs are taken in infants with suspicion of CPC to detect large dilatation of the pouch, the determination of the type of CPC is made during surgical exploration. Since large variations in the length of normal colon are present in the various types, management strategy options can be determined only at the time of surgery.

Objective.—The aim of this study was to review abdominal radiographs of children with congenital pouch colon (CPC) and evaluate their value in determining the type of CPC prior to surgical exploration to assist pre-operative planning.

Materials and Methods.—Over a 12-year period (1995–2007), CPC was documented in 80 children (52 boys and 28 girls, age range 1 day–9 years, median 2.4 days) and retrospective analysis of plain abdominal radiographs of 77 children at the time of presentation was performed. Radiographic findings were correlated with surgical findings.

Results.—Of 77 children, 5 were excluded from the study since the pouch colon was perforated. The direction of the pouch apex was correlated with surgical findings to determine the CPC type ($P<0.0001$, Fisher exact test). Type 1 (17/18) and type 2 CPC (18/18) were characterized by a single large pouch with the apex positioned in the left hypochondrium. In type 3 CPC (2/2) the pouch apex was directed towards the right hypochondrium. In type 4 CPC the apex of the pouch was directed towards the right hypochondrium (28/33); however in 5 children it was towards the left hypochondrium. In type 5 CPC ($n=1$) the radiograph was inconclusive.

Conclusion.—Plain abdominal radiographs have a predictive value in determining the type of CPC and obviating the need for an invertogram (Fig 6).

▶ One should always remember that a small but important percentage of infants with imperforate anus has no colon present beyond the cecum. These

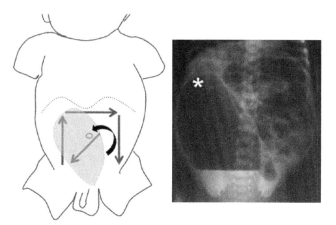

FIGURE 6.—Schematic view (*left*) shows the level of small bowel mesenteric attachment (*blue arrow*) and ascending/transverse/descending colon attachment (*red arrows*) in type 4 CPC with the position (*curved black arrow*) of the pouch (*grey*). Abdominal radiograph (*right*) of a 2-day-old male neonate shows apex of the pouch (*asterisk*) directed to the right hypochondrium with small bowel loop displaced to the left side. For interpretation of the references to color in this figure legend, the reader is referred to web version of this article. (Reprinted from Mathur P, Saxena AK, Bajaj M, et al. Role of plain abdominal radiographs in predicting type of congenital pouch colon. *Pediatr Radiol.* 2010;40:1603-1608, with permission from Springer-Verlag.)

cases are the prototype of what has become known as pouch colon and most typically a wide pouch (the cecum) with gas and fluid communicating via a fistula to the posterior bladder. However, not mentioned in this article are some cases in which the fistula is blocked by material such as meconium and other cases in which no bladder has developed, so that it cannot receive such a fistula. Among the interesting features emphasized in this report are the left or right abdominal location of the pouch (which usually has a gas-fluid level extending over 50% across the abdomen) and use of that information to predict the exact type of pouch in the Saxena-Mathur classification. For example, looking at Fig 6, I agree with their conclusion that an invertogram plain image is not necessary but do think that some horizontal beam plain image is helpful. Many cases of pouch colon or complete absence of the colon beyond cecum have been reported through the years, as early as 1912.[1] Some cases of sirenomelia, incidentally, have a pattern in the abdomen that falls within the rubric of pouch colon/complete agenesis of the colon beyond the cecum.

A. E. Oestreich, MD

Reference

1. Spriggs NI. Congenital intestinal occlusion. An account of twenty-four unpublished cases, with remarks based thereon and upon the literature of the subject. *Guy's Hosp Rep.* 1912;66:143-218.

Fetal gastrointestinal MRI: all that glitters in T1 is not necessarily colon
Colombani M, Ferry M, Garel C, et al (La Timone Children's Hosp, Marseille, France; Groupe Rennais d'Imagerie Médicale, Rennes, France; Hôpital d'Enfants Armand-Trousseau, Paris, France; et al)
Pediatr Radiol 40:1215-1221, 2010

Background.—It has been described that both the colon and distal ileum present with a physiological hypersignal on T1-weighted sequences during the second and third trimesters of pregnancy because of their protein-rich meconium content, it was unclear whether the normal characteristics that have been described on fetal MRI can be applied to gastrointestinal (GI) obstructions.

Objective.—To analyse the localisation value of T1 hypersignal within dilated bowel loops in fetuses with gastrointestinal tract obstruction.

Materials and Methods.—A retrospective 4-year multicentre study analysing cases of fetal GI obstruction in which MRI demonstrated T1 hypersignal content in the dilated loops. Data collected included gestational age (GA) at diagnosis, bowel appearance on US, CFTR gene mutations and amniotic levels of gastrointestinal enzymes. The suggested prenatal diagnosis was eventually compared to postnatal imaging and surgery.

Results.—Eleven patients were included. The median GA at US diagnosis was 23 weeks (range 13—32). In eight cases there was a single dilated loop, while several segments were affected in three. The median GA at

MRI was 29 weeks (range 23—35). One case presented with cystic fibrosis mutations. Final prenatally suspected diagnoses were distal ileal atresia or colon in nine cases and proximal atresia in two. Postnatal findings were proximal jejunal atresia in nine cases and meconium ileus in two. In five cases the surgical findings demonstrated short bowel syndrome.

Conclusion.—In cases of fetal occlusion, T1 hypersignal should not be considered as a sign of distal ileal or colonic occlusion. The obstruction may be proximal, implying a risk of small bowel syndrome, which requires adequate parental counselling.

▶ Prenatal ultrasound (US) has been valuable in identifying problems during pregnancy, often in conjunction with prenatal MRI used to clarify suspected abnormalities and perhaps reveal other significant findings. When the MRI finding, in this instance high T1 in bowel loop or loops, does not follow conventional wisdom, or current knowledge, it is most valuable to have an article such as this both to describe the exceptions and to attempt explanation. A good example is the obstruction responsible for the bright T1 loop shown in Fig 3. Apparently, normal prenatal gastrointestinal tract meconium has the biochemical make-up to cause the usually encountered bright signal on T1; the biochemical makeup of bowel content (small or large bowel) proximal to intrauterine obstruction must share features that cause T1 brightness. As the authors suggest, trying to interpret both US and MRI together may predict the surgically important diagnosis lurking behind the bright T1. Perhaps meconium in other situations, unless it has already calcified, may also yield a potentially confusing bright T1 signal, such as meconium that has escaped into the peritoneum of the fetus secondary to perforation. However, once meconium

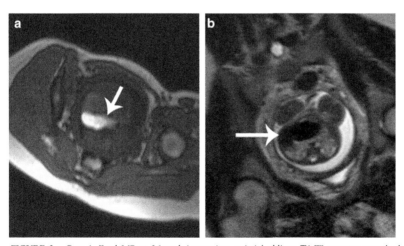

FIGURE 3.—Case 1. Fetal MR at 26 weeks' gestation. **a** Axial oblique T1-W sequence reveals the hypersignal content of the dilated loop (*arrow*). The anterior abdominal wall looks normal. **b** Axial oblique T2-W sequence demonstrates the same bowel lesion with low T2 signal intensity (*arrow*). (With kind permission from Springer Science and Business Media: Colombani M, Ferry M, Garel C, et al. Fetal gastrointestinal MRI: all that glitters in T1 is not necessarily colon. *Pediatr Radiol.* 2010;40:1215-1221.)

is bathed in peritoneal fluid or urine (via a fistula) sufficiently long, it will calcify and thus not have high T1 signal.

A. E. Oestreich, MD

Point-of-care ultrasound diagnosis of pediatric cholecystitis in the ED
Tsung JW, Raio CC, Ramirez-Schrempp D, et al (Bellevue Hosp Ctr/NYU School of Medicine, NY; Northshore Univ Hosp, Manhasset, NY; Boston Med Ctr, MA; et al)
Am J Emerg Med 28:338-342, 2010

Objective.—The diagnosis of cholecystitis or biliary tract disease in children and adolescents is an uncommon occurrence in the emergency department and other acute care settings. Misdiagnosis and delays in diagnosing children with cholecystitis or biliary tract disease of up to months and years have been reported in the literature. We discuss the technique and potential utility of point-of-care ultrasound evaluation in a series of pediatric patients with suspected cholecystitis or biliary tract disease.

Methods.—We present a nonconsecutive case series of pediatric and adolescent patients with abdominal pain diagnosed with cholecystitis or biliary tract disease using point-of-care ultrasound. The published sonographic criteria is 3 mm or less for the upper limits of normal gallbladder wall thickness and is 3 mm or less for normal common bile duct diameter (measured from inner wall to inner wall) in children. Measurements above these limits were considered abnormal, in addition to the sonographic presence of gallstones, pericholecystic fluid, and a sonographic Murphy's sign.

Results.—Point-of care ultrasound screening detected 13 female pediatric patients with cholecystitis or biliary tract disease when the authors were on duty over a 5-year period. Diagnoses were confirmed by radiology imaging or at surgery and surgical pathology.

Conclusions.—Point-of-care ultrasound to detect pediatric cholecystitis or biliary tract disease may help avoid misdiagnosis or delays in diagnosis in children with abdominal pain.

▶ Just so we understand, point-of-care ultrasound refers to imaging done by emergency (or other) physicians personally at the time of a patient visit. Indeed, many of the patients in this study were later sent for radiology ultrasound examination for confirmation of abnormality and further imaging evaluation. In this turf-sensitive arena, note that this article is authored by emergency room physicians plus 1 pediatrician. But looking beyond who does or should do the imaging, the results are impressive. In this world of increasing obesity, cholecystitis and gallstones seem to be increasing in incidence. If a subject is overly stout, the 3.5 to 5-MHz transducers successfully used by the authors might not suffice. Their patients' age ranged from 18 months to 15 years. None of their patients had all of the classic triad of fever: elevated white blood cell count, and an acute abdomen on physical examination. Delay in diagnosis (with point-of-care imaging) ranged from greater than 2 months to 5 years. Should such a patient happen to have had an abdominal radiograph, recall that in about half of children with gallstones, unlike adults, the stones are radiodense enough to be visualized on plain images.[1]

A. E. Oestreich, MD

Reference

1. Henschke CI, Teele RL. Cholelithiasis in children: recent observations. *J Ultrasound Med.* 1983;2:481-484.

Transient reticular gallbladder wall thickening in severe dengue fever: a reliable sign of plasma leakage
Oliveira GA, Machado RC, Horvat JV, et al (Nossa Senhora da Gloria Children's Hosp, Vitoria, Brazil; Federal Univ of Espirito Santo, Vitoria, Brazil)
Pediatr Radiol 40:720-724, 2010

Background.—Dengue fever (DF) is an acute infection caused by a flavivirus. Although most patients present mild symptoms, some progress to a severe condition characterized by hypovolemic shock and hemorrhagic phenomena. The main feature of this severe form of DF is plasma leakage. Gallbladder wall thickening (GBWT), ascites and pleural effusion represent the sonographic triad of plasma leakage in DF.

Objective.—To evaluate the plasma leakage triad in severe DF with emphasis on the GBWT.

Materials and Methods.—Thirty-seven children with severe DF underwent abdominal US on the day of admittance and on the day of discharge, or 7 days after the first examination if the child was still hospitalized.

Results.—Of the 37 children, 33 (89.2%) presented GBWT, 29 (78.4%) ascites and 26 (70.3%) pleural effusion. All of these findings had resolved by the second examination. Of the 33 GBWTs, 29 (87.9%) presented a reticular pattern, which could be considered typical of plasma leakage in patients with severe DF.

Conclusion.—GBWT, ascites and pleural effusion are transient findings in DF. The authors have described a typical reticular pattern of GBWT that can be used to diagnose and follow up on patients with severe DF and should not be considered an acalculous cholecystitis.

▶ It's about time to include the scourge of dengue fever in our selections. A pattern of gallbladder wall abnormality on ultrasound, typified by Fig 2, is newly reported as characteristic of the severe version of the disease. The vector is the *Aedes aegypti* mosquito. The mosquito and the flavivirus were spread among the tropics and subtropics by classic travelers such as Columbus, da Gama, and Magellan. Characteristic is rapid onset of fever and malaise followed by rash. Perhaps 20 million persons are infected yearly. A repeat infection tends to be more severe, with increase of vascular permeability, and this form of

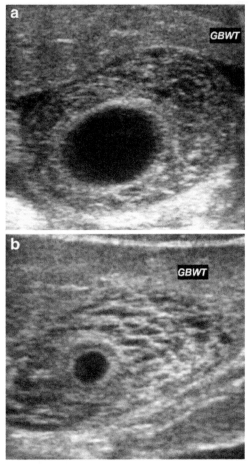

FIGURE 2.—Reticular pattern in GBWT. **a, b** Multiple interlaced echogenic lines demonstrate the reticular pattern in a 10-year-old boy and in a 6-year-old girl with DHF/DSS. (With kind permission from Springer Science and Business Media: Oliveira GA, Machado RC, Horvat JV, et al. Transient reticular gallbladder wall thickening in severe dengue fever: a reliable sign of plasma leakage. *Pediatr Radiol.* 2010;40:720-724.)

dengue fever is known as dengue hemorrhagic fever or dengue shock syndrome and features plasma leakage. In the significant Brazilian 2009 outbreak of dengue, US evaluation of most children with the severe form revealed the characteristic reticular gallbladder wall thickening, reported here with several illustrative images. The pattern is important to learn, to distinguish from other forms of gallbladder disease, and for radiologic contribution to diagnosis, especially in epidemics. Meanwhile, workers are investigating possible preventative measures.[1] The dengue fever we all (hopefully) studied in medical school is still with us today, so be aware.

A. E. Oestreich, MD

Reference

1. Brandler S, Ruffie C, Najburg V, et al. Pediatric measles vaccine expressing a dengue tetravalent antigen elicits neutralizing antibodies against all four dengue viruses. *Vaccine*. 2010;28:6730-6739.

Urogenital

Ultrasonographic Patterns of Reproductive Organs in Infants Fed Soy Formula: Comparisons to Infants Fed Breast Milk and Milk Formula

Gilchrist JM, Moore MB, Andres A, et al (Univ of Arkansas for Med Sciences, Little Rock, AR; et al)

J Pediatr 156:215-220, 2010

Objective.—To determine if differences exist in hormone-sensitive organ size between infants who were fed soy formula (SF), milk formula (MF), or breast milk (BF).

Study Design.—Breast buds, uterus, ovaries, prostate, and testicular volumes were assessed by ultrasonography in 40 BF, 41 MF, and 39 SF infants at age 4 months.

Results.—There were no significant feeding group effects in anthropometric or body composition. Among girls, there were no feeding group differences in breast bud or uterine volume. MF infants had greater ($P < .05$) mean ovarian volume and greater ($P < .01$) numbers of ovarian cysts per ovary than did BF infants. Among boys, there were no feeding group differences in prostate or breast bud volumes. Mean testicular volume did not differ between SF and MF boys, but both formula-fed groups had lower volumes than BF infants.

Conclusions.—Our data do not support major diet-related differences in reproductive organ size as measured by ultrasound in infants at age 4 months, although there is some evidence that ovarian development may be advanced in MF-fed infants and that testicular development may be slower in both MF and SF infants as compared with BF. There was no evidence that feeding SF exerts any estrogenic effects on reproductive organs studied.

▶ For those of us who spend a portion of our working day measuring the size of gonads and uteri in a variety of diagnostic situations, some further insight into the size of those organs should be of interest. Breastfeeding has many advantages in most infants (with exceptions for conditions such as galactosemia, hereditary lactase deficiency, and secondary lactose intolerance, as mentioned by the authors). Nonetheless, mothers choose alternatives for bottle-feeding. The study seeks to investigate (and perhaps allay) the fears of some investigators that soy-based formulas may have estrogen-related deleterious effects. They believe they found no adverse effects, but for us measurers it is of interest that milk formula-fed baby girls had significantly greater mean ovarian volume and ovarian cyst number than breast-fed baby girls, and testicular volumes were lower in bottle-fed baby boys than breast-fed baby boys. Nonetheless, all fell within normal range. So it seems that it's all right to bottle-feed, even soy formula, from a volume of end organ point of view, but it might be of interest to the ultrasound imagers to ask about method of feeding when conducting their studies.

A. E. Oestreich, MD

Prevalence of Testicular Adrenal Rest Tissue in Neonates
Bouman A, Hulsbergen-van de Kaa C, Claahsen-van der Grinten HL (Radboud Univ Nijmegen Med Centre, The Netherlands)
Horm Res Paediatr 2010 [Epub ahead of print]

Background.—Infertility is a serious complication among male congenital adrenal hyperplasia (CAH) patients which is often caused by testicular adrenal rest tumors (TART). TART are already present in childhood and early infancy in CAH patients. The incidence of TART in neonates without CAH has not yet been described in detail before.

Objective.—To study the prevalence of testicular adrenal rests in non-CAH neonates.

Design.—Descriptive study.

Setting.—Radboud University Nijmegen Medical Centre, The Netherlands.

Patients and Methods.—115 testis samples of 89 male infants without CAH who died within the neonatal period were histologically examined.

Main Outcome Measures.—Prevalence of adrenal rest tissue in the neonatal testes.

Results.—Adrenal rests were found in 4 samples (3.5%). These adrenal nodules were all located within the epididymis; only in 1 sample a nodule was found close to the rete testis but still within the caput of the epididymis. No nodules were found within the testes. Of the 4 children with adrenal rests, 3 had urological malformations.

Conclusion.—The incidence of testicular adrenal rests in non-CAH neonates is low. Further studies are necessary to study the incidence of TART in CAH infants and detect typical risk factors in this patient group.

▶ Congenital adrenal rests in the testis, tartly named testicular adrenal rest tumors, are found typically in children and adults with congenital adrenal hyperplasia. On ultrasound (US), they appear as relatively hypoechoic rounded or oval lesions within the testis. Excellent US illustrations may be found in another recent article.[1] This current article extends knowledge relevant to the pediatric ultrasonographer with regard to such adrenal rests in boys without congenital adrenal hyperplasia. Although the incidence in babies was low, it was nonnegligible, and, interestingly, the rests were found at postmortem pathology in the epididymis rather than the testis proper. Based on the histological sections in the current article, it seems reasonable to assume that such rests in the epididymis would similarly appear on US as low-echogenic round/ovoid lesions. Histologically, the rests are of adrenal cortical morphology. From this cited article, then, we extend the anatomic locations of this US lesion that could otherwise be confused with leukemia of the testis or other malignancies.

A. E. Oestreich, MD

Reference

1. Claahsen-van der Grinten HL, Sweep FC, Blickman JG, Hermus AR, Otten BJ. Prevalence of testicular adrenal rest tumours in male children with congenital adrenal hyperplasia due to 21-hydroxylase deficiency. *Eur J Endocrinol.* 2007;157:339-344.

Posterior cloaca—further experience and guidelines for the treatment of an unusual anorectal malformation
Peña A, Bischoff A, Breech L, et al (Cincinnati Children's Hosp Med Ctr, OH)
J Pediatr Surg 45:1234-1240, 2010

Introduction.—The term *posterior cloaca* refers to a malformation in which the urethra and vagina are fused, forming a urogenital sinus that deviates posteriorly to open in the anterior rectal wall or immediately anterior to the anus.

Methods.—A retrospective review of 411 patients diagnosed with cloaca was performed to identify the ones with a posterior cloaca. Special emphasis was placed on anatomy, diagnosis, associated anomalies, and outcome in terms of urinary and fecal continence. Surgical treatment was a total urogenital mobilization with a transrectal approach.

Results.—Twenty-nine patients were diagnosed with a posterior cloaca. Of these, 15 had a single orifice at the normal location of the anus with the urogenital sinus opening in the anterior rectal wall. Fourteen had the urogenital sinus opening immediately anterior to the normally located anal opening (2 orifices), which we considered a posterior cloaca variant. Nineteen patients (65%) had hydrocolpos. Twenty-seven patients (93%) had associated urologic anomalies, 12 patients (41%) had gynecologic anomalies, and vertebral malformations occurred in 41% of cases. Other anomalies included gastrointestinal (7 patients), cardiac (5), and tethered cord (2). Late diagnosis occurred in 2 patients. Twenty patients were available for long-term follow-up: 17 are fecally continent, 3 are fecally incontinent, 11 are urinary continent, 5 are dry with intermittent catheterization, and 4 have dribble urine.

Conclusion.—The most important characteristic of the posterior cloaca is the high frequency of a normal anus, which differentiates this malformation from the classic cloaca. Often, many associated malformations are present and therefore should be suspected and diagnosed. The main goal during the operation should be to not mobilize the anus and thereby preserve the anal canal. A total urogenital mobilization, transperineally or with a transanorectal approach, is ideal for the repair (Figs 1 and 3).

▶ This is a report of twenty-nine cases of an almost unheard of female anorectal malformation, with an important message to be delivered by the savvy

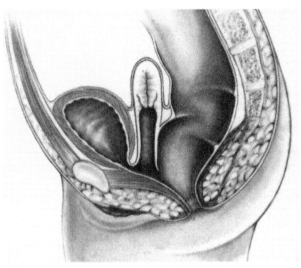

FIGURE 1.—Artistic diagram of a posterior cloaca. (Reprinted from Peña A, Bischoff A, Breech L, et al. Posterior cloaca—further experience and guidelines for the treatment of an unusual anorectal malformation. *J Pediatr Surg*. 2010;45:1234-1240, with permission from Elsevier.)

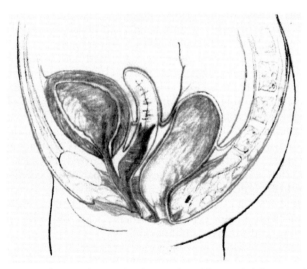

FIGURE 3.—Artistic diagram of a posterior cloaca variant with urogenital sinus posteriorly deviated, opening immediately anterior to the anus. (Reprinted from Peña A, Bischoff A, Breech L, et al. Posterior cloaca—further experience and guidelines for the treatment of an unusual anorectal malformation. *J Pediatr Surg*. 2010;45:1234-1240, with permission from Elsevier.)

radiologist to the surgeon—namely, preserve the anus to preserve bowel function! The anatomy of the posterior cloaca entity is nicely summarized in Figs 1 and 3, each type having been encountered in about half of the patients. The authors appropriately emphasize associated findings including, in a majority, hydrometrocolpos. Our prenatal imaging colleagues have diagnosed posterior cloaca in fetuses; ideally, when such a case is so identified, arrangements would be made for birth to occur at a center with specialist pediatric anorectal surgeons. In the only 3 fecally incontinent long-term follow-up patients in the authors' series of 20, one had sacral agenesis and one had tethered cord associated. One other finding of interest to radiologists—and a clue to diagnosis—is a prominent overgrowth of the pubic bones (which the authors wonder might be cause or effect of the malformation). Although posterior cloaca has been described under other names, it is the message proclaimed in this article that is key, although the name posterior cloaca seems quite logical to use uniformly.

A. E. Oestreich, MD

Effect of Rectal Distention on Lower Urinary Tract Function in Children
Burgers R, Liem O, Canon S, et al (Emma Children's Hosp/Academic Med Ctr, Amsterdam, The Netherlands; Nationwide Children's Hosp, Columbus, OH)
J Urol 184:1680-1685, 2010

Purpose.—We investigated the effect of rectal distention on lower urinary tract function.

Materials and Methods.—Children were assigned to a constipation and lower urinary tract symptoms group or to a lower urinary tract symptoms only group. The definition of constipation was based on pediatric Rome III criteria. Standard urodynamics were done initially and repeated during simultaneous barostat pressure controlled rectal balloon distention and after balloon deflation. We evaluated the effects of rectal balloon inflation and deflation on urodynamic parameters. Colonic transit time measurement, anorectal manometry and the Parenting Rating Scale of child behavior were also used.

Results.—We studied 7 boys and 13 girls with a median age of 7.5 years who had constipation and lower urinary tract symptoms, and 3 boys and 3 girls with a median age of 7.5 years who had lower urinary tract symptoms only. Urodynamic patterns of response to rectal distention were inhibitory in 6 children and stimulatory in 12, and did not change in 8. In 54% of the cases balloon deflation reversed balloon inflation changes while in 46% balloon inflation changes persisted or progressed. No significant differences were noted in children with vs without constipation and no clinical symptom or diagnostic study predicted the occurrence, direction or degree of bladder responses.

Conclusions.—In almost 70% of children with lower urinary tract symptoms rectal distention significantly but unpredictably affected bladder capacity, sensation and overactivity regardless of whether the children had constipation, and independent of clinical features and baseline urodynamic findings. Urodynamics and management protocols for lower urinary tract symptoms that fail to recognize the effects of rectal distention may lead to unpredictable outcomes.

▶ The mutual effects of the rectum and the bladder have always been a matter of interest. For that reason, it behooves the pediatric imager to observe and perhaps mention the degree of distention of the rectum or rectosigmoid when roentgen or ultrasound imaging is done for the bladder. Similarly, distention of the bladder ought to be mentioned when discussing the imaging appearance of the rectum. This article delves into dynamic and imaging effects of rectal distention. Other examples of the relationship would be the megacystis micro-colon syndrome. The occasional patient with severe osteogenesis in whom bilateral protrusio acetabuli[1] causes rectal narrowing and thus potential consti-pation is an example of a skeletal/rectal clinically significant relationship. This article would suggests that such patients with osteogenesis imperfecta need to have their urinary dynamics investigated as well.

A. E. Oestreich, MD

Reference

1. Violas P, Fassier F, Hamdy R, Duhaime M, Glorieux FH. Acetabular protrusion in osteogenesis imperfecta. *J Pediatr Orthop.* 2002;22:622-625.

Role of spinning top urethra in dysfunctional voiding
Kutlu O, Koksal IT, Guntekin E, et al (Akdeniz Univ, Antalya, Turkey)
Scand J Urol Nephrol 44:32-37, 2010

Objective.—The role of spinning top urethra (STU) in children with dysfunctional voiding was evaluated retrospectively.

Material and Methods.—From 1995 to 2002, the records of 154 chil-dren with dysfunctional voiding were reviewed retrospectively. Of the chil-dren 110 (71%) were girls and 44 (29%) were boys (mean age 8 years, range 4—14). All children were neurologically normal and no exhibited physical signs of occult spinal dysraphism. Patients were divided into two groups according to their width of proximal urethra: group I had STU and the group II had normal urethral width. The groups were compared with each other for gender, voiding symptoms, urinary tract infection (UTI), vesicoureteral reflux (VUR) and urodynamic observations.

Results.—There were 84 children (mean age 8.3 ± 2.2 years, range 4—14) in group I and 70 (mean age 8.0 ± 2.1 years, range 4—14) in group II; no significant age difference was found between the two groups $(p = 0.4674)$. Group I consisted of 66 (71%) girls and 18 (29%) boys and group II 44 (63%) girls and 26 (37%) boys. STU was observed more in girls than boys in group I $(p = 0.0316)$. UTI was observed in 57 patients (68%) in group I and 34 (49%) in group II $(p = 0.0154)$. Mean duration of symptoms was 42 ± 24 months (range 6—118) and 39 ± 23 (range 3—120) months in groups I and II, respectively $(p = 0.6302)$. Postvoid residual urine (PVR) more than 10% of expected bladder capacity was detected in 15 patients (18%) in group I and seven (10%) in group II. No association was found between the meaningful PVR and STU ($p = 0.1653$). The presence of detrusor overactivity during filling was observed in 54 patients (64%) in group I and 42 (60%) in group II ($p = 0.4676$). Diminished bladder compliance (<10 ml/cm H_2O) was detected in 34 patients (40%) in group I and 17 (24%) in group II ($p = 0.0335$). The mean voiding pressure was measured as 56 ± 29 cm H_2O in group I, which was significantly higher than in group II (49 ± 25 cm H_2O) ($p = 0.0373$). The mean flow rate during the emptying phase of urodynamics was 16 ± 8 and 15 ± 6 ml/s in groups I and II, respectively (not significant, $p = 0.2686$). VUR was detected in 16 patients (19%) in group I and two (3%) in group II ($p = 0.0018$).

Conclusions.—STU was related to recurrent UTIs, VUR, poor bladder compliance and more serious functional urinary obstruction. Furthermore, STU may be a consequence of a neurogenic maturation defect in detrusor—sphincter coordination resembling that of urofacial syndrome, because development of this situation was found to be independent of the duration of symptoms (Fig 1).

▶ Here comes that spinning top again! When I grew up in pediatric radiology, I only knew of spinning top urethra (STU) in girls; this article also discusses cases in males. Indeed, the male equivalent of STU has been discussed,[1] but I would consider radish urethra, with a long root, as a more apt description. Kutlu et al describe dysfunctional voiding as a common clinical problem, which is a urodynamic entity characterized by an intermittent and/or fluctuating urine flow rate because of involuntary contractions of the striated muscle of the external urethral sphincter or pelvic floor during voiding in neurologically normal individuals. That definition is not gender specific. Fig 1 nicely shows the correlation of imaging and function (electromyogram). Among bothersome symptoms more prevalent with STU was daytime incontinence, at least in girls.

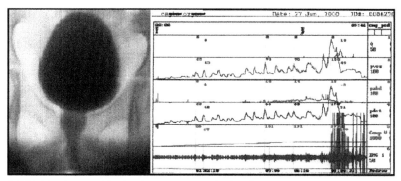

FIGURE 1.—A 6-year-old girl with spinning top urethra had detrusor overactivity, diminished bladder compliance, high voiding pressure and low flow rate with electromyographic activity. (Reprinted from Kutlu O, Koksal IT, Guntekin E, et al. Role of spinning top urethra in dysfunctional voiding. *Scand J Urol Nephrol.* 2010;44:32-37, with permission from Informa UK Ltd.)

Endoscopic incision was particularly successful treatment in some involved boys, including all of Hoebeke's cases.[1]

A. E. Oestreich, MD

Reference

1. Hoebeke PB, Van Laecke E, Raes A, Vande Walle J, Oosterlinck W. Membrano-bulbo-urethral junction stenosis. Posterior urethra obstruction due to extreme caliber disproportion in the male urethra. *Eur Urol*. 1997;32:480-484.

Assessment of Parental Satisfaction in Children Undergoing Voiding Cystourethrography Without Sedation

Sandy NS, Nguyen HT, Ziniel SI, et al (Children's Hosp Boston and Harvard Med School, MA)
J Urol 185:658-662, 2011

Purpose.—Approximately 50,000 children undergo voiding cystourethrography annually. There is a recent trend toward using sedation or delaying voiding cystourethrography due to the anticipated distress to the patient. We hypothesized that with adequate preparation and proper techniques to minimize anxiety, voiding cystourethrography can be performed without sedation. We assessed parental satisfaction associated with patient and parent experience of voiding cystourethrography without sedation.

Materials and Methods.—We used a 33-question survey to evaluate parental satisfaction with patient and parent experience of voiding cystourethrography without sedation. Children were divided into 3 groups according to toilet training status. Statistical analysis was performed using Stata®.

Results.—A total of 200 surveys were completed. Of the children 54% were not toilet trained. Of the parents 90% reported adequate preparation. More than half of parents classified the experience of voiding cystourethrography as equivalent to or better than a physical examination, immunization, ultrasound and prior catheterization. Most parents were satisfied with the ability of the child to tolerate the procedure and considered the experience better than expected. Children in the process of toilet training had the most difficulty with the procedure, correlating with lower levels of parental satisfaction.

Conclusions.—Voiding cystourethrography performed with adequate preparation and support can be tolerated without sedation. Children in the process of toilet training and females tolerate the procedure least.

▶ Voiding cystourethrography (VCUG) is no fun. That holds for nuclear and ultrasound methods as well as X-ray fluoroscopy. When this procedure can be avoided or should be avoided, especially when radiation is involved, the unhappiness and the risks are obviated. The value of this article is in emphasizing that if a voiding cystourethrogram is indeed indicated, then parents and children benefit from pretesting preparation. Child Life and similar professional presence before and during the procedure can indeed alleviate anxiety. A corollary implication might be that if VCUG needs to be done, it should be done in a facility specialized in the care of children and staffed with health care professionals trained to assist. However, the more specialized centers might be more likely to understand when a lack of indication exists for this bothersome investigation. In addition, I support avoiding sedation, especially because VCUG should be evaluating the quality of voiding in the natural (unsedated) state if indeed it is performed.

A. E. Oestreich, MD

Functional analysis in MR urography — made simple
Khrichenko D, Darge K (The Children's Hosp of Philadelphia, PA)
Pediatr Radiol 40:182-199, 2010

MR urography (MRU) has proved to be a most advantageous imaging modality of the urinary tract in children, providing one-stop comprehensive morphological and functional information, without the utilization of ionizing radiation. The functional analysis of the MRU scan still requires external post-processing using relatively complex software. This has proved to be a limiting factor in widespread routine implementation of MRU functional analysis and use of MRU functional parameters similar to nuclear medicine. We present software, developed in a pediatric radiology department, that not only enables comprehensive automated functional analysis, but is also very user-friendly, fast, easily operated by the average radiologist or MR technician and freely downloadable at www. chop-fmru.com. A copy of IDL Virtual Machine is required for the installation, which is obtained at no charge at www.ittvis.com. The analysis software, known as "CHOP-fMRU," has the potential to help overcome the obstacles to widespread use of functional MRU in children.

▶ The authors describe this important methodology as user friendly—always a questionable claim. When presented in person by Khrichenko and Kassa, it indeed flows without difficulty. That said, they offer an important tool that makes the functional abilities of MR urography widely available and thus contribute to the vanquishing of necessity for radiation-using technology urography. The term one-stop shopping to describe MR urography becomes more applicable when one secures mastery of this program offered generously by the authors. Electronic supplementary material to the article further elucidates us of their method. Their method cuts down the time of extensive calculations and allows easy to grasp displays of the results for imagers and clinicians alike, as demonstrated in their Fig 6. It is worth the effort to obtain the materials offered in the article to avoid radiographic urography and nuclear function

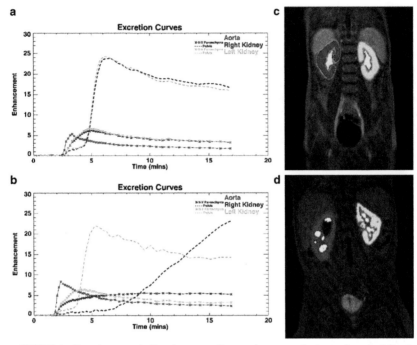

FIGURE 6.—Excretion curves (a, b) and corresponding sample segmentation images from the 3-D series (c, d) in bilateral normal kidneys (a, c) and in a case with a right-side (blue) dilatation (c, d). (With kind permission from Springer Science and Business Media: Khrichenko D, Darge K. Functional analysis in MR urography — made simple. *Pediatr Radiol.* 2010;40:182-199.)

imaging, yet obtain the information needed to treat children with abnormalities of the urinary tract.

A. E. Oestreich, MD

The Swedish Reflux Trial in Children: IV. Renal Damage

Brandström P, Nevéus T, Sixt R, et al (Univ of Gothenburg, Göteborg, Sweden; Uppsala Univ Children's Hosp, Sweden)
J Urol 184:292-297, 2010

Purpose.—We compared the development of new renal damage in small children with dilating vesicoureteral reflux randomly allocated to antibiotic prophylaxis, endoscopic treatment or surveillance as the control group.

Materials and Methods.—Included in the study were 128 girls and 75 boys 1 to younger than 2 years with grade III–IV reflux. Voiding cystourethrography and dimercapto-succinic acid scintigraphy were done before randomization and after 2 years. Febrile urinary tract infections were recorded during followup. Data analysis was done by the intent to treat principle.

Results.—New renal damage in a previously unscarred area was seen in 13 girls and 2 boys. Eight of the 13 girls were on surveillance, 5 received endoscopic therapy and none were on prophylaxis (p = 0.0155). New damage was more common in children with than without febrile recurrence (11 of 49 or 22% vs 4 of 152 or 3%, p <0.0001).

Conclusions.—In boys the rate of new renal damage was low. It was significantly higher in girls and most common in the control surveillance group. There was also a strong association between recurrent febrile UTIs and new renal damage in girls.

▶ What is the purpose of (repeated) imaging of the urinary tract in young children if we really cannot get a hang on the relationships between reflux (on voiding cystourethrogram) and renal damage and renal health? An ambitious and well-organized pan-Swedish clinical and imaging clinical trial has faced this question and given some answers that might guide the radiologist as to the efficacy of our imaging. The *Journal of Urology* and the authors divided the results into 5 consecutive articles, one of which I here select. In girls with moderately severe reflux, the trend is clearly to suggest that prophylactic antibiotics are helpful (in the prevention of new renal damage), and therefore clinicians need to know if such reflux is present. In boys, it seemed that treatment has little influence on the incidence of the few new scars that occurred. If then imaging is necessary to determine the moderately severe reflux in young girls, hopefully we in the United States will be permitted to use ultrasound contrast material so that such imaging will be done without radiation.

A. E. Oestreich, MD

Neurologic/Vertebral

Improved Delineation of Ventricular Shunt Catheters Using Fast Steady-State Gradient Recalled-Echo Sequences in a Rapid Brain MR Imaging Protocol in Nonsedated Pediatric Patients

Miller JH, Walkiewicz T, Towbin RB, et al (Phoenix Children's Hosp, AZ)
AJNR Am J Neuroradiol 31:430-435, 2010

Background and Purpose.—Rapid brain MR imaging is often substituted for head CT in multiply imaged patients with shunted hydrocephalus. Fast TSE-T2 sequences are commonly used in these protocols. One limitation of TSE-T2 sequences is the decreased catheter delineation compared with CT. The aim of this study was to compare fast TSE-T2 with rapid SS-GRE sequences in the evaluation of intracranial shunt catheter delineation as part of a rapid nonsedated pediatric brain MR imaging protocol.

Materials and Methods.—We evaluated the findings from 179 consecutive patients who underwent routine clinical imaging according to the rapid nonsedated pediatric brain MR imaging protocol. Comparison of the quality of intracranial shunt catheter localization on SS-GRE versus TSE-T2 was performed.

Results.—Of the total of 179 rapid nonsedated pediatric brain MR images that were reviewed, 62 (35%) had an intracranial shunt catheter. The shunt catheter tip was better localized on the SS-GRE than on the TSE-T2 images in 49/62 (79%) of these patients. Of the remaining 13/62 (21%), the TSE-T2 was either better or equivalent in localizing the shunt catheter tip.

Conclusions.—Our study shows that rapid SS-GRE sequences can provide better delineation of standard intracranial shunt catheters than standard rapid MR imaging protocols containing only fast TSE-T2 sequences.

▶ Whether we call it ALARA or Image Gently, the message is now well and truly out there: particularly in pediatric imaging, we should do our utmost to minimize patient exposure to ionizing radiation. Head CT is used to depict shunt catheter tips in children with hydrocephalus. This group of children may be subject to multiple imaging; therefore, limiting the number of CT scans or even eliminating them altogether would considerably reduce population radiation exposure.

MRI may be the solution. Aware of the limitations of standard fast T2 turbo spin-echo (TSE-T2) sequences, the authors have attempted to introduce and optimize a rapid steady-state gradient recalled-echo (SS-GRE) sequence. However, I do not fully agree with their conclusion as stated in the abstract. The 21% of cases in which TSE-T2 was better than or equivalent to SS-GRE is not an insignificant minority (TSE-T2 was found to be better, particularly in cases with at least moderate hydrocephalus with a well-positioned catheter). For the time being (and yes, I know it prolongs scan times), I wonder whether it might not be more sensible to include both sequences rather than replacing one with the other.

Another approach indirectly alluded to by the authors is to develop catheter materials that allow optimum depiction using currently available rapid MR sequences. Now that would be a clever solution, wouldn't it?

A. C. Offiah, BSc, MBBS, MRCP, FRCR, PhD

Comparison of neonatal MRI examinations with and without an MR-compatible incubator: Advantages in examination feasibility and clinical decision-making
Rona Z, Klebermass K, Cardona F, et al (Semmelweis Univ, Budapest, Hungary; Med Univ of Vienna, Austria)
Eur J Paediatr Neurol 14:410-417, 2010

Purpose.—To assess the utility of an MRI-compatible incubator (INC) by comparing.

1. The frequency of MR examinations done in 18 months periods each in unstable newborns with suspect central-nervous system (CNS) problems,
2. The respective expenditure of time, and
3. The amount of necessary sedatives with and without the INC.

Methods.—In a retrospective study, the clinical and radiological aspects of 129 neonatal MRI examinations during a 3 year period were analyzed. Routine protocols including fast spin-echo T2-weighted (w) sequences, axial T1w, Gradient-echo, diffusion sequences, and 3D T1 gradient-echo sequences were performed routinely, angiography and spectroscopy were added in some cases. Diffusion-tensor imaging was done in 50% of the babies examined in the INC and 26% without INC. Sequences, adapted from fetal MR-protocols were done in infants younger than 32 gestational weeks. Benefit from MR-information with respect to further management was evaluated.

Results.—The number of the examinations increased (30–99), while the mean age (43–38, 8 weeks of gestational age) and weight (3308–2766 g) decreased significantly with the use of the MR-compatible incubator. The mean imaging time (34, 43–30, 29 min) decreased, with a mean of one additionally performed sequence in the INC group. All infants received sedatives according to our anaesthetic protocol preceding imaging, but a repeated dose was never necessary (10% without INC) using the INC. Regarding all cases, MR-based changes in clinical management were initiated in 58%, while in 57% of cases the initial ultrasound diagnosis was changed or further specified.

Conclusions.—The use of the INC enables the MR access of unstable infants with suspect CNS problems to the management, of whom is improved by MR information to significantly higher percentage, than without INC (Table 1).

▶ The earliest reports on MR-compatible incubators for imaging preterm infants and neonates were published in 2003 and 2004 (by Erberich et al,[1] by my own colleagues in Sheffield,[2] and by Bluml et al[3]); therefore, the MR-compatible incubator cannot be described as new technology.

However, I have chosen to include this article under the theme of technical report because there are very few articles published on the impact of these machines and there are pediatric centers at which MR-compatible incubators are not available. Although used in specialist centers, articles such as this help to keep the general pediatric radiologist up-to-date.

TABLE 1.—Clinical and Imaging Data

	All Patients			Patients Under 2000 g		
	INC ($n=99$)	No INC ($n=30$)	p Value	INC ($n=28$)	No INC ($n=5$)	p Value
Mean age (GA)	38.82	43.03	$p=0.015$	34.0	33.0	$p=0.66$
Mean weight (g)	2766	3308	$p=0.017$	1750	1761	$p=0.88$
Mean imaging time (min)	30.29	34.43	$p=0.113$	30.79	33.20	$p=0.013$
Mean sequences	10.63	9.67	$p=0.231$	11.61	12.40	$p=0.45$
Ventilation necessary during examination	36%	20%	$p=0.077$	53.6%	80%	$p=0.28$
Critically ill infants	48%	30%	$p=0.074$	53.6%	100%	$p=0.05$
Incomplete imaging procedure	0%	10%	$p=0.001$	0%	20%	$p=0.015$

Results of this article further support the use of an MR-compatible incubator (Table 1). While the 4-minute reduction in imaging time may not appear particularly significant, more importantly, the average overall time this group of (unstable) infants was away from the neonatal unit reduced by 24 minutes because of decreased handling times. That has got to be a good thing.

A word of caution, however—the relative ease of performing scans with the MR-compatible incubator may lead to a rise in the number of scans individual patients are exposed to. The long-term effects (if any) of MR imaging on the extremely premature brain are not known. In this regard, the study by Dyet et al[4] is therefore reassuring, and I think it is fair to say, as in the words of the current authors, "...MR imaging with the use of the INC is a safe and clinically informative examination even in the most unstable, critically ill premature infant."

A. C. Offiah, BSc, MBBS, MRCP, FRCR, PhD

References

1. Erberich SG, Friedlich P, Seri I, Nelson MD Jr, Blüml S. Functional MRI in neonates using neonatal head coil and MR compatible incubator. *Neuroimage*. 2003;20:683-692.
2. Whitby EH, Griffiths PD, Lonneker-Lammers T, et al. Ultrafast magnetic resonance imaging of the neonate in a magnetic resonance-compatible incubator with a built-in coil. *Pediatrics*. 2004;113:e150-e152.
3. Blüml S, Friedlich P, Erberich S, Wood JC, Seri I, Nelson MD Jr. MR imaging of newborns by using an MR-compatible incubator with integrated radiofrequency coils: initial experience. *Radiology*. 2004;231:594-601.
4. Dyet LE, Kennea N, Counsell SJ, et al. Natural history of brain lesions in extremely preterm infants studied with serial magnetic resonance imaging from birth and neurodevelopmental assessment. *Pediatrics*. 2006;118:536-548.

Nerve Root Enhancement on Spinal MRI in Pediatric Guillain-Barré Syndrome

Mulkey SB, Glasier CM, El-Nabbout B, et al (Univ of Arkansas for Med Sciences, Little Rock; Via Christi Health Network, Wichita, KS)
Pediatr Neurol 43:263-269, 2010

Guillain-Barré syndrome diagnosis is based on clinical presentation and supportive diagnostic testing. In its early stage, no single, reliable diagnostic test is available. However, a finding of nerve root enhancement on spinal magnetic resonance imaging may be useful. We evaluated the frequency of nerve root enhancement on spinal magnetic resonance imaging in children with Guillain-Barré syndrome. At a single tertiary pediatric center, we conducted a retrospective chart review of children with Guillain-Barré syndrome who had complete spinal or lumbosacral spinal magnetic resonance imaging with gadolinium administration from January 2002-January 2009. Twenty-four consecutive patients were identified. Spinal nerve root enhancement with gadolinium was present in 92% (22/24) of children with Guillain-Barré syndrome on initial spinal magnetic resonance imaging (95% confidence interval, 0.745-0.978). This finding increased to 100% of patients, after two patients underwent repeat spinal magnetic resonance imaging that did reveal nerve root enhancement. Patterns of enhancement were variable, but involved the thoracolumbar nerve roots in all patients. Enhancement of nerve roots with gadolinium on initial spinal magnetic resonance imaging was frequently present in these children with Guillain-Barré syndrome. Spinal magnetic resonance imaging is a sensitive diagnostic test and should be considered an additional diagnostic tool in select cases (Fig 2).

▶ In this retrospective study, the authors highlight the high prevalence of nerve root enhancement (92%) on initial postcontrast spinal MRI in 24 children with clinically suspected Guillain-Barré syndrome. Follow-up scan results were positive in the remaining 8% (2 patients). Thoracolumbar nerve root enhancement was seen in 22 of the 24 children, whereas cervical nerve root enhancement was seen in only 2 of the 20 children in whom the cervical spine was imaged. Nerve root enhancement was seen as early as 2 days after the onset of symptoms.

The diagnosis of Guillain-Barré syndrome is mainly clinical. However, this is an important sign to look for in children with atypical clinical presentations or when the results of other tests (cerebrospinal fluid protein levels, nerve conduction studies) are unavailable, equivocal, or negative. Postcontrast spinal MR has the further advantage of excluding transverse myelitis.

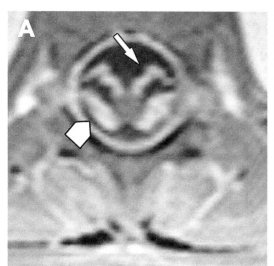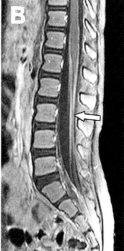

FIGURE 2.—Patient 24, a 4-year-old girl, was nonambulatory at admission and exhibited a very diffuse pattern of contrast enhancement in her spinal nerve roots on T_1 postcontrast axial (A) and sagittal (B) images with fat suppression. Thin arrow indicates ventral nerve roots. (A) Thick arrow indicates dorsal nerve roots. (B) Nerve roots in the cauda equina (arrow). (Reprinted from Mulkey SB, Glasier CM, El-Nabbout B, et al. Nerve root enhancement on spinal MRI in pediatric Guillain-Barré syndrome. *Pediatr Neurol.* 2010;43:263-269.)

Like many other radiological signs, nerve root enhancement is not pathognomonic of a particular disorder, and as the authors caution us, it may also be seen in a variety of other conditions; therefore, as always, dialogue with our clinical colleagues is required.

Unfortunately, a control group of MRI scans was not included in the study, and therefore, the authors were not able to provide us with sensitivity, specificity, or predictive values. They did, however, attempt to assess patterns of enhancement (Fig 2) that were variable. Sometimes I think we have a tendency to complicate issues. Until larger studies or meta-analyses are performed, the key fact to remember is that thoracolumbar nerve root enhancement is an early feature of Guillain-Barré syndrome in at least 90% of affected children.

A. C. Offiah, BSc, MBBS, MRCP, FRCR, PhD

Imaging—Genetics Applications in Child Psychiatry
Pine DS, Ernst M, Leibenluft E (Natl Inst of Mental Health Intramural Res Program, Bethesda, MD)
J Am Acad Child Adolesc Psychiatry 49:772-782, 2010

Objective.—To place imaging—genetics research in the context of child psychiatry.

Method.—A conceptual overview is provided, followed by discussion of specific research examples.

Results.—Imaging—genetics research is described linking brain function to two specific genes, for the serotonin-reuptake-transporter protein and a monoamine oxidase enzyme. Work is then described on phenotype selection in imaging genetics.

Conclusions.—Child psychiatry applications of imaging genetics are only beginning to emerge. The approach holds promise for advancing understandings of pathophysiology and therapeutics (Fig 2).

▶ Many of us will be aware of phenotype-genotype correlation studies, whether it is mutations in a single gene causing several distinct phenotypes, mutations in the diastrophic dysplasia sulfate transporter gene causing diastrophic dysplasia, atelosteogenesis type II[1] and autosomal recessive multiple epiphyseal dysplasia, or mutations in different genes leading to characteristic imaging findings of specific disorders such as different patterns of muscle involvement on MR in the rigid spine muscular dystrophies.[2]

However, if like me you have come across but not properly understood what is meant by imaging genetics, particularly in the context of child psychiatry, then you could do worse than reading through this review article, which not only highlights the potential but also emphasizes the limitations of this exciting cohesion of genetic and imaging technologies.

The authors review some interesting ideas. For instance, individual differences related to genes and to diagnosis may shape amygdala response to threats in youth (Fig 2). The technique holds promise for the development of novel treatments for child psychiatric disorders in the not-too-distant future.

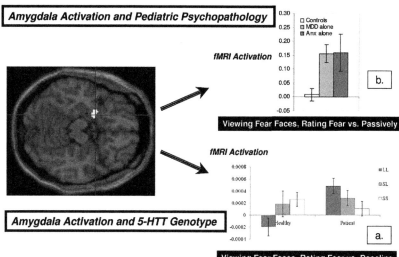

FIGURE 2.—5-HTT imaging–genetics in adolescents. Note: Illustrated are findings from two studies on relations among amygdala function, 5-HTT genotype, and developmental psychopathology. Amygdala topography is displayed on the lefthand side, in an axial slice. (a) Data from an imaging–genetics study in adolescents.[30] Levels of amygdala activation are shown for six groups, comprising three groups of healthy adolescents on the left-hand side and three groups of patients with anxiety disorders or major depressive disorder (MDD) on the right-hand side. Each of these three groups is formed based on the level of 5-HTT function (low [S, S], medium [S, L], high [L, L]) associated with the three genotypes, with L_G and S carriers being classified together. These data are for a functional magnetic resonance imaging (fMRI) contrast of fear-face–viewing events, viewed while fear levels are rated compared with a low-level, null-event baseline. Amygdala activity in healthy subjects is highest for the SS/SL$_G$ low-activity-allele group, whereas amygdala activity in patients is highest for the high-activity L$_A$/L$_A$ allele group. (b) Data from an imaging study focused on adolescent psychopathology,[29] which includes the subjects shown in panel a. Levels of amygdala activation are shown in healthy adolescents, nonanxious adolescents with MDD, and euthymic adolescents with anxiety for a contrast of fear-face–viewing events, viewed while fear levels are rated compared with events where these same faces are passively viewed. Anx = anxiety. (Reprinted from Pine DS, Ernst M, Leibenluft E. Imaging–genetics applications in child psychiatry. *J Am Acad Child Adolesc Psychiatry*. 2010;49:772-782, with permission from American Academy of Child and Adolescent Psychiatry.)

However, the authors caution that researchers are much further away when it comes to changing how disorders are diagnosed or classified.

The concepts within the article are not necessarily easy to grasp, but I do think it's worth reading, particularly for those who have an interest in functional MRI.

A. C. Offiah, BSc, MBBS, MRCP, FRCR, PhD

References

1. Dwyer E, Hyland J, Modaff P, Pauli RM. Genotype-phenotype correlation in DTDST dysplasias: Atelosteogenesis type II and diastrophic dysplasia variant in one family. *Am J Med Genet A*. 2010;152A:3043-3050.
2. Mercuri E, Clements E, Offiah A, et al. Muscle magnetic resonance imaging involvement in muscular dystrophies with rigidity of the spine. *Ann Neurol*. 2010;67:201-208.

Thoracic/Airway

Hand-Carried Ultrasound Devices in Pediatric Cardiology: Clinical Experience with Three Different Devices in 110 Patients

Dalla Pozza R, Loeff M, Kozlik-Feldmann R, et al (Ludwig-Maximilians-Univ, Munich, Germany)
J Am Soc Echocardiogr 23:1231-1237, 2010

Background.—The aims of this study were to determine the usefulness of hand-carried ultrasound devices in pediatric cardiology and to compare the performance of three different hand-carried ultrasound devices in a pediatric cardiology outpatient clinic and intensive care unit.

Methods.—One hundred ten patients (49 male; mean age, 6.4 ± 5.2 years; range 0.1−38 years) with congenital heart defects or innocent heart murmurs were examined using Siemens Acuson P10, Siemens Acuson P50, and Philips CX 50 systems. The quality of images and the accuracy of B-mode measurements were compared with those obtained using a standard echocardiographic system (Philips iE33).

Results.—Fifty-nine patients were examined with the Siemens Acuson P10, 29 with the Siemens Acuson P50, and 22 with the Philips CX 50 system. There were no significant differences in B-mode measurements. The Acuson P10 system, however, showed significantly lower image quality, with 64.54% of all studies considered of excellent quality compared with 92.83% with the Acuson P50 and 95.52% with the CX 50 ($P < .05$) and a mean quality score (1 = fair, 5 = excellent) of 3.5 versus 4.57 with the Acuson P50 and 4.86 with the CX 50 ($P < .05$). This was attributed to the limited capacity for accurate diagnosis in children with body weights <10 kg and complex heart defects.

Conclusion.—Hand-carried ultrasound devices represent a valuable alternative to standard echocardiographic systems in pediatric cardiology. In particular, systems including all echocardiographic modalities offer unlimited versatility in outpatient and intensive care (Figs 1-4).

▶ Anyone who has had to maneuver ultrasound machines such as the Phillips iE33 from imaging department to neonatal unit (for example) and back will share my frustration that this is not infrequently the most difficult part of the entire examination, unless of course he or she is trying to position the machine satisfactorily enough to perform the scan once the patient's bedside has been reached. Either way, reports such as this in which handheld devices have been tested and found to be useful alternatives are most welcome.

Such devices are in more widespread use in the adult population and are not limited to cardiac imaging. I suspect that they will become increasingly popular for imaging of children, and therefore, this article is particularly helpful, comparing as it does 3 handheld models, with the Philips iE33 serving as gold standard. It is a pity that each child was only scanned with one of the handheld devices (cooperation was obviously an issue, but scans could have

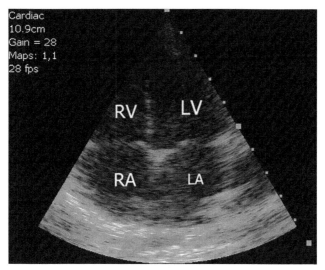

FIGURE 1.—Four-chamber view of a child using the Siemens Acuson P10 system. *LA*, Left atrium; *LV*, left ventricle; *RA*, right atrium; *RV*, right ventricle. (Reprinted from the Journal of the American Society of Echocardiography, Dalla Pozza R, Loeff M, Kozlik-Feldmann R, et al. Hand-carried ultrasound devices in pediatric cardiology: clinical experience with three different devices in 110 patients. *J Am Soc Echocardiogr.* 2010;23:1231-1237, copyright © 2010 with permission from the American Society of Echocardiography.)

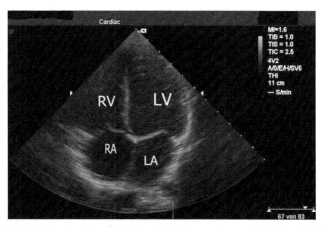

FIGURE 2.—Four-chamber view of a child using the Siemens Acuson P50 system. *LA*, Left atrium; *LV*, left ventricle; *RA*, right atrium; *RV*, right ventricle. (Reprinted from the Journal of the American Society of Echocardiography, Dalla Pozza R, Loeff M, Kozlik-Feldmann R, et al. Hand-carried ultrasound devices in pediatric cardiology: clinical experience with three different devices in 110 patients. *J Am Soc Echocardiogr.* 2010;23:1231-1237, copyright © 2010 with permission from the American Society of Echocardiography.)

been performed on different days particularly in the older age group). Nevertheless, the variation in image quality between the machines is readily apparent (Figs 1-4).

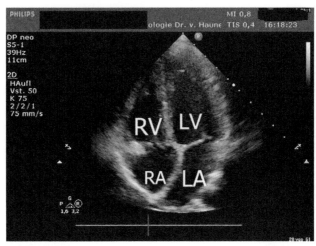

FIGURE 3.—Four-chamber view of a child using the Philips CX 50 system. *LA*, Left atrium; *LV*, left ventricle; *RA*, right atrium; *RV*, right ventricle. (Reprinted from the Journal of the American Society of Echocardiography, Dalla Pozza R, Loeff M, Kozlik-Feldmann R, et al. Hand-carried ultrasound devices in pediatric cardiology: clinical experience with three different devices in 110 patients. *J Am Soc Echocardiogr.* 2010;23:1231-1237, copyright © 2010 with permission from the American Society of Echocardiography.)

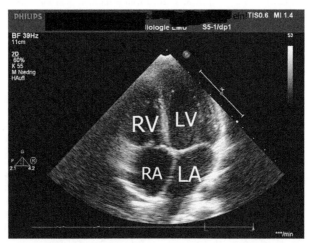

FIGURE 4.—Four-chamber view of a child using the Philips iE33 system. *LA*, Left atrium; *LV*, left ventricle; *RA*, right atrium; *RV*, right ventricle. (Reprinted from the Journal of the American Society of Echocardiography, Dalla Pozza R, Loeff M, Kozlik-Feldmann R, et al. Hand-carried ultrasound devices in pediatric cardiology: clinical experience with three different devices in 110 patients. *J Am Soc Echocardiogr.* 2010;23:1231-1237, copyright © 2010 with permission from the American Society of Echocardiography.)

Be wary if selecting one of the tested machines for your hospital. Given the rapid pace of technological advancement, newer improved handheld ultrasound devices were in existence by the time this article had been published. At end of their article, the authors indicate this by stating, "The capabilities of portable echocardiographic devices, and their performance, is a 'moving target.'"

Moving target? In an article about cumbersome machines, handheld portable devices, and cardiac imaging—in children?!

If the authors wanted to raise an ironic smile, they certainly got one out of me!

A. C. Offiah, BSc, MBBS, MRCP, FRCR, PhD

An unusual mature thyroid teratoma on CT and [99]Tcm scintigraphy imaging in a child

Zhang Y-Z, Li W-H, Zhu M-J, et al (Shanghai Jiaotong Univ School of Medicine, China)

Pediatr Radiol 40:1831-1833, 2010

We report the imaging findings of a mature thyroid teratoma in a 5-year-old girl. Nuclear imaging showed a decrease in [99]Tcm uptake in the right lobe of the thyroid gland. CT scan showed a slightly lobulated soft-tissue mass without calcification, fat or cystic components. Histological analysis showed that the tumor was composed of mature neural tissue, cartilaginous, and epithelial elements. This case study provides new insights into the CT appearance of mature thyroid teratomas (Fig 3).

▶ How rare can it get? The 5-year-old girl in this case report presented with atypical radiological features of a relatively uncommon pediatric tumor occurring at an unusual site.

The incidence of teratoma is 1 per 20 000 to 40 000 people; the most common sites are the gonads, while the neck and abdominal viscera are the least common. Even when they do occur in the neck (7%-9% of all teratomas[1]), location within the thyroid gland is rare. Teratomas originate from stem cells, and because they consist of elements derived from all 3 germ cell layers, the typical radiological features include calcification/ossification (including teeth), hair, cystic elements,

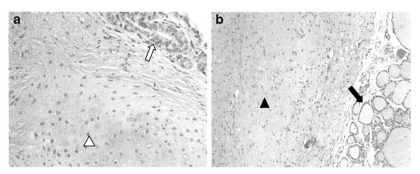

FIGURE 3.—High-power photomicrograph (hematoxylin-eosin, 200×). **a** The tumor components of mature epithelial elements (*white arrow*) and cartilaginous tissue (*white triangle*) can be seen. **b** Image shows neural tissue (brain) (*black triangle*) and thyroid tissue (at the periphery, *black arrow*). (With kind permission from Springer Science and Business Media: Zhang Y-Z, Li W-H, Zhu M-J, et al. An unusual mature thyroid teratoma on CT and [99]Tcm scintigraphy imaging in a child. *Pediatr Radiol.* 2010;40:1831-1833, with permission from Springer-Verlag.)

and fat. Thyroid masses in children are most commonly benign adenomas or carcinoma (medullary, follicular, or papillary).

The radionuclide scan and ultrasound performed in this child should have been sufficient imaging investigations, usually followed by fine needle aspiration biopsy and/or surgical resection. It is unclear why a CT scan was performed; ultrasound had already confirmed a hypoechoic solid mass and should have excluded calcific and fatty components. The limited role of CT (and MR) in the face of a thyroid nodule/mass is well illustrated by this report. Note that features suggestive of malignancy are detectable by ultrasound.[2]

Although radiological investigations were nonspecific, histopathology clinched the diagnosis by demonstrating the presence of mature epithelial elements, cartilage, and neural tissue within the mass (Fig 3).

For an overview of neck tumors in children (and adults), readers are directed to the article by Imhof et al,[1] while Babcock[2] provides a useful review of thyroid disease in the pediatric patient.

A. C. Offiah, BSc, MBBS, MRCP, FRCR, PhD

References

1. Imhof H, Czerny C, Hörmann M, Krestan C. Tumors and tumor-like lesions of the neck: from childhood to adult. *Eur Radiol.* 2004;14:L155-L165.
2. Babcock DS. Thyroid disease in the pediatric patient: emphasizing imaging with sonography. *Pediatr Radiol.* 2006;36:299-308.

Comparison of Haller index values calculated with chest radiographs versus CT for pectus excavatum evaluation
Khanna G, Jaju A, Don S, et al (Washington Univ School of Medicine, St Louis, MO; et al)
Pediatr Radiol 40:1763-1767, 2010

Background.—Pectus excavatum is a common chest wall anomaly in children. Pre-operative imaging for pectus excavatum is performed with CT, which is used to calculate the Haller index to determine the severity of pectus excavatum.

Objective.—To determine the correlation between Haller index values calculated with two-view chest radiographs and those calculated with CT and to determine, with CT as the reference standard, the diagnostic performance of radiographic Haller index for identifying cases that meet imaging criteria for surgical correction of pectus excavatum.

Materials and Methods.—For the period 2001–2009, our radiology information system was searched to identify all children who had undergone CT for Haller index calculation. Children who had also undergone two-view chest radiography (CXR) within 6 months of the CT were included in this retrospective study. Two radiologists independently calculated CT Haller index and radiographic Haller index. Data distributions were tested for normality with the Shapiro-Wilk W test. The associations between CT Haller index and radiographic Haller index were determined with the Spearman coefficient of rank correlation. Differences between CT Haller index and radiographic Haller index were tested with the Wilcoxon signed rank test. Haller index values were dichotomized into positive (>3.2) and negative (≤3.2) cases. Using CT as the reference standard, the sensitivity, specificity, and accuracy of radiographic Haller index in identifying children who meet imaging criteria for surgery were calculated.

Results.—CT and CXR for evaluation of pectus excavatum were available for 32 children (25 male; median age 14.5 years). With CT, the median Haller indices for observers 1 and 2 were 3.4 and 3.5 and with CXR 3.5 and 3.5. There were statistically significant correlations between the radiographic Haller index and CT Haller index estimated by the two observers [Spearman correlation coefficient (95% confidence interval) for observer 1=0.71 (0.48—0.85, *P*<0.01) and for observer 2=0.77 (0.52—0.88, *P*<0.01)]. A statistically significant correlation was found between the radiographic Haller index calculated by the two observers [Spearman correlation coefficient=0.98 (0.95—0.99, *P*<0.01)]. Using CT Haller index as the reference standard, radiographic Haller index had a sensitivity of 0.95 (0.75—0.99), specificity of 0.75 (0.43—0.94), and accuracy of 0.88 (0.72—0.95) for observer 1, and a sensitivity of 0.95 (0.75—0.99), specificity of 0.67 (0.35—0.90), and accuracy of 0.84 (0.68—0.93) for observer 2.

Conclusion.—Radiographic Haller index correlates strongly with CT Haller index, has good interobserver correlation, and has a high diagnostic accuracy for pre-operative evaluation of pectus excavatum. We suggest that a CT of the chest is not required for pre-operative evaluation of pectus excavatum, and a two-view chest radiograph is sufficient for preoperative imaging of pectus excavatum.

▶ In 2009, I provided a short commentary on an article by Mueller et al[1] in which they investigated the use of chest radiography as the primary modality for the investigation of pectus excavatum. The results were impressive, but the study was small (only 12 patients), and I recommended that the study be repeated. Well, now it has been, though I claim no credit!

Khanna et al enrolled 32 patients and came to the same conclusion as Mueller et al: the 2-view chest radiograph is sufficient for preoperative assessment of pectus excavatum. Diagnostic accuracy and interobserver reliability were high. In addition, the authors presented radiation dose calculations for a 15-year-old teenager weighing between 46 kg and 54 kg. Depending on technical factors, the effective dose for CT ranged from 1.1 mSv to 4.1 mSv, compared to only 0.0198 mSv for both anteroposterior and lateral chest radiographs.

Quod erat demonstrandum.

Some questions remain unanswered; there is more work to be done. In the words of the authors, "... there have been no prospective studies to validate the use of Haller index in differentiating patients with pectus excavatum who have a deformity severe enough to require surgery from those who do not need surgical intervention. It remains unclear whether this objective index for assessing pectus correlates with the patient's subjective symptoms. In addition,

there are no data on whether breath-holding or phase of respiration can result in a significant difference in estimation of Haller index."
Quidquid Latine dictum sit altum videtur!

A. C. Offiah, BSc, MBBS, MRCP, FRCR, PhD

Reference

1. Mueller C, Saint-Vil D, Bouchard S. Chest x-ray as a primary modality for preoperative imaging of pectus excavatum. *J Pediatr Surg.* 2008;43:71-73.

Vitamin A Deficiency in an Infant With PAGOD Syndrome

Gavrilova R, Babovic N, Lteif A, et al (Mayo Clinic, Rochester, MN)
Am J Med Genet A 149A:2241-2247, 2009

PAGOD syndrome is a rare condition characterized by multiple congenital anomalies including pulmonary artery and lung hypoplasia, agonadism, diaphragmatic abnormalities, cardiac defects, omphalocele, and various genital anomalies. The etiology of this condition is unknown but the spectrum of birth defects is similar to the developmental anomalies observed in vitamin A deficiency animal models. We describe an infant with PAGOD syndrome phenotype. The patient had a normal male karyotype and no copy number changes were seen on chromosome genomic hybridization (CGH) microarray. Endocrine evaluation was consistent with primary hypogonadism. The testes and Müllerian structures were absent by imaging studies, raising the possibility of arrest of early gonadogenesis. The plasma free vitamin A was low, consistent with moderate to severe vitamin A deficiency; the maternal plasma vitamin A level was normal. During pregnancy maternal vitamin A is taken up by retinol binding protein 4 (RBP4) which is expressed in the embryonic visceral endoderm from pregastrulational stages. This transport is mediated via the specific membrane receptor for RBP, stimulated by retinoic acid 6 (STRA6). STRA6 is widely expressed inhuman organ systems including the placenta during embryonic development. Mutations in the *STRA6* gene result in Matthew–Wood syndrome, which demonstrates significant phenotypic overlap with PAGOD syndrome. Sequencing of *STRA6* coding regions in our patient, revealed no mutations. We present a case of PAGOD syndrome with a review of the literature, posing the hypothesis that a vitamin A metabolic defect, other than transport mediated by STRA6 receptor, might have an etiological role in the development of this multiple congenital anomalies syndrome (Table 1).

▶ SPONASTRIME, RAPADILINO, CAMFAK, PAGOD...
The acronym aside, in these days when fewer and fewer are being accepted for publication, I have selected this single case report demonstrating as it does how animal models of disease help us to better understand their human counterparts. Although it has previously been recognized that offspring born to

TABLE 1.—Characteristic Clinical Features in Common Between PAGOD Syndrome, Fetal Vitamin A Deficiency (VAD) Syndrome, and Matthew—Wood Syndrome (RBP-Receptor Gene STRA6 Mutations)

Clinical Characteristics	PAGOD Syndrome	Fetal VAD Syndrome	Matthew—Wood Syndrome
Anophthalmia		+	+
Diaphragmatic eventration	+	+	+
Great vessels			
Aortic hypoplasia	+	+	+
PA hypoplasia/atresia	+	+	+
Heart			
ASD	+	+	+
Left ventricular hypoplasia	+	+	+
VSD	+	+	+
Hypo/agonadism	+	+	
Lung hypoplasia/agenesis	+	+	+
Maldevelopment/retention of Wolffian and Mullerian duct structures	+	+	
Poor survival (death <2 years of age)	+	+	+

ASD, atrial septal defect; PA, pulmonary artery; VSD, ventral septal defect.

animals with vitamin A deficiency have similar findings to humans with pulmonary and pulmonary artery hypoplasia, agonadism, omphalocele, diaphragmatic defect, and dextrocardia (PAGOD) syndrome, this is in fact the first time that vitamin A deficiency has been demonstrated in a case of PAGOD syndrome.

Table 1 provides a useful comparison of overlapping conditions. An interesting aspect of this syndrome is the unilateral pulmonary hypoplasia with which it is associated. It appears that vitamin A is important for lung morphogenesis and differentiation of lung epithelium. The authors explain the heterogeneity of findings (eg, their patient had no eye problems) by postulating that severity is related to the gestational age at which vitamin A deficiency occurs. Does vitamin A play a role in isolated cases of pulmonary hypoplasia?

Although it is rare (11 reported cases including the current), we cannot make diagnoses of conditions that we are unaware of. Dextrocardia, hypogonadism, and eye problems may occur in other disorders, in particular the fairly diverse group of disorders known as the ciliopathies (eg, Kartagener, Bardet-Biedl, short rib—polydactyly syndromes) spring to mind. Together, however, the constellation of findings that constitute PAGOD syndrome is relatively unusual. Until I read this article, I had not come across the syndrome. Now I wonder whether vitamin A levels should be checked in any newborn presenting with at least 2 of the described features. I feel the answer should be, "yes."

ICOCBW (I could of course be wrong)!

A. C. Offiah, BSc, MBBS, MRCP, FRCR, PhD

Development of Low-Dose Protocols for Thin-Section CT Assessment of Cystic Fibrosis in Pediatric Patients

O'Connor OJ, Vandeleur M, McGarrigle AM, et al (Univ College Cork and Cork Univ Hosp, Wilton, Ireland)
Radiology 257:820-829, 2010

Purpose.—To develop low-dose thin-section computed tomographic (CT) protocols for assessment of cystic fibrosis (CF) in pediatric patients and determine the clinical usefulness thereof compared with chest radiography.

Materials and Methods.—After institutional review board approval and informed consent from patients or guardians were obtained, 14 patients with CF and 11 patients without CF (16 male, nine female; mean age, 12.6 years ± 5.4 [standard deviation]; range, 3.5−25 years) who underwent imaging for clinical reasons underwent low-dose thin-section CT. Sections 1 mm thick (protocol A) were used in 10 patients, and sections 0.5 mm thick (protocol B) were used in 15 patients at six levels at 120 kVp and 30−50 mA. Image quality and diagnostic acceptability were scored qualitatively and quantitatively by two radiologists who also quantified disease severity at thin-section CT and chest radiography. Effective doses were calculated by using a CT dosimetry calculator.

Results.—Low-dose thin-section CT was performed with mean effective doses of 0.19 mSv ± 0.03 for protocol A and 0.14 mSv ± 0.04 for protocol B (*P* < .005). Diagnostic acceptability and depiction of bronchovascular structures at lung window settings were graded as almost excellent for both protocols, but protocol B was inferior to protocol A for mediastinal assessment (*P* < .02). Patients with CF had moderate lung disease with a mean Bhalla score of 9.2 ± 5.3 (range, 0−19), compared with that of patients without CF (1.1 ± 1.4; *P* < .001). There was excellent correlation between thin-section CT and chest radiography (*r* = 0.88−0.92; *P* < .001).

Conclusion.—Low-dose thin-section CT can be performed at lower effective doses than can standard CT, approaching those of chest radiography. Low-dose thin-section CT could be appropriate for evaluating bronchiectasis in pediatric patients, yielding appropriate information about lung parenchyma and bronchovascular structures.

▶ All radiologists are aware of the trade off between radiation dose and image quality; however, we may choose to define the latter!

The subjectivity associated with determining the quality of an image was well expressed by Barnhard,[1] "...image quality is in the eye of the beholder..." However, the key requirement of medical imaging is that a (correct) diagnosis should be reached, hence Rossman's[2] definition of image quality as, "...that attribute of the image which affects the certainty with which diagnostically useful detail can be detected visually by the radiologist..." Along the same vein, Martin et al[3] state that the purpose of diagnostic radiology is to, "Obtain images which are adequate for the clinical purpose with the minimum radiation dose to the patient."

This principle is well demonstrated in the article by O'Connor et al. The authors have shown that although it scored lower for image quality, a 26% reduction in effective radiation dose had no adverse effect on diagnosis of bronchiectasis in children with cystic fibrosis. Given the number of children who will have serial chest CT throughout their lives (and the authors state that there is now 80% probability of affected patients surviving up to 40 years), this is a significant individual and population radiation dose saving—which all imaging departments are instantly able to implement.

With increased awareness of the complications of radiation, there have been a vast array of similar articles, related to many specialties and all imaging modalities that use ionizing radiation. Awareness of the ALARA principle and the more recent Image Gently campaign will ensure that such studies continue, for we are all now beginning to understand, to paraphrase Rossman's[2] 1969 statement that, "A medical image is of the highest quality if it does not adversely affect the diagnosis."

A. C. Offiah, BSc, MBBS, MRCP, FRCR, PhD

References

1. Barnhard HJ. Image quality standards. *Radiology.* 1982;143:275-276.
2. Rossman K. Image quality. *Radiol Clin N Am.* 1969;7:418-433.
3. Martin CJ, Sharp PF, Sutton DG. Measurement of image quality in diagnostic radiology. *Appl Radiat Isot.* 1999;50:21-38.

Other

Developing participatory research in radiology: the use of a graffiti wall, cameras and a video box in a Scottish radiology department

Mathers SA, Anderson H, McDonald S, et al (Aberdeen Royal Infirmary, UK; Royal Aberdeen Children's Hosp, UK; et al)
Pediatr Radiol 40:309-317, 2010

Background.—Participatory research is increasingly advocated for use in health and health services research and has been defined as a 'process of producing new knowledge by systematic enquiry, with the collaboration of those being studied'. The underlying philosophy of participatory research is that those recruited to studies are acknowledged as experts who are 'empowered to truly participate and have their voices heard'. Research methods should enable children to express themselves. This has led to the development of creative approaches of working with children that offer alternatives to, for instance, the structured questioning of children by researchers either through questionnaires or interviews.

Objective.—To examine the feasibility and potential of developing participatory methods in imaging research.

Materials and Methods.—We employed three innovative methods of data collection sequentially, namely the provision of: 1) a graffiti wall;

2) cameras, and 3) a video box for children's use. While the graffiti wall was open to all who attended the department, for the other two methods children were allocated to each 'arm' consecutively until our target of 20 children for each was met.

Results.—The study demonstrated that it was feasible to use all three methods of data collection within the context of a busy radiology department. We encountered no complaints from staff, patients or parents. Children were willing to participate but we did not collect data to establish if they enjoyed the activities, were pleased to have the opportunity to make comments or whether anxieties about their treatment inhibited their participation. The data yield was disappointing. In particular, children's contributions to the graffiti wall were limited, but did reflect the nature of graffiti, and there may have been some 'copycat' comments. Although data analysis was relatively straightforward, given the nature of the data (short comments and simple drawings), the process proved to be extremely time-consuming. This was despite the modest amount of data collected.

Conclusions.—Novel methods of engaging with children have been shown to be feasible although further work is needed to establish their full potential (Figs 2 and 3).

▶ I do not know about other countries, but certainly in the United Kingdom, there is increasing emphasis by the government and funding bodies to involve

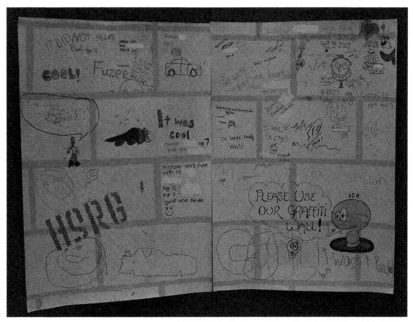

FIGURE 2.—Completed graffiti wall. (With kind permission from Springer Science and Business Media: Mathers SA, Anderson H, McDonald S, et al. Developing participatory research in radiology: the use of a graffiti wall, cameras and a video box in a Scottish radiology department. *Pediatr Radiol.* 2010;40:309-317, with permission from Springer-Verlag.)

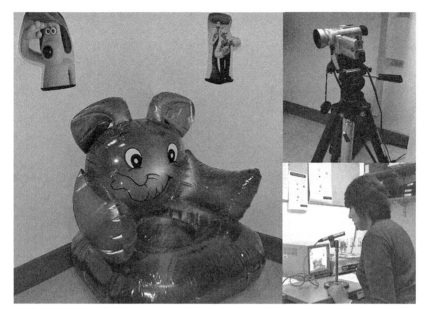

FIGURE 3.—Pictures showing configuration of the video box. (With kind permission from Springer Science and Business Media: Mathers SA, Anderson H, McDonald S, et al. Developing participatory research in radiology: the use of a graffiti wall, cameras and a video box in a Scottish radiology department. *Pediatr Radiol.* 2010;40:309-317, with permission from Springer-Verlag.)

patients in research, not simply as subjects on whom a hypothesis or novel investigation is to be tested but as intelligent individuals with their own expectations and ideas about research and how it might be conducted, that is, participatory research or patient and public involvement (PPI).

In a recent grant application, in which I recruited 2 adult lay members to the advisory committee, the review panel recommended that I also include 1 member under the age of 16 years, as this represented the age group I would be recruiting from. In the event, I included 2 (additional) lay members both younger than 16 years to the satisfaction of the panel.

In the United Kingdom, support for participatory research/PPI is available from the various Research Design Services. Useful publications and advice can also be obtained by contacting INVOLVE (a national advisory group sponsored by the National Institute for Health Research) or by visiting their Web site (http://www.invo.org.uk/).

Despite the increasing emphasis on participatory research and PPI, methods of including children in radiologic research have thus far only been scantily investigated. In this article, 3 novel methods are researched: cameras, to allow children to take photographs and record their experiences within the radiology department; a video box akin to that used in the popular television show Big Brother (Fig 3); and my own personal favorite, a graffiti wall (Fig 2).

Despite their efforts, the authors were disappointed by the relatively poor response rate. They discuss reasons why this might have been and possible methods of increasing response to future studies, including patient involvement at the design stage.

Whether we like it or not, as might be found on a graffiti wall, "PPI is here to stay. OK." For this reason, I have categorized this article as a 3-star article, that is, within the top 10% of importance for all articles in 2010. We all need to take steps to incorporate participatory research into our own studies, and ideas from this article make a good starting point.

A. C. Offiah, BSc, MBBS, MRCP, FRCR, PhD

Musculoskeletal

Clinical impact of gadolinium in the MRI diagnosis of musculoskeletal infection in children

Kan JH, Young RS, Yu C, et al (Vanderbilt Univ, Nashville, TN)
Pediatr Radiol 40:1197-1205, 2010

Background.—The incremental value of gadolinium in the diagnosis of musculoskeletal infection by MRI is controversial.

Objective.—To compare diagnostic utility of noncontrast with contrast MRI in the evaluation of pediatric musculoskeletal infections.

Materials and Methods.—We reviewed 90 gadolinium-enhanced MRIs in children with suspected musculoskeletal infection. Noncontrast and contrast MRI scans were evaluated to determine sensitivity and specificity in the diagnosis of musculoskeletal infection and identification of abscesses.

Results.—Pre- and post-contrast diagnosis of osteomyelitis sensitivity was 89% and 91% ($P=1.00$) and specificity was 96% and 96% ($P=1.00$), respectively; septic arthritis sensitivity was 50% and 67% ($P=1.00$) and specificity was 98% and 98% ($P=1.00$), respectively; cellulitis/myositis sensitivity was 100% and 100% ($P=1.00$) and specificity was 84% and 88% ($P=0.59$), respectively; abscess for the total group was 22 (24.4%) and 42 (46.6%), respectively ($P<0.0001$). Abscesses identified only on contrast sequences led to intervention in eight additional children. No child with a final diagnosis of infection had a normal pre-contrast study.

Conclusion.—Intravenous gadolinium should not be routinely administered in the imaging work-up of nonspinal musculoskeletal infections, particularly when pre-contrast images are normal. However, gadolinium contrast significantly increases the detection of abscesses, particularly small ones that might not require surgical intervention.

▶ The authors of this article question the need for routine administration of gadolinium in children with suspected musculoskeletal infection. They cite American College of Radiology guidelines and "recent review articles" as continuing to support the use of intravenous gadolinium, despite the lack of research on its effect on diagnostic accuracy.

I have put "recent review articles" in quotation marks because first, one of the articles[1] was published in 1995 (hardly recent and MR image quality has since markedly improved), and second, the authors cite a review article by a certain

Dr A. C. Offiah. In this article,[2] I merely point out the advantages of intravenous gadolinium and do not illustrate its use in any patient with normal precontrast MR or other imaging.

But these are minor quibbles that should not detract from the need for and quality of this study, the results of which indicate that in the context of suspected musculoskeletal infection in children, intravenous gadolinium is not required if the precontrast scan is normal.

Charles Kettering held the view that, "If you have always done it that way, it is probably wrong."

Many imaging departments will have a standard protocol for MR scans for suspected musculoskeletal infection in a child, which will include the administration of contrast. This bypasses the need for an experienced radiologist to check precontrast scans in a busy department. Scans may be performed because of previously identified radiographic or ultrasound abnormality, thus pre-empting the abnormal precontrast MR. Another quibble, I know, but the authors do not tell us how many of their patients had previously normal findings and how many had some abnormality on imaging (radiography, ultrasound, even CT) performed before the MR. Finally, performing MR in children may require either sedation or general anesthetic. Particularly in the latter situation, all involved are reluctant to have to bring the child back to administer previously omitted contrast.

The routine use of gadolinium covers all eventualities (except of course complications related to the gadolinium itself, which are rare). Scans will have been performed with routine contrast for as long as staff in some departments can remember. This does not of course make it right, but to paraphrase Mr Kettering, I would say, "If you have always done it that way, it is probably convenient."

While it will almost certainly change what authors say in their review articles, I hope that in addition, the results of this article are compelling enough to cause departments to reconsider and possibly change their current practice.

A. C. Offiah, BSc, MBBS, MRCP, FRCR, PhD

References

1. Jaramillo D, Treves ST, Kasser JR, Harper M, Sundel R, Laor T. Osteomyelitis and septic arthritis in children: appropriate use of imaging to guide treatment. *AJR Am J Roentgenol*. 1995;165:399-403.
2. Offiah AC. Acute osteomyelitis, septic arthritis and discitis: differences between neonates and older children. *Eur J Radiol*. 2006;60:221-232.

Breast fibroadenomas in the pediatric population: common and uncommon sonographic findings

Sanchez R, Ladino-Torres MF, Bernat JA, et al (Univ of Michigan Health System, Ann Arbor)

Pediatr Radiol 40:1681-1689, 2010

Background.—Sonography is usually requested to evaluate palpable pediatric breast lumps, and solid masses are almost always fibroadenomas.

Lack of familiarity with the findings of fibroadenomas can lead to diagnostic uncertainty and sometimes unnecessary biopsy and excision. We sought to review the spectrum of sonographic findings in our cases of pathology proven pediatric fibroadenomas.

Objective.—The purpose of this retrospective study was to describe the sonographic appearances of pathologically proven pediatric breast fibroadenomas.

Materials and methods.—A query of the Department of Radiology database at our institution was performed for all patients younger than 19 years who underwent breast US from January 2001 to June 2009. A total of 332 patients were identified: 282 girls (85%) and 50 boys (15%). Ninety-one girls and no boys had a solid breast mass based on US findings. Forty-three children had a total of 49 pathologically proven breast masses with the diagnoses of fibroadenoma (44), hamartoma (1), non-Hodgkin lymphoma (1), tubular adenoma (1), pseudoangiomatous stromal hyperplasia (1) and lactation changes (1). Reviews of medical records, histological results and sonographic examinations of all pathology-proven fibroadenomas were performed. US findings were characterized according to location, multiplicity, size, shape, echogenicity and homogeneity, definition of margins, posterior acoustic features and Doppler vascularity.

Results.—The vast majority of solid breast masses in girls are histologically benign. Fibroadenomas accounted for 91% of the pathologically proven solid breast masses. Common findings on US imaging are an oval shape, hypoechoic echo pattern, posterior acoustic enhancement and internal Doppler signal. Lobulations were found in 57% of the masses. Less common findings are absent internal vascular flow and complex echo pattern, while isoechoic echo pattern, posterior shadowing and angular margins are rare or unusual.

Conclusion.—Fibroadenomas represent the most common solid mass in the breasts of girls. Sonographic appearances are usually characteristic and do not significantly differ from those found in adults. The radiologist must be aware of common and uncommon sonographic appearances of fibroadenomas in the pediatric age group and should be cautious when recommending histological confirmation based on imaging findings, as breast malignancy is extremely rare.

▶ Compared with adults, the greater relative amount of fibroglandular breast tissue in girls means that mammography is a less suitable method of investigating breast masses. There is also, of course, the issue of unwanted exposure to ionizing radiation; therefore, in children, ultrasound is the imaging modality of choice for investigating breast lesions.

The vast majority of breast lesions in children are benign, and in this article, the authors seek to reduce the number of unnecessary surgical procedures (biopsies and excisions may cause disfigurement) that are performed by characterizing the ultrasound appearance of histologically confirmed fibroadenomas.

The authors performed a 9.5-year retrospective review, and although breast masses were seen as early as the neonatal period, the youngest child with proven fibroadenoma was just 11.8 years old. It is reassuring to note that in the majority of cases, the fibroadenomas had characteristic ultrasound features.

Interestingly, however, I selected this article for what it did *not* set out to demonstrate rather than for what it did. Of the 50 boys who underwent breast ultrasound in the authors' department over the study period, not one had a solid breast mass on ultrasonography. This was the group I was interested in.

Breast lesions in boys are rare but include gynecomastia, galactoceles, mastitis, intraductal papilloma, intramammary lymph nodes, hemangioma, and carcinoma. If like me you are also interested, then you might like to read the article by Chung et al for a comprehensive review of breast masses in children and adolescents.[1]

A. C. Offiah, BSc, MBBS, MRCP, FRCR, PhD

Reference

1. Chung EM, Cube R, Hall GJ, González C, Stocker JT, Glassman LM. From the archives of the AFIP: breast masses in children and adolescents: radiologic-pathologic correlation. *Radiographics*. 2009;29:907-931.

The Impact of Laser Doppler Imaging on Time to Grafting Decisions in Pediatric Burns
Kim LHC, Ward D, Lam L, et al (Children's Hosp Burns Res Inst, New South Wales, Australia; The Univ of Sydney, New South Wales, Australia)
J Burn Care Res 31:328-332, 2010

Early definitive treatment of burns facilitates optimal results by reducing the risk of subsequent hypertrophic scarring. Laser Doppler imaging (LDI) has been shown to assist in predicting burn wound healing potential. This study sought to determine whether use of LDI in pediatric burn patients has led to earlier decision making for grafting. The study cohort were patients who underwent a skin grafting procedure for a burn wound at a single institution, a state referral center for all major pediatric burns, between June 2006 and December 2007. Patients were divided into two groups: those who underwent LDI scanning and those who were only assessed clinically. Time of burn injury to time of decision making for the grafting procedure was calculated in days. Forty-nine percent of 196 patients underwent LDI. The mean time from the date of injury to decision making for graft procedure was 8.9 days in those patients who had an LDI scan vs 11.6 days in the group assessed by clinical observation alone. This trend for earlier decision for grafting procedure in the LDI group was statistically significant ($P = .01$). There was no significant difference between those patients who were scanned and those only assessed clinically in relation to gender, age, mechanism of injury, percentage BSA burnt, and wound culture results. There was a significant reduction in time to grafting decision in the LDI group. This would potentially lead to reduced length of stay, reduced number of hospital visits, and stream-lined care for the patient and their family.

▶ An effective use of laser Doppler imaging (LDI) in clinical care of pediatric burn patients is described and evaluated. The judgment when to perform skin graft after major body burns has up to now relied on clinical judgment, especially of estimated burn depth, as to the best time for performing the graft to cover an area but at the same time avoiding the dreaded complication of hypertrophic scarring. LDI uses a relatively expensive machine to measure cutaneous blood flow, in perfusion units, assessed by the power spectrum frequency shift on reflected laser light. The analogy to ultrasound Doppler should be clear. The advantages shown in this study in terms of earlier decision making for operative intervention (averaged 3 days), and then earlier surgery as well as definitive care, seem to justify the cost of the technology in a busy burn center. Previous similar time-saving with LDI reported in adults[1] are reflected in the current population of children ranging up to 15 years in age. Good show, mates.

A. E. Oestreich, MD

Reference

1. Jeng JC, Bridgeman A, Shivnan L, et al. Laser Doppler imaging determines need for excision and grafting in advance of clinical judgment: a prospective blinded trial. *Burns.* 2003;29:665-670.

Clinical and Magnetic Resonance Imaging Findings Associated With Little League Elbow

Wei AS, Khana S, Limpisvasti O, et al (Rebound Orthopedics and Neurosurgery, Vancouver, WA; Radnet Inc, Los Angeles, CA; Kerlan Jobe Orthopedic Clinic, Los Angeles, CA; et al)
J Pediatr Orthop 30:715-719, 2010

Background.—Valgus overload in the skeletally immature elbow can lead to medial epicondyle apophysitis, or Little League elbow. The skeletal manifestations have been well described through radiographic studies. The involvement of surrounding structures, including the ulnar collateral ligament, remains unclear. The purpose of this study is to better characterize the involvement and relationship of medial elbow structures in Little League elbow through magnetic resonance (MR) imaging.

Methods.—Institutional review board approval was obtained. Nine Little Leaguers, 8 to 13 years, with clinical diagnosis of Little League elbow were enrolled. Play history questionnaire (including age, position, pitching history, duration of symptoms, and Kerlan Jobe Orthopedic Clinic shoulder elbow score), clinical examination, radiograph, and MRI of both elbows were obtained for analysis. Evaluation of radiographs and MRIs were performed by 2 radiologists blinded to clinical findings.

Results.—A majority of the players reported compliance with pitch count recommendations. Four out of 9 players, however, were throwing breaking pitches at an average age of 11 years. Radiographic abnormalities were present in 4 players. MRI abnormalities were present in 6 players. All patients demonstrated normal ulnar collateral ligament (UCL) on MRI. The distance from UCL origin to the medial epicondyle physis were measured in both injured and healthy elbows. No significant differences were found. This distance ranged from 0 to 4 mm.

Conclusions.—MRI of Little League elbow demonstrated more abnormalities compared with radiographs. The increased number of findings,

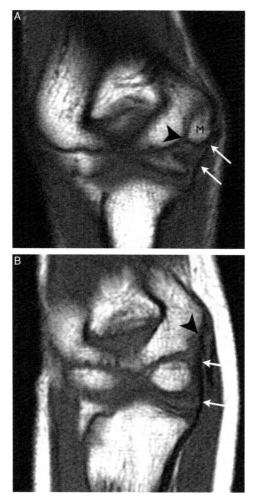

FIGURE 3.—A, Ulnar collateral ligament originating from medial epicondyle apophysis. The anterior band of the ulnar collateral ligament (arrows) originates medial to the physis (arrowhead) from the medial epicondyle (M). B, Ulnar collateral ligament originating from medial epicondyle physis. The anterior band of the ulnar collateral ligament (arrows) originates on the medial physis (arrowhead). The anterior edge of the medial epicondyle apophysis is partially visualized medial to the physis. (Reprinted from Wei AS, Khana S, Limpisvasti O, et al. Clinical and magnetic resonance imaging findings associated with little league elbow. *J Pediatr Orthop*. 2010;30:715-719, with permission from Lippincott Williams & Wilkins.)

however, does not change clinical management. MR evaluation of the ulnar collateral ligament demonstrates no role for reconstruction in Little League elbow. In addition, given the close proximity of the ligament to the physis, any surgical procedure involving the UCL origin should be performed with caution (Fig 3).

▶ In skeletally mature athletes, repetitive valgus extension forces associated with overhead throwing cause ulnar collateral ligament (UCL) and flexor-pronator injuries. By comparison, in the skeletally immature athlete, the same forces cause a medial condylar apophysitis with characteristic radiographic features. The suggested explanation for this is that medially, the weakest part of the skeletally immature elbow is the medial apophysis. Therefore, while UCL surgery for major league elbow syndrome leads to a good outcome,[1] its role in little league elbow syndrome is less certain. Despite this uncertainty, the authors of the current article mention anecdotal reports of UCL surgery for little league elbow.

Of course being anecdotes, we do not know the specifics of these cases, and it may be that surgery *was* indicated. We cannot comment. What is known is that we (physicians, surgeons, radiologists, etc) must, as far as is possible, practice evidence-based medicine.

The 2 questions asked by this article, answers to which might change our practice are:

1. Does elbow MRI have a routine role in little league elbow?
2. Does UCL abnormality in little league elbow suggest that surgery for this condition is indicated?

While MRI did pick up more abnormality than radiographs, the additional findings had no bearing on clinical management. On the other hand, although the origin of the UCL varied between patients (Fig 3), in no patient was abnormality of the UCL itself demonstrated.

The answer to question 1 is a confident, "No".

Unfortunately only 9 patients were recruited in the study; therefore, the answer to question 2 ranges from a confident "No" via a more cautious "Probably not" to a doubtful "Possibly." Until results from larger studies are available, current results indicate that anybody who finds they are considering surgery, should proceed with caution and not without first performing an MRI.

A. C. Offiah, BSc, MBBS, MRCP, FRCR, PhD

Reference

1. Gibson BW, Webner D, Huffman GR, Sennett BJ. Ulnar collateral ligament reconstruction in major league baseball pitchers. *Am J Sports Med.* 2007;35:575-581.

Biphasic threat to femoral head perfusion in abduction: arterial hypoperfusion and venous congestion
Yousefzadeh DK, Jaramillo D, Johnson N, et al (Comer Children's Hosp, Chicago, IL; Children's Hosp of Philadelphia, PA; Cincinnati Children's Hosp, OH; et al)
Pediatr Radiol 40:1517-1525, 2010

Background.—Hip abduction can cause avascular necrosis (AVN) of the femoral head in infants.

Objective.—To compare the US perfusion pattern of femoral head carti-lage in neutral position with that in different degrees and duration of abduction, testing the venous congestion theory of post-abduction ischemia.

Materials and Methods.—In 20 neonates, the Doppler flow characteris-tics of the posterosuperior (PS) branch of the femoral head cartilage feeding vessels were evaluated in neutral and at 30°, 45°, and 60° abduc-tion. In three neonates the leg was held in 45-degree abduction and flow was assessed at 5, 10, and 15 min.

Results.—Male/female ratio was 11/9 with a mean age of 1.86 ± 0.7 weeks. The peak systolic velocities (PSV) declined in all three degrees of abduction. After 15 min of 45-degree abduction, the mean PSV declined and showed an absent or reversed diastolic component and undetectable venous return. No perfusion was detected at 60-degree abduction.

Conclusion.—Abduction-induced femoral head ischemia is biphasic and degree- and duration-dependent. In phase I there is arterial hypoperfusion and in phase II there is venous congestion. A new pathogeneses for femoral head ischemia is offered (Figs 5, 8 and 9).

▶ In this very interesting article, the authors elegantly demonstrate the effects of varying degrees and duration of hip abduction on femoral head perfusion in a cohort of normal African American neonates (maximum age was 11 weeks).

The authors include an array of figures (14 in total) in their article. Of these, I have selected 3 showing the effects of abduction on posterosuperior (PS) Doppler waveform.

As far as the authors (and I) are aware, this is the first time that the possible role of venous congestion in the etiology of avascular necrosis (AVN) following hip abduction therapy for developmental hip dysplasia (DDH) has been demonstrated. However, the authors go even further than this; they postulate a cause: compression of the PS branch of the medial circumflex artery by the lower edge of the labrum as the hip is abducted.

The selection of only African American patients reminds me of the very low rates of DDH in Africans, ascribed to carrying babies astride their mothers' backs. On the other hand, it has been shown[1] that the acetabulums of African neonates is deeper than those of Caucasians. Might this not also explain why, if the findings of this study are accepted, there is not a higher rate of AVN among

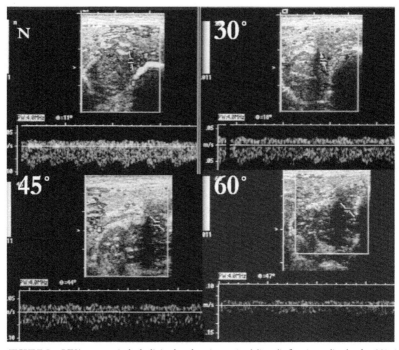

FIGURE 5.—PSV is progressively declining but there is sustained diastolic flow immediately after 30°, 45° and 60° of abduction. (With kind permission from Springer Science and Business Media: Yousefzadeh DK, Jaramillo D, Johnson N, et al. Biphasic threat to femoral head perfusion in abduction: arterial hypoperfusion and venous congestion. *Pediatr Radiol.* 2010;40:1517-1525, with permission from Springer-Verlag.)

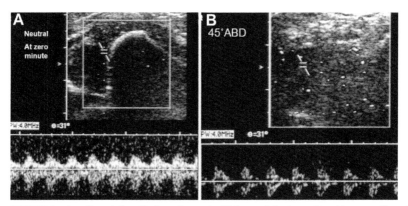

FIGURE 8.—Systolic and diastolic flow changes in 45-degree abduction. a Broad-base systolic and sustained diastolic flow (below the baseline) in neutral position. b Dampened PSV with a narrower base than in neutral position (A) and loss of diastolic flow 15 min after 45-degree abduction. (With kind permission from Springer Science and Business Media: Yousefzadeh DK, Jaramillo D, Johnson N, et al. Biphasic threat to femoral head perfusion in abduction: arterial hypoperfusion and venous congestion. *Pediatr Radiol.* 2010;40:1517-1525, with permission from Springer-Verlag.)

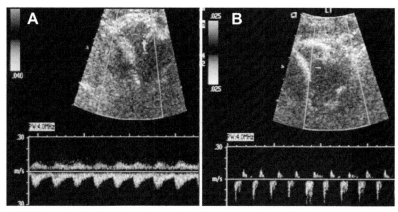

FIGURE 9.—Systolic, diastolic and venous flow changes at 45-degree abduction. a Broad-base systolic and sustained diastolic flow in neutral position, below the baseline, and sluggish and wavy venous return above the baseline. b Narrowed systolic base, needle-point PSV below the baseline, and reversed diastolic flow above the baseline. The venous return was no longer detectable. (With kind permission from Springer Science and Business Media: Yousefzadeh DK, Jaramillo D, Johnson N, et al. Biphasic threat to femoral head perfusion in abduction: arterial hypoperfusion and venous congestion. *Pediatr Radiol.* 2010;40:1517-1525, with permission from Springer-Verlag.)

Africans? Or is it that the degree of hip abduction associated with the cultural positioning of African babies is such that it does not interfere with blood flow? Or both?

Many nations have developed (or are developing) screening programs aimed at early detection of DDH.

When diagnosed before 6 months of age, abduction treatment (Pavlik harness) is standard.[2] Since the rate of AVN has been shown to be 8% of affected hips in one study[3] and 7% of affected hips and 2.9% of contralateral normal hips in another,[4] the potential implications of this study are significant. It may be that the routine (and simple) use of power Doppler interrogation of the femoral head to optimize the degree of abduction in individual patients will reduce the numbers developing AVN.

As an aside, the results of this study are also of relevance to designers of baby slings.

A. C. Offiah, BSc, MBBS, MRCP, FRCR, PhD

References

1. Skirving AP, Scadden WJ. The African neonatal hip and its immunity from congenital dislocation. *J Bone Joint Surg Br.* 1979;69-B:339-341.
2. Kaplan K. Developmental dysplasia of the hip. http://www.orthopaedia.com/display/Main/Developmental+dysplasia+of+the+hip. Accessed March 24, 2011.
3. Suzuki S, Kashiwagi N, Kashara Y, Seto Y, Futami T. Avascular necrosis and the Pavlik harness. The incidence of avascular necrosis in three types of congenital dislocation of the hip as classified by ultrasound. *J Bone Joint Surg Br.* 1996;78: 631-635.
4. Pap K, Kiss S, Shisha T, Marton-Szucs G, Szöke G. The incidence of avascular necrosis of the healthy, contralateral femoral head at the end of the use of Pavlik harness in unilateral hip dysplasia. *Int Orthop.* 2006;30:348-351.

Intraoperative Arthrography for the Evaluation of Closed Reduction and Percutaneous Fixation of Displaced MacFarland Fractures: An Alternative to Open Surgery

Duran JA, Dayer R, Kaelin A, et al (Univ of Geneva Hosp, Switzerland)
J Pediatr Orthop 31:e1-e5, 2011

Background.—MacFarland fracture is a joint fracture of the ankle in children involving the medial malleolus (Salter-Harris type III or IV). These fractures are acknowledged to have poor prognosis because of the risk of misalignment due to the development of an epiphysiodesis bridge. Current recommended treatment for a displacement of ≥ 2 mm is open reduction through an arthrotomy with screw fixation. This study aimed to evaluate functional and radiologic results of a less-invasive surgical technique consisting of closed reduction, arthrographic control of fracture reposition, and percutaneous screw fixation.

Methods.—Retrospective analysis of 12 cases of children with MacFarland fractures who underwent percutaneous screw fixation with intraoperative arthrography. Data collected for each child included age, sex, radiologic Salter-Harris classification of medial and lateral malleolus fractures, fracture gap before and after treatment, intraoperative and postoperative complications, and length of follow up. Results were evaluated according to the 3 outcome categories according to the classification by Gleizes and based on clinical and radiologic criteria.

Results.—There were 7 boys and 5 girls with an age range of 10 to 15 years (average, 12 y 6 mo). Average follow-up was 18 months (range: 9 to 57 mo). Medial malleolus fracture was Salter-Harris type III in 7 patients and type IV in 5. There were 9 Salter-Harris type I fractures and 1 type II at the level of the distal fibular physis. The mean preoperative gap was 2.8 mm (1.9 to 4 mm). Fracture fixation was performed with 2 screws in 9 patients and 1 screw in 3 patients. Mean surgical time was 58 minutes (45 to 75 min). The mean postoperative articular gap was 0 mm in 8 patients, inferior to 1 mm in 3 patients, and 2 mm in 1 patient. At the time of last follow-up, the outcome was considered good in all but 1 patient.

Conclusions.—Closed reduction combined with ankle arthrography followed by percutaneous osteosynthesis is an interesting and less invasive safe surgical alternative to classic open reduction and internal fixation of displaced MacFarland fractures.

Level of Evidence.—Therapeutic study, level IV (Fig 1).

► The premise of this article is praiseworthy if further results support the conclusions: The use of a diagnostic imaging study to change a surgical operation from an open technique to a closed technique. This benefit is akin to the use of ultrasound and other imaging methods to obviate open surgery of the abdomen. As demonstrated in Fig 1, the arthrography may have a side benefit of demonstrating or confirming additional ankle fracture, in that case a medial fracture of the distal fibula epiphysis. What the article does not address is the

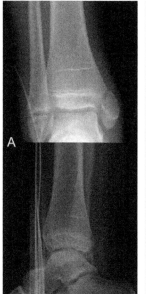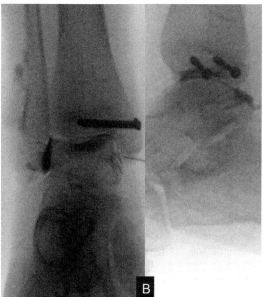

FIGURE 1.—A, Preoperative radiographs showing a Salter-Harris type III fracture of the medial malleolus in a 12-year-old girl. B, Arthrographic control after percutaneous osteosynthesis with 2 partially threaded cannulated screws showed an anatomic reduction of the fracture, as shown by the absence of contrast leakage through the fracture line in images on the intensifier screen. An associated fracture of the distal fibular physis was observed, as illustrated by contrast leakage at this level. (Reprinted from Duran JA, Dayer R, Kaelin A, et al. Intraoperative arthrography for the evaluation of closed reduction and percutaneous fixation of displaced MacFarland fractures: an alternative to open surgery. *J Pediatr Orthop.* 2011;31:e1-e5, with permission from Lippincott Williams & Wilkins.)

additional diagnostic and surgery-planning information that can be gained from ankle CT.[1] Although one should avoid unnecessary CT, the cited article[1] revealed many clinically significant findings not seen with plain images (at least in the authors' experience). Nonetheless, intraoperative arthrography (with immediate diagnostic interpretation) has the potential of helping avoid potential complications attendant on open versus closed surgery.

A. E. Oestreich, MD

Reference

1. Lemburg SP, Lilienthal E, Heyer CM. Growth plate fractures of the distal tibia: is CT imaging necessary? *Arch Orthop Trauma Surg.* 2010;130:1411-1417.

Fetal MRI of clubfoot associated with myelomeningocele

Servaes S, Hernandez A, Gonzalez L, et al (The Children's Hosp of Philadelphia, PA)
Pediatr Radiol 40:1874-1879, 2010

Background.—The sensitivity and specificity of evaluating clubfoot deformity by MR in high-risk fetuses is currently unknown.

Objective.—To correlate fetal MRI with US in the assessment of clubfoot and to identify the MRI features most characteristic of clubfoot.

Materials and methods.—With IRB approval and informed consent, the presence of fetal clubfoot was prospectively evaluated in mothers referred for MRI for a fetus with myelomeningocele. Two radiologists blind to the US results independently reviewed the MRI for the presence of clubfoot. MRI results were compared with US results obtained the same day and birth outcomes.

Results.—Of 20 patients enrolled, there were 13 clubfeet. Interobserver agreement for the presence of clubfoot was 100%. The sensitivity of the MRI exam was 100% and the specificity 85.2%. A dedicated sagittal imaging plane through the ankle region allowed the most confident diagnosis; medial deviation of the foot relative to the leg was seen in all 13 fetuses with clubfoot.

Conclusion.—The correlation of fetal MRI with US in the evaluation of clubfoot yields a sensitivity of 100% and specificity of 85.2%. The sagittal plane provided the most useful information (Figs 1 and 4).

▶ Johann Wolfgang Von Goethe said, "Every day we should hear at least one little song, read one good poem, see one exquisite picture, and, if possible,

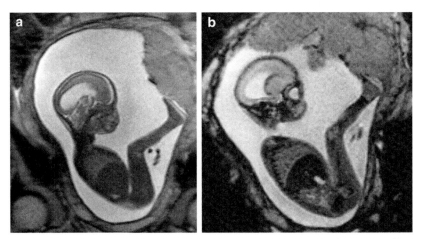

FIGURE 1.—Normal right lower extremity, 24 weeks' gestational age. a HASTE. b EPI. Notice dilatation of ventricle. (Reprinted from Servaes S, Hernandez A, Gonzalez L, et al. Fetal MRI of clubfoot associated with myelomeningocele. *Pediatr Radiol.* 2010;40:1874-1879, with permission from Springer-Verlag.)

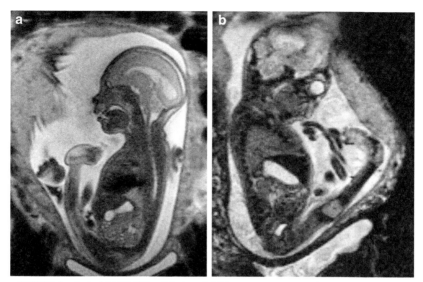

FIGURE 4.—Sagittal (a) HASTE and (b) EPI of clubfoot. Note extension of extremity in this 21-week gestation fetus. (Reprinted from Servaes S, Hernandez A, Gonzalez L, et al. Fetal MRI of clubfoot associated with myelomeningocele. *Pediatr Radiol.* 2010;40:1874-1879, with permission from Springer-Verlag.)

speak a few sensible words." I am assuming that MR images count as pictures and refer you to Figs 1 and 4 of the article by Servaes et al—exquisite indeed!

I don't know about speaking "a few sensible words," but if a picture is worth a thousand words, I can end my commentary right here. Of course I won't, because we know that our job is not about obtaining pretty pictures, but about making correct diagnoses. MRI will never replace routine dating and anomaly screening ultrasound scans, so what's the fuss?

Well, the point is that aided by what we tell them, clinicians must offer advice to parents of a fetus in which abnormality has been detected. The decision whether to continue with or terminate the pregnancy is often a difficult one. It will depend on the extent and severity of abnormalities detected. Fetal MR (particularly of the central nervous system) is used to further characterize the abnormality detected on ultrasound. However, involvement of other systems (eg, lung volumes, kidneys, gastrointestinal tract) is increasingly being assessed with fetal MR. Additionally, with more rapid sequences (eg, half-Fourier acquisition single-shot turbo spin-echo and echoplanar imaging) as used in this study, images of high-enough quality are now being obtained of the musculoskeletal system to allow the impressive results achieved by the authors.

In skeletal dysplasias and other syndromic conditions, multiple anomalies often coexist. As MR technology advances, we are able to more correctly identify these abnormalities and reach more precise conclusions as to diagnosis and prognosis. When an abnormality is detected, the decision has to be made whether or not to continue with the pregnancy. Why shouldn't we work toward easing the decision process—by doing what we can to paint a full picture?

A. C. Offiah, BSc, MBBS, MRCP, FRCR, PhD

Stüve–Wiedemann syndrome: long-term follow-up and genetic heterogeneity

Jung C, Dagoneau N, Baujat G, et al (Université Paris Descartes, France; et al)
Clin Genet 77:266-272, 2010

Stüve–Wiedemann syndrome (SWS, OMIM 601559) is a severe auto-somal recessive condition caused by mutations in the leukemia inhibitory receptor (*LIFR*) gene. The main characteristic features are bowing of the long bones, neonatal respiratory distress, swallowing/sucking difficulties and dysautonomia symptoms including temperature instability often leading to death in the first years of life. We report here four patients with SWS who have survived beyond 36 months of age with no *LIFR* mutation. These patients have been compared with six unreported SWS survivors carrying null *LIFR* mutations. We provide evidence of

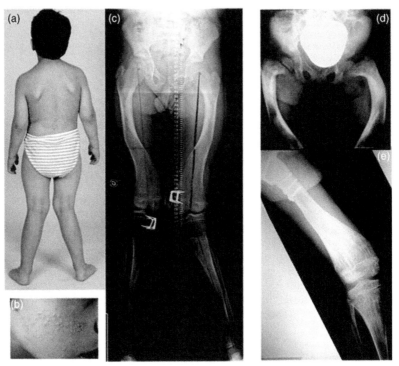

FIGURE 1.—Clinical and radiological manifestations in patients 1 and 6. Patient 1: (a) general habitus; (b) cutaneous milia; (c) lower limb X-rays at 9 years old. Note the major deformation of the lower limbs with genu valgum, wide metaphyses and abnormal trabecular pattern. Patient 6: (d) and (e) lower limb X-rays at five years of age. Note the bowing of the lower limbs with the internal cortical thickening, and the abnormal trabecular pattern with radiolucent metaphyses. (Reprinted from Jung C, Dagoneau N, Baujat G, et al. Stüve–Wiedemann syndrome: long-term follow-up and genetic heterogeneity. *Clin Genet.* 2010;77:266-272, with permission from John Wiley & Sons A/S.)

clinical homogeneity of the syndrome in spite of the genetic heterogeneity (Fig 1).

▶ Now and then it seems worthwhile to alert radiologists to characteristic radiologic findings in newly defined genetic syndromes; this time it's Stüve-Wiedemann syndrome. Often the disease is fatal early because of respiratory disease or the temperature instability of the accompanying dysautonomia. Radiologic findings, highlighted by bowing of the long bones, are summarized by the findings in Fig 1. Previous reports have mentioned short (bowed) and long bones, prominent joints with restricted joint mobility, severe spinal deformities, and spontaneous fractures. Sucking and swallowing difficulties occur early in life. Criteria for inclusion in the current group of patients included internal cortical thickening of bones and wide metaphyses. Age range was 3 to 14 years. Also encountered were camptodactyly, clubfoot, and dental abnormalities. Dislocations of patellae and proximal radius were common. This report, besides summarizing the relatively homogeneous clinical pattern, details some of the genetic heterogenicity, raising questions concerning mutations in the leukemia inhibitory receptor gene. The original report of Stüve and Wiedemann appeared in 1971.[1]

A. E. Oestreich, MD

Reference

1. Stüve A, Wiedemann HR. Congenital bowing of the long bones in two sisters. *Lancet.* 1971;2:495.

Wolf-Hirschhorn syndrome: diagnosis using hand radiograph performed for bone age
Beluffi G, Savasta S (Fondazione IRCCS Policlinico S. Matteo, Pavia, Italy)
Pediatr Radiol 40:1580, 2010

Background.—Delayed bone age is a common radiological finding in 4p- deletion or Wolf-Hirschhorn syndrome (WHS). A child with growth and weight delay was evaluated radiologically to clarify the diagnosis.

Case Report.—Boy, 4 years 10 months, was evaluated for generalized hypotonia, seizures, gait impairment, and an abnormal facial appearance, specifically, frontal bossing, epicanthus, and irregularly shaped and low-set ears. Examination revealed hypospadia with undescended testes, bilateral clubfoot, and fourth-toe clinodactyly. A bone age hand radiograph was obtained, demonstrating severely delayed skeletal maturation. Only two carpal centers were seen. There were also basal pseudoepiphyses of the second, fourth, and fifth metacarpals, distal pseudoepiphysis of the first metacarpal, and an unusual malformation of the distal aspects of the proximal and middle phalanges that resembled a tongue joint.

Conclusions.—The diagnosis of WHS was clarified by obtaining the bone age radiograph of the hand. The tongue-joint malformation and multiple basal pseudoepiphyses are uncommon presentations in WHS. Other common signs seen radiographically include skull malformation and skeletal anomalies, including fused vertebrae, underdeveloped cervical spine, small pelvis with small or missing pubic bones, clavicles shaped like a bottle opener, and sternal ossification anomalies (Fig 1).

▶ A picture is often worth 1000 words (or at least the 150 expected minimum in this commentary), and such is the case with Fig 1 of a bone age image in this

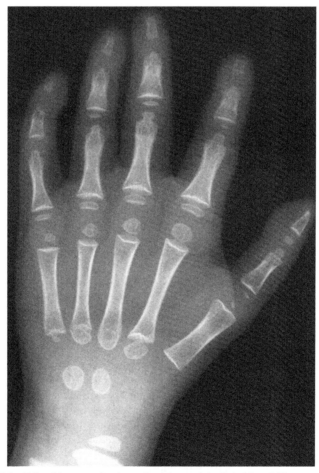

FIGURE 1.—Delayed bone age; basal pseudoepiphyses of the 2nd, 4th and 5th metacarpals; distal pseudoepiphysis of the 1st metacarpal bone; and tongue-joint like malformation of the distal ends of the proximal and middle phalanges. (Reprinted from Beluffi G, Savasta S. Wolf-Hirschhorn syndrome: diagnosis using hand radiograph performed for bone age. *Pediatr Radiol*. 2010;40:1580, with permission from Springer-Verlag.)

succinct, but important, contribution. Among skeletal malformation syndromes, one worth knowing is the 4p- deletion syndrome known as Wolf-Hirschhorn syndrome. Moreover, it is always satisfying, as the article's full title implies, when one can make a diagnosis merely from a bone age hand wrist radiograph. Several other conditions have prominent pseudoepiphyses of the proximal end of the second metacarpal, including cleidocranial dysplasia/dysostosis, but the rest of the pattern is different. Beluffi and Savasta have chosen to describe the other highly specific finding in Wolf-Hirschhorn syndrome, at the distal ends of proximal and middle phalanges, as tongue-joint like, an apt term for those readers who are adept at carpentry. The distal ends look also a bit like the tops of bishops in the classic wooden chess sets. I resolved to select this article after I prospectively saw a bone age image earlier this week with the same specific findings (pseudoepiphyses and tongue-joints), although we do not have genetic confirmation yet. If I am correct, it should be safe to call the pattern pathognomonic. This same pattern in Wolf-Hirschhorn syndrome was shown in the hand text of Andy Poznanski and originally in an article[1] from 1971 but without description of the distal ends of proximal and middle phalanges, which are, however, clearly demonstrated. A pattern to be remembered!

A. E. Oestreich, MD

Reference

1. Poznanski AK, Garn SM, Holt JF. The thumb in the congenital malformation syndromes. *Radiology.* 1971;100:115-129.

5 Economics, Research, Education, and Quality

Introduction

Another interesting year in the world of safety, quality, and clinical practice management!

Perhaps the largest focus of the year was the increasing attention among radiologists and other health care providers toward minimizing radiation exposure for patients undergoing diagnostic studies. Although there remains justifiable skepticism in the scientific community as to whether x-irradiation in very low doses indeed causes cancer, the cautious approach has been to assume that it does and act accordingly. In this section you will find several interesting articles, including exposure risks from airport scanners to whole-body CT. Coupled with this increased attention to radiation exposure is the appropriateness of various imaging studies, which is now important not only from an economic point of view, but from a health risk point of view as well.

Hopefully you will find something among these diverse articles that will both interest you and improve the way you practice radiology.

Allen D. Elster, MD

Contrast Agents

Intravenous Contrast Medium—induced Nephrotoxicity: Is the Medical Risk Really as Great as We Have Come to Believe?
Katzberg RW, Newhouse JH (Univ of California-Davis Med Ctr, Sacramento; Columbia Univ Med Ctr, NY)
Radiology 256:21-28, 2010

From the multiple perspectives described, it is our belief that the risk of CIN with CE CT has been exaggerated. Clinical rates and adverse outcomes from cardiac catheterization and intervention cannot be extrapolated to the clinical experience with CE CT. It appears that all currently used nonionic CM have similar safety profiles.

We believe that modern CM pose only a small risk to renal function and that thresholds of creatinine above which CM are withheld for CT should be increased to improve the accuracy of CT examinations. The population of patients with mild to moderate renal dysfunction who would then receive CM should be analyzed carefully to determine whether the thresholds subsequently can be increased further. International radiologic professional organizations, such as the American College of Radiology, should revisit the basis of their practice guidelines to reduce their implications about the danger of CIN with CE CT (Fig 1).

▶ Always the skeptic myself, I particularly appreciate papers that challenge conventional wisdom, in this case, long-held beliefs concerning the risks of contrast-induced nephropathy (CIN) in patients undergoing iodine contrast–enhanced computed tomography (CT) scans. This article is not original research but an editorial and critical review of the existing literature.

The authors are not saying there is no risk of CIN after CT; quite the contrary, the risk is very real. What they conclude, however, is that this risk has been

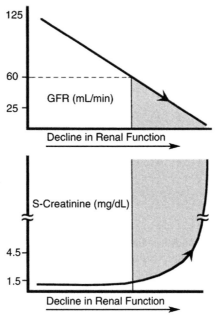

FIGURE 1.—Graphs show the relationship between GFR, which serves as the measure of renal function, and SCr level. Top: There is a linear relationship between GFR and renal function. Bottom: There is a well-known nonlinear relationship between SCr *(S-Creatinine)* level and renal function. With a decline in renal function and a low GFR (shaded region), there is an exponential increase in the SCr level. (Reprinted from Katzberg RW, Newhouse JH. Intravenous contrast medium–induced nephrotoxicity: is the medical risk really as great as we have come to believe? *Radiology.* 2010;256:21-28. Copyright by the Radiological Society of North America.)

exaggerated by incorrectly extrapolating data from studies and reasoning by analogy, rather than hard science.

The major limitations of most published studies include (1) controls for concurrent disease have been almost completely lacking; (2) use of serum creatinine as the endpoint, whereas there is a strong nonlinear relationship between this value and the degree of renal impairment as measured by glomerular filtration rate (Fig 1); (3) variation in serum creatinine levels has been interpreted as indicating nephrotoxicity even though such variation occurs without CM administration; and (4) the risks of intravenous CM injection and intra-arterial CM injection during angiocardiography have been unjustifiably equated. In angiocardiography, a high dose of intra-arterial contrast hits the kidneys in one tight bolus, potentially injuring the nephrons more than a more dilute exposure from venous injection.

A. D. Elster, MD

Acute Adverse Reactions to Gadopentetate Dimeglumine and Gadobenate Dimeglumine: Experience With 32,659 Injections

Abujudeh HH, Kosaraju VK, Kaewlai R (Massachusetts General Hosp and Harvard Med School, Boston)

AJR Am J Roentgenol 194:430-434, 2010

Objective.—The purpose of this study was to retrospectively assess the frequency, manifestations, and severity of acute adverse reactions associated with administration of two gadolinium-based contrast agents to patients who underwent MRI at a single large academic institution.

Materials and Methods.—Data from continuous quality assurance records on the number of administrations of and acute adverse reactions to gadopentetate dimeglumine and gadobenate dimeglumine at our institution October 2007 to December 2008 were tabulated and analyzed. During the investigation period, 32,659 administrations of gadolinium-based contrast agents were performed for MRI examinations. Of these, 27,956 administrations were gadopentetate dimeglumine, and 4,703 administrations were gadobenate dimeglumine. Data were collected on the frequency and severity of acute adverse reactions.

Results.—A total of 51 acute adverse reactions occurred in 50 patients (16 men, 34 women; mean age, 48 years), accounting for 0.16% of all administrations (51/32,659). Thirty-eight reactions (38/27,956, 0.14%) were associated with gadopentetate dimeglumine, and 13 (13/4,703, 0.28%) were associated with gadobenate dimeglumine. Forty-three reactions were mild, six were moderate, and two were severe. The severe reactions occurred with the use of gadobenate dimeglumine.

Conclusion.—The rates of acute adverse reactions to gadopentetate dimeglumine and gadobenate dimeglumine were 0.14% and 0.28%, respectively. The overall adverse reaction rate was 0.16% in our patient sample. Direct comparison of adverse reaction rates of the two agents

TABLE 2.—Adverse Reactions Categorized by Severity and Agent

Agent	No. of Administrations	Mild	Moderate	Severe	Total
			No. of Adverse Reactions		
Gadopentetate dimeglumine	27,956	36	2	0	38 (0.14)
Gadobenate dimeglumine	4,703	7	4	2	13 (0.28)
Total	32,659	43	6	2	51 (0.16)

Note—Values in parentheses are percentages.

was not possible because of the retrospective uncontrolled study design (Table 2).

▶ Although a number of studies over the past 20 years have evaluated the incidence of reactions to gadolinium-based contrast agents (and found it to be low), room always exists for re-evaluation, particularly as new agents become available. This article thus looks not only at gadopentetate dimeglumine, the oldest such agent in widespread clinical use, but also the newer agent gadobenate dimeglumine. The database is large and appears complete, with over 32 000 subjects, the vast majority of whom received gadopentetate dimeglumine.

The incidence of reactions to gadopentetate dimeglumine was in the 0.14% range, consistent with many previous postmarketing surveillance studies of this agent. The surprising result from this study was a 2 fold higher incidence of reaction to gadobenate dimeglumine (0.28%, Table 2). Moreover, what appears to be a significantly higher number of moderate and severe reactions occurred with the latter agent.

Brief descriptions are provided for the half-dozen patients with moderate or severe reactions to gadobenate, which are frankly a little frightening. These include significant bronchospasm in several cases, a seizure/convulsion requiring transfer to the emergency room, and full-blown cardiopulmonary arrest with pulseless electrical activity.

While the uncontrolled and retrospective nature of the study prohibits true statistical significance of these different reaction rates from being calculated, there is enough evidence here to at least suggest the safety profile of gadobenate dimeglumine, while still excellent, may not be as good as the older agent gadopentetate dimeglumine. Larger controlled studies will be necessary in the future to evaluate this possibility more thoroughly.

A. D. Elster, MD

Change in Use of Gadolinium-Enhanced Magnetic Resonance Studies in Kidney Disease Patients After US Food and Drug Administration Warnings: A Cross-sectional Study of Veterans Affairs Health Care System Data From 2005-2008
Kim K-H, Fonda JR, Lawler EV, et al (State Univ of New York at Stony Brook; VA Boston Healthcare System, MA; et al)
Am J Kidney Dis 56:458-467, 2010

Background.—Exposure to gadolinium in patients with kidney disease has been linked to risk of developing nephrogenic systemic fibrosis. The US Food and Drug Administration (FDA) has issued warnings against the use of gadolinium in this population. We studied the impact of these warnings on the use of gadolinium-enhanced magnetic resonance (GE-MR) studies in patients with decreased estimated glomerular filtration rate (eGFR) and the practice of measuring serum creatinine before gadolinium exposure.

Study Design.—Cross-sectional study of patients who had undergone MR studies from October 2002 to September 2008.

Setting & Participants.—Patients receiving medical care in the US Department of Veterans Affairs Health Care System.

Predictor.—Date of MR imaging, serum creatinine level, and eGFR using the 4-variable Modification of Diet in Renal Disease (MDRD) Study equation.

Outcomes & Measurements.—The rate of MR studies performed with and without gadolinium from July 2005 to September 2008 in patients with different stages of kidney disease, defined using eGFR. The proportion of GE-MR studies with a screening serum creatinine level.

Results.—There was a 71% decrease in the rate of GE-MR use in patients with GFR <30 mL/min/1.73 m^2 2 years after the release of the first public health advisory, although studies continued to be performed in patients with stages 4 and 5 chronic kidney disease. The proportion of GE-MR studies with serum creatinine measured within 1 month before the study increased by 99%.

Limitations.—Data available up to September 30, 2008. Indications for the GE-MR studies were not assessed. The accuracy of *Current Procedural Terminology* and *International Classification of Diseases, Ninth Revision* coding was not assessed.

Conclusion.—There was a large decrease in the use of GE-MR studies in patients with GFR <30 mL/min/1.73 m^2 and a large but not universal increase in the practice of measuring serum creatinine before GE-MR after the release of the FDA warnings.

▶ Nephrogenic systemic fibrosis (NSF) is a rare but potentially lethal condition diagnosed much more frequently in the last decade in parallel with the increasing use of gadolinium-containing contrast agents in patients with renal failure or insufficiency. In 2007, the US Food and Drug Administration (FDA) issued a black box warning concerning the risk of these agents in this population.

The authors of this study set out to determine (1) whether decreased use of gadolinium-enhanced examinations have occurred after the FDA advisories; (2) whether such a decrease has occurred in patients with impaired renal function; and (3) whether the FDA notices have increased the practice of obtaining a screening serum creatinine level before gadolinium exposure.

The answer to all 3 questions is yes. The FDA warnings and associated press induced a substantial change in radiologic practice in each dimension analyzed. As such, the number of new cases of NSF have virtually disappeared during the last 1 to 2 years, suggesting that this iatrogenic disease is now firmly in control.

A. D. Elster, MD

Food and Drug Administration Requirements for Testing and Approval of New Radiopharmaceuticals
Harapanhalli RS (PAREXEL Consulting, Bethesda, MD)
Semin Nucl Med 40:364-384, 2010

In March 2004, the Food and Drug Administration (FDA) published a report entitled *Challenge and Opportunity on the Critical Path to New Medical Products* in which it explained the critical path to medical product development and called for a nationwide effort to modernize the critical-path sciences with the aim of moving medical product development and patient care into the 21st century. The report identified medical imaging and imaging biomarkers as potential clinical development tools to facilitate medical product development and to help minimize drug attritions and development timelines. Also, in recent years, basic research on receptor-based imaging has led to an increase in the new investigational radiopharmaceuticals, many of which are in basic research stages in academic institutions. It is therefore an opportune time to review the FDA requirements for testing and approval of new radiopharmaceuticals to further the cause of development and approval of newer medical imaging and therapeutic agents. Although the radiopharmaceutical-development process aligns well with the drug-development process for conventional pharmaceuticals, it has its own challenges and unique considerations. For example, unique issues surrounding short-lived positron emission tomography drugs have necessitated revisions and refinements to the existing regulations. The FDA Modernization Act mandate has finally resulted in the publication of new cGMPs (current good manufacturing practice) for positron emission tomography drugs. Often, the radiopharmaceutical community is not well-informed about the regulatory pathways and scientific basis for the regulations they are subjected to. Questions, such as (1) "Do I need an investigational new drug (IND) or can I do my investigation under an RDRC (radioactive drugs research committee) oversight?" (2) "What type of information on radiopharmaceutical product quality is needed for an IND?" (3) "What level of cGMPs I am expected to operate under?" (4) "Do I need a traditional IND or can I perform studies under an exploratory IND?" (5) "What

TABLE 4.—Applicable PDUFA Fee Structures for Radiopharmaceuticals (FY210)

Fee Category	Fee Rate for FY 2010	Comments*
Application requiring clinical data	$1,405,500	Unless qualified for a fee waiver, all radiopharmaceutical NDA applications are required to pay this fee
Application not requiring clinical data	$702,750	Unless qualified for a fee waiver, all radiopharmaceutical NDA applications are required to pay this fee
Supplemental application requiring clinical data	$702,750	Unless qualified for a fee waiver, all radiopharmaceutical NDA applications are required to pay this fee
Establishments	$457,200 (Non-PET commercial radiopharmaceuticals)	Section 736(a)(2)(C) of the Act provides for special rules for the assessment of establishment fees for PET products.
	$76,200 (commercial PET radiopharmaceuticals)	If an establishment is shared by multiple applicants, the establishment fee is equally divided and assessed among the applicants whose products are manufactured by the establishment during the fiscal year.
Products	$79,720	The fee will be waived as soon as an ANDA is approved for the same RLD.

*Waivers from the application fee, establishment fee, and product fee are possible for qualified applicants.

are the IND-enabling pharmacology and toxicology studies?" (6) "Is my practice consistent with pharmacy compounding or do I need to file an application with the FDA?", for example, are a source of confusion to the radiopharmaceutical community. This review provides an overview of FDA's drug development and approval process with special emphasis on radiopharmaceuticals and attempts to clarify many regulatory issues and questions by providing appropriate discussion and FDA references.

► This review article is not for everyone. But if you would really like to have some insight into the process by which new radiopharmaceuticals undergo testing and ultimately receive approval for human use, this is the best source I can imagine.

Perhaps the most interesting table is Table 4, which lists the fees that pharmaceutical companies must pay to begin the approval process. For applications requiring submission of clinical data, the basic fee is just over $1.4 million!

A. D. Elster, MD

Radiation Exposure and Risks

Cancer Risks After Radiation Exposure in Middle Age

Shuryak I, Sachs RK, Brenner DJ (Columbia Univ Med Ctr, NY; Univ of California, Berkeley)

J Natl Cancer Inst 102:1628-1636, 2010

Background.—Epidemiological data show that radiation exposure during childhood is associated with larger cancer risks compared with exposure at older ages. For exposures in adulthood, however, the relative risks of radiation-induced cancer in Japanese atomic bomb survivors generally do not decrease monotonically with increasing age of adult exposure. These observations are inconsistent with most standard models of radiation-induced cancer, which predict that relative risks decrease monotonically with increasing age at exposure, at all ages.

Methods.—We analyzed observed cancer risk patterns as a function of age at exposure in Japanese atomic bomb survivors by using a biologically based quantitative model of radiation carcinogenesis that incorporates both radiation induction of premalignant cells (initiation) and radiation-induced promotion of premalignant damage. This approach emphasizes the kinetics of radiation-induced initiation and promotion, and tracks the yields of premalignant cells before, during, shortly after, and long after radiation exposure.

Results.—Radiation risks after exposure in younger individuals are dominated by initiation processes, whereas radiation risks after exposure at later ages are more influenced by promotion of preexisting premalignant cells. Thus, the cancer site—dependent balance between initiation and promotion determines the dependence of cancer risk on age at radiation exposure. For example, in terms of radiation induction of premalignant cells, a quantitative measure of the relative contribution of initiation vs promotion is 10-fold larger for breast cancer than for lung cancer. Reflecting this difference, radiation-induced breast cancer risks decrease with age at exposure at all ages, whereas radiation-induced lung cancer risks do not.

Conclusion.—For radiation exposure in middle age, most radiation-induced cancer risks do not, as often assumed, decrease with increasing age at exposure. This observation suggests that promotional processes in radiation carcinogenesis become increasingly important as the age at exposure increases. Radiation-induced cancer risks after exposure in middle age may be up to twice as high as previously estimated, which could have implications for occupational exposure and radiological imaging (Fig 2).

▶ This is yet another mathematical modeling of exposure of Japanese patients to radiation during atomic bomb blasts in 1945. Although you might think this data base has been exhaustively studied, there are still some pearls to be gained. Here, the focus is on cancers induced in middle-aged adults—a category

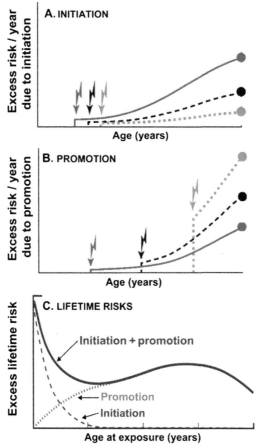

FIGURE 2.—Schematic illustrating the dominant factors determining the variation in radiation-induced cancer risk with age at exposure. **Jagged arrows** indicate different times of radiation exposure, and the **solid circles** represent risks at a given attained age (eg, 80 years). **A)** Excess risk per year due to radiation initiation; for an exposure at a younger age, initiated cells have longer to exploit their growth advantage over normal cells. **B)** Excess risk per year due to radiation promotion; people irradiated at older ages, when there are more premalignant cells for promotion to act upon, are expected to have larger promotion-driven risks. **C)** Excess lifetime risks due to radiation-induced initiation and promotion. Initiation and promotion result in very different variations in cancer risk as a function of age at exposure; the downturn in excess lifetime risk shown in (C) for very old ages at exposure is due mainly to competing risks. (Reprinted from Shuryak I, Sachs RK, Brenner DJ. Cancer risks after radiation exposure in middle age. *J Natl Cancer Inst.* 2010;102:1628-1636, The Author 2010. Published by Oxford University Press.)

previously considered to be relatively spared from the most severe effects of ionizing radiation.

The model of radiation carcinogenesis used in this study allows ionizing radiation to act not only as an initiator of premalignant clones but also as a promoter of preexisting premalignant damage. Promotion is the process by which an initiated cell (radiation-induced initiation or otherwise) clonally expands, proportionately increasing the preexisting average number of premalignant stem cells per clone. As shown in Fig 2, initiation processes would be expected to result in decreasing excess lifetime cancer risks with increasing ages at exposure. Conversely, promotional processes can result in increasing excess lifetime cancer risks with increasing ages at exposure because the number of preexisting premalignant clones on which promotional processes can act increases with age. Overall, because initiation effects are expected to dominate radiation-induced premalignant clone production at younger ages at exposure, whereas promotional effects will dominate for older ages at exposure, a combination of these 2 effects would produce cancer risk patterns as a function of age at radiation exposure that would not be immediately apparent otherwise.

If we can believe this model, cancer risks after exposure in middle age may be up to twice as high as previously estimated.

A. D. Elster, MD

Multidetector CT Dose: Clinical Practice Improvement Strategies From a Successful Optimization Program
Wallace AB, Goergen SK, Schick D, et al (Australian Radiation Protection and Nuclear Safety Agency, Yallambie, Australia; Monash Med Centre, Clayton, Australia; Queensland Health Dept, Brisbane, Australia; et al)
J Am Coll Radiol 7:614-624, 2010

Purpose.—The aims of this study were to collect data relating to radiation dose delivered by multidetector CT scanning at 10 hospitals and private practices in Queensland, Australia, and to test methods for dose optimization training, including audit feedback and didactic, face-to-face, small-group teaching of optimization techniques.

Methods.—Ten hospital-based public and private sector radiology practices, with one CT scanner per site, volunteered for the project. Data were collected for a variety of common adult and pediatric CT scanning protocols, including tube current—time product, pitch, collimation, tube voltage, the use of dose modulation, and scan length. A one-day feedback and optimization training workshop was conducted for participating practices and was attended by the radiologist and medical imaging technologist responsible for the project at each site. Data were deidentified for the workshop presentation. During the feedback workshop, a detailed analysis and discussion of factors contributing to dose for higher dosing practices for each protocol occurred. The postoptimization training data collection phase allowed changes to median and spread of doses to be measured.

Results.—During the baseline survey period, data for 1,208 scans were collected, and data from 1,153 scans were collected for the postoptimization dose survey for the 4 adult protocols (noncontrast brain CT, CT pulmonary angiography , CT lumbar spine, and CT urography). A mean decrease in effective dose was achieved with all scan protocols. Average reductions of 46% for brain CT, 28% for CT pulmonary angiography, 29% for CT lumbar spine, and 24% CT urography were calculated.

It proved impossible to collect valid pediatric data from most sites, because of the small numbers of children presenting for multidetector CT, and phantom data were acquired during the preoptimization and postoptimization phase. Substantial phantom dose reductions were demonstrated at all sites.

Conclusion.—Audit feedback and small-group teaching about optimization enabled clinically meaningful dose reduction for a variety of common adult scans. However, access to medical radiation physicists, assistance with time-consuming data collection, and technical support from a medical imaging technologist were costly and critical to the success of the program.

▶ Is it possible to reduce patient dose significantly using multidetector computed tomography (CT) beyond current levels, giving attention to scanning parameters only and not buying specific dose-reduction software? The answer from this study is yes.

The study describes the results of a concerted effort by 10 hospitals and imaging centers in Queensland, Australia, to reduce patient dose on multidetector CT from September 2008 through May 2009. As listed in the abstract, very remarkable dose reductions (ranging from 24%-46%) were obtained, the highest being in brain CT. Key elements of their success included (1) buy-in from the participating institutions, (2) a formal workshop where protocols were discussed, (3) sharing best practices protocols among the groups, and (4) distribution of a step-by-step "how to do it" dose optimization sheet prepared after the workshop and distributed to participating sites.

This project demonstrates that through focused efforts and peer pressure, radiation dose to patients can be reduced significantly.

A. D. Elster, MD

Airport Full-Body Scanners
Mahesh M (Johns Hopkins Univ, Baltimore, MD)
J Am Coll Radiol 7:379-381, 2010

Background.—"Full-body scanners" are used at airports to screen travelers. They can employ either millimeter radio wave technology or backscatter technology. The former uses no x-rays. The latter uses a narrow x-ray beam to scan persons at high speed in a raster pattern. The backscattered x-rays are captured by large detectors that create back and front images within seconds. The relatively low energy x-rays used penetrate through clothing and may even penetrate through the body, but the most bounce off the skin surface. This allows them to detect objects hidden under clothing or taped to the skin but does not detect objects hidden deep inside the body. Transmission x-rays are needed for that. It is likely that mandatory screening of travelers using full-body scanners will become routine. The radiation exposure from backscatter x-ray full-body scanners was explored along with exposures to medical x-rays and other issues.

Exposure.—The backscatter systems currently used for security scans deliver effective doses of <0.10 μSv and can yield doses as low as 0.05 μSv. To receive a dose equivalent to that of a medical chest x-ray a traveler would have to have 1000 to 2000 backscatter scans. Air travelers are also exposed to radiation from atmospheric and other sources, which differ with altitude, flight path, and other factors. The scan dose is about what is received during 2 to 10 minutes of an average flight.

The National Council on Radiation Protection and Measurements defines a negligible individual dose (NID) as equal to the level of average annual excess risk of fatal health effects caused by exposure to radiation below which no efforts to reduce the exposure are required. An individual would have to undergo between 100 and 200 backscatter scans to reach the NID annual effective dose of 10 μSv. The annual limit imposed by the Nuclear Regulatory Commission and other regulatory agencies is 1000 μSv from all sources and 250 μSv from a single source or practice. A traveler would have to have 2500 to 5000 scans each year to reach this limit, which is highly unlikely to occur for a single person.

Other Issues.—A key concern especially in countries where maintenance may be unpredictable or absent is the long-term stability of the scanner to deliver low dose x-rays that permit sufficient image quality. A routine maintenance and quality assurance program conducted by properly trained individuals should be in place to verify that the radiation dose delivered does not exceed recommended limits.

Privacy is another issue because the images reveal anatomic details of the person scanned. To address this concern, the image viewing stations are set up at remote locations rather than adjacent to the scanners, the systems do not save the images once the individual is cleared to proceed, and software packages modify the images so they are less intrusive, appear more generic in form, and lack personal details.

Conclusions.—The backscatter scans conducted at security checkpoints in airports increase the likelihood that persons carrying dangerous devices will not be permitted on airplanes. The scanners deliver an acceptably low dose of radiation and are safe for general use even in infants, children, pregnant women, and persons with a genetic sensitivity to radiation. Their benefits outweigh any risks.

▶ If you have ever been to an airport and subjected to whole body scanning by one of the new x-ray backscatter devices, you may be interested to know how this technology works and how it compares to conventional radiography. If so, this 2-page article is for you!

Unlike the conventional transmission x-ray systems used in medical radiography, backscatter systems use x-rays that are backscattered or bounce off the subject (Fig 1). Narrow beams scan subjects at high speeds using a raster pattern with low-energy x-rays. These x-rays can penetrate through the clothing, and a few may even pass through the body. However, the majority bounce off the skin surface to be recorded on large flat-plate detectors. They

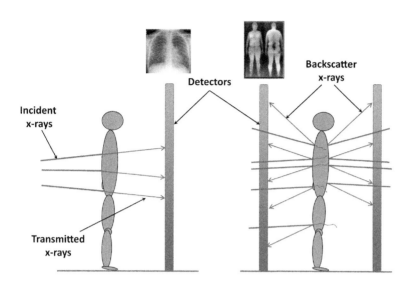

Transmission X-rays as in Medical Imaging **Backscatter X-rays as in Airport Full Body Scanners**

FIGURE 1.—Basic principles of transmission x-ray systems (medical x-rays) and backscatter x-ray systems (airport full-body scanners). (Reprinted from Mahesh M. Airport full-body scanners. *J Am Coll Radiol.* 2010;7:379-381, with permission from the American College of Radiology.)

TABLE 1.—Radiation Doses From Backscatter Systems and Number of Backscatter Scans Equivalent to Doses From Various Sources of Radiation

| | | | Number of Scans Equivalent to Doses From Other Sources | | |
Radiation Dose From Backscatter Systems (μSv/scan)*	Chest X-Ray[†]	Annual Dose Limit for Public[‡]	1 Day of Natural Background Radiation ($\sim 10\ \mu$Sv/d)[§]	Negligible Individual Dose[‖]	Average Dose From Air Travel[¶]
0.1	1000	2500	100	100	40
0.05	2000	5000	200	200	80

Note: A dose of 0.1 μSv from backscatter scan is equivalent to about 10 minutes of background radiation and about 2 minutes of radiation received from average air travel. A dose of 0.05 μSv from backscatter scan is equivalent to about 20 minutes of background radiation and about 4 minutes of radiation received from average air travel.
*10 μSv = 1 mrem.
[†]Typical chest x-ray dose is about 100 μSv [4].
[‡]Annual permissible dose to the general public from a single source is about 250 μSv [9].
[§]Annual natural background radiation dose is about 3100 μSv [5] or about 2400 μSv [6].
[‖]Negligible individual dose is about 10 μSv [8].
[¶]Average radiation exposure during air travel is about 4 μSv/h [7].

are thus useful for identifying objects on the skin and hidden under the clothing but are not useful for detecting objects hidden deep inside the body.

The radiation dose is minimal, less than 1/1000 of a chest x-ray (Table 1). There should thus be no concern of health risks, even in infants, children, and pregnant women. In fact, during your hour-long airplane flight at high altitudes you will absorb substantially more cosmic radiation than you will from the whole body scanner.

A. D. Elster, MD

Contrast Medium—enhanced Radiation Damage Caused by CT Examinations
Grudzenski S, Kuefner MA, Heckmann MB, et al (Darmstadt Univ of Technology, Germany; Univ Hosp of Erlangen, Germany)
Radiology 253:706-714, 2009

Purpose.—To assess the effect of iodinated contrast medium (CM) on the induction and repair of DNA double-strand breaks (DSBs) in peripheral blood lymphocytes after computed tomographic (CT) examinations.

Materials and Methods.—This prospective study was approved by the institutional ethics committee; written informed patient consent was obtained from 37 patients. Venous blood samples were taken from patients before and at 30 minutes, 1 hour, 2.5 hours, and 5 hours after performing CT with ($n = 18$) or without ($n = 19$) intravenous administration of CM (iopromide or iomeprol). DSBs were assessed in lymphocytes by enumerating γH2AX foci. DSB levels after CT were compared with those obtained after in vitro irradiation. Cell culture experiments with peripheral lymphocytes and fibroblasts were performed with iopromide, iomeprol, or the control substance mannitol added before or immediately after x- or γ-ray irradiation. DSBs were assessed at 5 minutes, 30 minutes, 2.5 hours, and 5 hours after irradiation. Data were analyzed by using linear regression and the one-tailed Welch and paired sample t tests.

Results.—The presence of CM during CT increases DSB levels in peripheral lymphocytes by approximately 30%. Cell culture experiments confirmed this effect and further showed that CM administered prior to x-ray irradiation increases the initial DSB yield but has no effect if added after irradiation or when γ-rays are used instead of x-rays.

Conclusion.—The highly sensitive γH2AX foci assay shows that CM-enhanced radiation damage incurred in peripheral lymphocytes during CT. However, it is unknown whether long-term bioeffects of low-dose ionizing radiation from CT examinations, such as cancer, are increased by using CM.

▶ I found this article fascinating because it raised an intriguing possibility I had never considered—that the presence of iodinated contrast in the body might potentiate cellular damage due to radiation. My first impression was, "No way! Who came up with this crazy idea?" But after reading on, there may indeed be something to this idea.

The technique used to study this phenomenon is not likely familiar to radiologists. The authors measured the number of DNA double-strand breaks (DSBs) in peripheral lymphocytes as an index to biologic damage induced by ionizing radiation.[1] Specifically, they enumerated H2AX (a phosphorylated histone) foci, which are thought to be a relatively sensitive and specific approach to measure the induction and repair of DSBs after low radiation doses.

The basic result from the study is that contrast media appear to potentiate damage in DNA induced by low-dose radiation by about 30% compared with radiation alone. It is still a long way from benchtop to bedtop, so the conclusions about final effects in humans such as induction of cancer are far from certain. Still, it is an intriguing concept to keep in mind as we consider the harmful effects of radiation in the future.

A. D. Elster, MD

Reference

1. Rogakou EP, Boon C, Redon C, Bonner WM. Megabase chromatin domains involved in DNA double-strand breaks in vivo. *J Cell Biol.* 1999;146:905-916.

Estimates of lifetime attributable risk of cancer after a single radiation exposure from 64-slice computed tomographic coronary angiography
Faletra FF, D'Angeli I, Klersy C, et al (Fondazione Cardiocentro Ticino, Lugano, Switzerland; IRCCS Fondazione Policlinico San Matteo, Pavia, Italy; et al)
Heart 96:927-932, 2010

Aims.—To estimate the life attributable risk (LAR) of cancer incidence over a wide range of dose radiation exposure and a large spectrum of possible diagnostic computed tomographic coronary angiography (CTCA) scenarios.

Methods.—This study included 561 consecutive patients who underwent a successful prospective ECG-gating CTCA protocol (low-dose group) 64-slice CTCA and 188 patients who underwent retrospective ECG-gating CTCA with ECG-triggered dose modulation CTCA (high-dose group). LAR was computed, given the organ equivalent dose, for all cancers in both sexes. LAR was tabulated for each decile of dose-length product by 10-year age classes, separately for each sex.

Results.—Estimates of LAR of any cancer for an exposure at age ≤40 year were lower in males than in females for any given quantile. At age ≥50 years, LAR was similar between sexes only at the lowest exposure doses, whereas at higher dosage, it was, in general, higher for women. At the median age of this case series (62 years) and for a radiation exposure ranging from 1.33 to 3.81 mSv, LAR was 1 in 4329 (or 23.1 per 10^5 persons exposed) and 1 in 4629 (or 21.6 per 10^5 persons) in men and women, respectively. For an exposure ranging from 10.34 to 18.97 mSv at the same median age, the LAR of cancer incidence was 1 in 1336 (or 74.8 per 10^5 persons) in men and doubled (1 in 614 or 162.8 per 10^5 persons) in women.

Conclusions.—This study provided an estimate of the LAR of cancer in middle-aged patients of both sexes after a single diagnostic CTCA, providing an easy-to-read table.

▶ This study provides practical estimates for the life attributable risk (LAR) of cancer incidence (including breast cancer) using real 64-slice computed tomographic (CT) scanner readings. The data show that in a typical population who might undergo a 64-slice CT because of suspected coronary artery disease or as a follow-up after coronary intervention (typical age range, 40-70 years), the estimate of LAR of any cancer approximately ranges from 1:1500 to 1:4000 for an exposure of 3 to 5 mSv, which is the most frequent range of exposure of prospective electrocardiogram (ECG)-gated CT coronary arteriography. However, for retrospective ECG-gated techniques in which exposures typically range from 8 to 25 mSv, the risk increases to between 1:300 and 1:1800. Tables are provided that can be consulted by practitioners when considering or advising patients to have such a study.

Like all similar studies, the LARs are based upon cancer estimates from the Biological Effects of Ionising Radiation Seventh Report (BEIR VII) phase 2 model.[1] It is recognized that the BEIR VII tables are subject to several sources of uncertainty because of inherent limitations in epidemiological data and in the general understanding of how radiation exposure increases the risk of cancer. Additionally, the populations and exposures from Hiroshima and Nagasaki may not apply to modern non-Japanese populations receiving significantly lower doses. Linear no-threshold models applied in BEIR VII have also been questioned.[2] Despite these uncertainties, the BEIR VII model is the current favorite among those who know, so we would be safe to assume these risks, even if overstated.

A. D. Elster, MD

References

1. Committee to Assess Health Risks From Exposure to Low Levels of Ionizing Radiation; Nuclear and Radiation Studies Board, Division on Earth and Life, Studies, National Research Council of the National Academies. *Health Risks From Exposure to Low Levels of Ionizing Radiation: BEIR VII Phase 2.* Washington, DC: The National Academies Press; 2006.
2. Tubiana M. Dose-effect relationship and estimation of the carcinogenic effects of low doses of ionizing radiation: the joint report of the Académie des Sciences (Paris) and of the Académie Nationale de Médecine. *Int J Radiat Oncol Biol Phys.* 2005;63:317-319.

Appropriate Imaging

Is the Use of Pan-Computed Tomography for Blunt Trauma Justified? A Prospective Evaluation

Tillou A, Gupta M, Baraff LJ, et al (Univ of California, Los Angeles)
J Trauma 67:779-787, 2009

Objective.—Many trauma centers use the pan-computed tomography (CT) scan (head, neck, chest, and abdomen/pelvis) for the evaluation of blunt trauma. This prospective observational study was undertaken to determine whether a more selective approach could be justified.

Methods.—We evaluated injuries in blunt trauma victims receiving a pan-CT scan at a level I trauma center. The primary outcome was injury needing immediate intervention. Secondary outcome was any injury. The perceived need for each scan was independently recorded by the emergency medicine and trauma surgery service before patients went to CT. A scan was unsupported if at least one of the physicians deemed it unnecessary.

Results.—Between July, 1, 2007, and December, 28, 2007, 284 blunt trauma patients (average Injury Severity Score = 11) underwent a pan-CT after the survey form was completed. A total of 311 CT scans were judged to be unnecessary in 143 patients (27%), including scans of the head (62), neck (50), chest (116), and abdomen/pelvis (83). Of the 284 patients, 48 (17%) had injuries on 52 unsupported CT scans. An immediate intervention was required in 2 of the 48 patients (4%). Injuries that would have been missed included 5 of 62 unsupported head scans (8%), 2 of 50 neck scans (4%), 33 of 116 chest scans (28%), and 12 of 83 abdominal scans (14%). These missed injuries represent 5 of the 61 patients with closed head injuries (8%) in the series, 2 of the 23 with C-spine injuries (9%), 33 of the 112 with chest injuries (29%), and 12 of the 86 with abdominal injuries (14%). In 19 patients, none of the four CT scans was supported; nine of these had an injury identified, and six were admitted to the hospital (1 to the intensive care unit). Injuries that would have been missed included intraventricular and intracerebral hemorrhage (4), subarachnoid hemorrhage (2), cerebral contusion (1), C1 fracture (1), spinous and transverse process fractures (3), vertebral fracture (6), lung lacerations (1), lung contusions (14), small pneumothoraces (7), grade II—III liver and splenic lacerations (6), and perinephric or mesenteric hematomas (2).

Conclusions.—In this small sample, physicians were willing to omit 27% of scans. If this was done, two injuries requiring immediate actions would have been missed initially, and other potentially important injuries would have been missed in 17% of patients.

▶ For those who practice at level I trauma centers, the number of complex pan-CT scans for trauma seems to be ever increasing. Radiologists, concerned about reducing radiation dose to the population, may berate their emergency physician colleagues for ordering what appear to be unnecessary studies. This article tries to put the high utilization of CT in trauma patients into some perspective.

For the definition of this article, pan-CT included CT scans of the head, neck, chest, abdomen, and pelvis. The list of missed findings in 48 patients that would have occurred should more restrictive criteria been applied is impressive (Table 4 in the original article). I must admit that after reading this article, I am much less likely to be critical of our emergency physician colleagues for ordering these tests.

An additional benefit of pan-scans was that exclusion of injuries with the use of pan-scan allowed discharge of patients who otherwise might have been admitted for observation. More than 10% of patients for whom admission had been planned regardless of CT findings, and almost 40% of patients with admission status that was undecided before CT, were discharged from the emergency department after the pan-scan was negative.

A. D. Elster, MD

Evaluation of Coronary CTA Appropriateness Criteria® in an Academic Medical Center
Miller JA, Raichlin E, Williamson EE, et al (Mayo Clinic, Rochester, MN)
J Am Coll Radiol 7:125-131, 2010

Background.—The aim of this study was to evaluate published appropriateness criteria for CT angiography (CTA) at the authors' academic medical center.

Methods.—Two observers independently reviewed the medical records of 251 patients who had undergone dual-source coronary CTA from June 1 to December 31, 2007. Patients were assigned to indications from 1 of 7 tables from the American College of Cardiology Foundation and ACR Appropriateness Criteria®. Agreement between the two observers was assessed using κ statistics. Disagreements were resolved by consensus panel. The final numbers of appropriate, uncertain, inappropriate, and not classifiable indications were recorded.

Results.—Indications for testing were classified as appropriate in 69 patients (27%), inappropriate in 42 patients (17%), and uncertain in 25 patients (10%). One hundred fifteen indications for coronary CTA (46%) were not classifiable. Analysis of interobserver variability for overall appropriateness yielded a κ value of 0.31, which was considered to indicate fair agreement.

Conclusion.—The results of this study suggest that a significant proportion (46%) of the coronary CTA studies performed at the authors' institution are for indications that are not covered by the published appropriateness criteria. Modifications to these criteria could help decrease the number of studies that are not classifiable. Physician education could decrease the number of inappropriate studies.

▶ Growth in spending for medical imaging has increased dramatically in recent years, and coronary CT angiography (CTA) has frequently been cited as a test with a high potential for overuse. Several national organizations, including the American College of Cardiology Foundation (ACCF) and the American College of Radiology (ACR), have developed appropriateness criteria for cardiac CT and MRI.[1] This article from the Mayo Clinic reviews how well clinicians at their institution ordering coronary CTA follow these appropriate-use guidelines.

The answer is, "Not very well." Only in just over a quarter of cases (27%) were the studies considered to have met appropriateness criteria. And if they can't do it right at the Mayo Clinic, what hope does this hold for the rest of us?

Perhaps the most useful finding to emerge from this study is the recognition that nearly half of the indications were unclassifiable. The authors suggest modifications to the ACR/ACCF criteria that would make them more useful and understandable.

A. D. Elster, MD

Reference

1. American College of Radiology, Society of Cardiovascular Computed Tomography, Society for Cardiovascular Magnetic Resonance, American Society of Nuclear Cardiology, North American Society for Cardiac Imaging, Society for Cardiovascular Angiography and Interventions, Society of Interventional Radiology. ACCF/ACR/SCCT/SCMR/ASNC/NASCI/SCAI/SIR 2006 appropriateness criteria for cardiac computed tomography and cardiac magnetic resonance imaging. A report of the American College of Cardiology Foundation Quality Strategic Directions Committee Appropriateness Criteria Working Group. *J Am Coll Radiol.* 2006;3:751-771.

Socioeconomic Issues

Changes in the Use and Costs of Diagnostic Imaging Among Medicare Beneficiaries With Cancer, 1999-2006

Dinan MA, Curtis LH, Hammill BG, et al (Duke Univ School of Medicine, Durham, NC)
JAMA 303:1625-1631, 2010

Context.—Emerging technologies, changing diagnostic and treatment patterns, and changes in Medicare reimbursement are contributing to increasing use of imaging in cancer. Imaging is the fastest growing expense for Medicare but has not been examined among beneficiaries with cancer.

Objective.—To examine changes in the use of imaging and how those changes contribute to the overall cost of cancer care.

Design, Setting, and Patients.—Analysis of a nationally representative 5% sample of claims from the US Centers for Medicare & Medicaid Services from 1999 through 2008. Patients were Medicare beneficiaries with incident breast cancer, colorectal cancer, leukemia, lung cancer, non-Hodgkin lymphoma, or prostate cancer.

Main Outcome Measures.—Use and cost of imaging by modality, year, and cancer type.

Results.—There were 100 954 incident cases of breast cancer, colorectal cancer, leukemia, lung cancer, non-Hodgkin lymphoma, and prostate cancer from 1999 through 2006. Significant mean annual increases in imaging use occurred among all cancer types for positron emission tomography (35.9%-53.6%), bone density studies (6.3%-20.0%), echocardiograms (5.0%-7.8%), magnetic resonance imaging (4.4%-11.5%), and ultrasound (0.7%-7.4%). Conventional radiograph rates decreased or stayed the same. As of 2006, beneficiaries with lung cancer and beneficiaries with lymphoma incurred the largest overall imaging costs, exceeding a mean of $3000 per beneficiary within 2 years of diagnosis. By 2005, one-third of beneficiaries with breast cancer underwent bone scans and half of beneficiaries with lung cancer or lymphoma underwent positron emission tomography scans. Mean 2-year imaging costs per beneficiary increased at a rate greater than the increase in mean total costs per beneficiary for all cancer types.

Conclusion.—Imaging costs among Medicare beneficiaries with cancer increased from 1999 through 2006, outpacing the rate of increase in total costs among Medicare beneficiaries with cancer.

▶ The authors of this article obtained administrative claims data for a national 5% sample of Medicare beneficiaries for 1997 through 2008 from the Centers for Medicare & Medicaid Services. Their goal was to look at imaging costs for 8 modalities: plain radiography, positron emission tomography (PET), CT, MR, ultrasound, nuclear medicine, bone densitometry, and echocardiography. As would be predicted, imaging costs in these patients increased substantially over the period. PET imaging grew the most (36%-54%), while conventional radiograph rates were static. The greatest increases occurred in patients with lung cancer or lymphoma.

Even though these growth rates were substantial, it should be recognized that imaging costs constitute a relatively small fraction of the cost of cancer care (less than 6%). During that period, the overall costs of cancer treatment not related to imaging increased by 3%-4%. Singling out radiology as the bad guy contributing to skyrocketing medical costs seems unwarranted in this population.

A. D. Elster, MD

Use of Advanced Radiology During Visits to US Emergency Departments for Injury-Related Conditions, 1998-2007
Korley FK, Pham JC, Kirsch TD (Johns Hopkins Univ, Baltimore, MD)
JAMA 304:1465-1471, 2010

Context.—Excessive use of medical imaging increases health care costs and exposure to ionizing radiation (a potential carcinogen) without yielding significant benefits to all patients.

Objective.—To determine whether there has been a change in the prevalence of emergency department visits for injury-related conditions for which computed tomography (CT) or magnetic resonance imaging (MRI) was obtained and whether there has been a change in the diagnosis of life-threatening conditions and patient disposition.

Design, Setting, and Participants.—Retrospective cross-sectional analysis of emergency department visits using data from the National Hospital Ambulatory Medical Care Survey (1998-2007). Sampled visits were weighted to produce estimates for the United States.

Main Outcomes Measures.—Proportion of visits for injury-related conditions during which a CT or MRI was obtained, a life-threatening condition was diagnosed (eg, cervical spine fracture, skull fracture, intracranial bleeding, liver and spleen laceration), and which resulted in hospital and intensive care unit admission.

Results.—The prevalence of CT or MRI use during emergency department visits for injury-related conditions increased from 6% (95% confidence interval [CI], 5%-7%) (257 of 5237 visits) in 1998 to 15% (95% CI, 14%-17%) (981 of 6567 visits) in 2007 (*P*<.001 for trend). There was a small increase in the prevalence of life-threatening conditions (1.7% [95% CI, 1.2%-2.2%; 59 of 5237 visits] in 1998 and 2.0% [95% CI, 1.6%-2.5%; 142 of 6567 visits] in 2007; *P*=.04 for trend). There was no change in prevalence of visits during which patients were either admitted to the hospital (5.9% [95% CI, 4.9%-6.9%] in 1998 and 5.5% [95% CI, 4.7%-6.5%] in 2007; *P*=.50 for trend) or to an intensive care unit (0.62% [95% CI, 0.40%-1.00%] in 1998 and 0.80% [95% CI, 0.53%-1.21%] in 2007; *P*=.14 for trend). Visits during which CT or MRI was obtained lasted 126 minutes (95% CI, 123-131 minutes) longer than those for which CT or MRI was not obtained.

Conclusion.—From 1998 to 2007, the prevalence of CT or MRI use during emergency department visits for injury-related conditions increased significantly, without an equal increase in the prevalence of life-threatening conditions.

▶ Scarcely anyone providing radiology services to hospital emergency rooms over the last decade has failed to notice a dramatic increase in imaging workload. This article, a national sampling of approximately 5000 emergency department visits per year over a 10-year period, quantitatively confirms the common wisdom (Figure 1 in the original article).

In adults, an approximately 3-fold increase in the prevalence of computed tomography (CT) or magnetic resonance imaging (MRI) was observed during emergency department visits for injury-related conditions between 1998 and 2007, without an equal increase in the prevalence of the diagnosis of life-threatening conditions or a change in the disposition of patients. Increase in CT use accounted for the majority of the increased CT or MRI use. In children, the increased use was about 2-fold.

What makes this article interesting is not that the increases were observed in advanced imaging but that they were not tied to increased hospitalization or change in discharge disposition. A major limitation of this study is that the authors do not consider whether changes in management to admitted patients occurred as a result of the imaging. Such management changes most certainly occur, for example, if a multitrauma patient destined to be admitted also has a cervical spine fracture.

I do not expect this paper to change anyone's practice, but it is interesting to see that such trends are being appreciated by high-level medical journals like *JAMA*.

A. D. Elster, MD

Teleradiology interpretations of emergency department computed tomography scans

Platts-Mills TF, Hendey GW, Ferguson B (Univ of California San Francisco-Fresno)
J Emerg Med 38:188-195, 2010

Background.—Teleradiologist interpretation of radiographic studies during after-hours Emergency Department (ED) care has the potential to influence patient management.

Study Objectives.—We sought to characterize frequencies of discrepancies between teleradiology and in-house radiology interpretations for computed tomography (CT) scans.

Methods.—We conducted a prospective observational study comparing teleradiologist and in-house radiologist interpretations of CT scans obtained between 7:00 p.m. and 7:00 a.m. from the ED at a Level I trauma center. For each scan, discrepancies were characterized as major, minor, or no discrepancy. Follow-up data were used to characterize major discrepancies.

Results.—Of 787 studies sent to teleradiology, 550 were scans of the head, cervical spine, chest, or abdomen and pelvis. Major discrepancies were identified in 32 of 550 studies (5.8%; 95% confidence interval 4.1%–8.1%), including 7 of 160 head CT scans, 1 of 29 cervical spine CT scans, 3 of 64 chest CT scans, and 21 of 297 abdominopelvic CT scans. We attributed 8 of the 32 major discrepancies to a teleradiology misinterpretation, with one case leading to an adverse event.

Conclusions.—We identified major discrepancies due to teleradiologist misinterpretation in 8 of 550 studies, with one patient suffering an adverse event. Our findings support the cautious use of teleradiology interpretations.

▶ Teleradiology has become common practice for emergency department interpretations throughout the United States. In 2004 a survey found that 82% of private community emergency departments relied on teleradiology services for nighttime image interpretations.[1] This study compared teleradiology and in-house interpretations of 4 common CT procedures (CT Brain, CT C-spine, CT Chest, and CT abdomen/pelvis) for 787 studies over a 3-month period.

Major discrepancies in interpretations by teleradiologists and in-house radiologists occurred for approximately 6% of CT scans. Somewhat surprisingly, misinterpretations by teleradiologists and in-house radiologists occurred at a similar frequency. Certain types of pathology commonly resulted in a major discrepancy in CT interpretation. These included intraparenchymal cerebral contusion or hemorrhage (6 cases), pulmonary embolism (2 cases), small bowel pathology (5 cases), and renal calculi (2 cases).

In summary, the teleradiologists in this study performed at error rates equal to the in-house radiologists. Both the teleradiologists and in-house radiologists were all American trained and Board Certified. The 6% major error rate seems a little high, as other studies have estimated the frequency of major discrepancies ranging from 1.5% to 5%.[2,3] It will be interesting to see whether these percentages hold up as similar observational studies are performed across a wide range of practices, including smaller emergency departments and academic centers.

A. D. Elster, MD

References

1. Saketkhoo DD, Bhargavan M, Sunshine JH, Forman HP. Emergency department image interpretation services at private community hospitals. *Radiology.* 2004; 231:190-197.
2. Gale ME, Vincent ME, Robbins AH. Teleradiology for remote diagnosis: a prospective multi-year evaluation. *J Digit Imaging.* 1997;10:47-50.
3. Robinson PJ, Wilson D, Coral A, Murphy A, Verow P. Variation between experienced observers in the interpretation of accident and emergency radiographs. *Br J Radiol.* 1999;72:323-330.

A Prior Authorization Program of a Radiology Benefits Management Company and How It Has Affected Utilization of Advanced Diagnostic Imaging

Levin DC, Bree RL, Rao VM, et al (Thomas Jefferson Univ Hosp and Jefferson Med College, Philadelphia, PA; HealthHelp, Inc, Houston, TX)

J Am Coll Radiol 7:33-38, 2010

Radiology benefits management companies have evolved in recent years to meet the need to control the rapid growth in advanced diagnostic imaging. The Obama administration and other key policymakers have proposed using them as a cost-control mechanism, but little is known about how they operate or what results they have produced. The main tool they use is prior authorization. The authors describe the inner workings of the call center of one radiology benefits management company and how its prior authorization program seems to have slowed the growth in the utilization of MRI, CT, and PET in the large markets of one commercial payer (Table 1).

▶ This article provides a nice review of how radiology benefits management companies (RBMs) operate and have affected access to imaging. RBMs are independent companies that contract with commercial insurers to serve as gatekeepers for obtaining prior authorization for imaging procedures. Currently 5 major companies dominate this market: HealthHelp, National Imaging Associates, American Imaging Management, MedSolutions, and Care Core National.

Several previous reports have suggested that RBMs are modestly effective in limiting the use of high-tech studies.[1,2] In this study as well as others, utilization rates tend to flatten out or decline initially after prior authorizations through RBMs are instituted, but may then resume an upward trend. As a result of the RBM process, about 4% of cases were either cancelled or changed to more

TABLE 1.—Results from the Radiology Benefits Management Call Center During 2008

	Requests (n)	Approved (%)	Request Withdrawn*	Examination Changed[†]	No Callback[‡]	No Consensus[§]	Referred to Next Tier
Tier 1	404,612	299,961 (74%)	4,164 (1%)	—	—	—	100,487 (25%)
Tier 2	100,487	82,598 (82%)	4,468 (4%)	1,736 (2%)	1,849 (2%)	—	9,836 (10%)
Tier 3	9,836	6,406 (65%)	1,261 (13%)	397 (4%)	1,620 (16%)	152 (2%)	—

Source: HealthHelp, Inc (Houston, Texas).
Note: Tier 1 is staffed by clinical service representatives, tier 2 by nurses, and tier 3 by subspecialized radiologists.
*The ordering physician agreed to withdraw the request for the study.
[†]The ordering physician agreed to change to a more appropriate imaging study.
[‡]A message was left, but the ordering physician or a staff member failed to return the call within 48 hours.
[§]The ordering physician and the subspecialized radiologist did not agree.

appropriate studies (Table 1). An overall decline in requests for imaging tests was seen and ascribed to a gatekeeper or sentinel effect.

A. D. Elster, MD

References

1. Iglehart JK. Health insurers and medical-imaging policy. *N Engl J Med*. 2009;360: 1030-1037.
2. Mitchell JM, LaGalia RR. Controlling the escalating use of advanced imaging: the role of radiology benefit management programs. *Med Care Res Rev*. 2009;66: 339-351.

Clinical Practice

Radiologist Report Turnaround Time: Impact of Pay-for-Performance Measures
Boland GWL, Halpern EF, Gazelle GS (Massachusetts General Hosp and Harvard Med School, Boston)
AJR Am J Roentgenol 195:707-711, 2010

Objective.—Expedited finalized radiologist report turnaround times (RTAT) are considered an important quality care metric in medicine. This study was performed to evaluate the impact of a radiologist pay-for-performance (PFP) program on reducing RTAT.

Materials and Methods.—A radiologist PFP program was used to assess its impact on RTAT for all departmental reports from 11 subspecialty divisions. Study periods were 3 months before (baseline period) and immediately after (immediate period) the introduction of the program and 2 years later after the program had terminated (post period). Three RTAT components were evaluated for individual radiologists and for each radiology division: examination completion (C) to final signature (F), C to preliminary signature (P), and P to F.

Results.—Eighty-one radiologists met the inclusion criterion for the study and performed a final signature on 99,959 reports during the baseline period, 104,673 reports during the immediate period, and 91,379 reports during the post period. Mean C–F, C–P, and P–F for all reports decreased significantly from baseline to immediate to post period ($p < 0.0001$), with the largest effect on the P–F component. Similarly, divisional C–F, C–P, and P–F also significantly decreased ($p < 0.0001$) for all divisions except the C–F for nuclear and neuro-vascular radiology from baseline to immediate period and the C–P component from baseline to post period for cardiac radiology.

Conclusion.—A radiologist PFP program appears to have a marked effect on expediting final report turnaround times, which continues after its termination.

▶ This is an interesting study using cash incentives to encourage radiologists to reduce turnaround time for signing their reports. Although performed at another hospital, we had a similar experience at our institution over the last 5 years where we also used a relatively small cash incentive to accomplish the same effect.

What is fascinating to me is how even for very highly paid faculty members, a small additional cash incentive (less than 5%) of their total income is sufficient to induce lasting changes in their behavior that persists even when the cash incentive is reduced or withdrawn. What we may be seeing is not the effect of the incentive alone, but a cultural change in departmental ethos, wherein individual physicians began to realize that reduced turnaround times were good for patient care and the operations of the department.

In our medical center, we found peer pressure to be an important factor as well. Each month, every faculty member sees the turnaround times of every other faculty member, including me (the Chair). So we are all on the line every month to keep the reports turning out in an efficient fashion.

A. D. Elster, MD

The Impact of an Early-Morning Radiologist Work Shift on the Timeliness of Communicating Urgent Imaging Findings on Portable Chest Radiography
Kaewlai R, Greene RE, Asrani AV, et al (Massachusetts General Hosp and Harvard Med School, Boston)
J Am Coll Radiol 7:715-721, 2010

Purpose.—The aim of this study was to assess the potential impact of staggered radiologist work shifts on the timeliness of communicating urgent imaging findings that are detected on portable overnight chest radiography of hospitalized patients.

Methods.—The authors conducted a retrospective study that compared the interval between the acquisition and communication of urgent findings on portable overnight critical care chest radiography detected by an early-morning shift for radiologists (3 AM to 11 AM) with historical experience with a standard daytime shift (8 AM to 5 PM) in the detection and communication of urgent findings in a similar patient population a year earlier.

Results.—During a 4-month period, 6,448 portable chest radiographic studies were interpreted on the early-morning radiologist shift. Urgent findings requiring immediate communication were detected in 308 (4.8%) studies. The early-morning shift of radiologists, on average, communicated these findings 2 hours earlier compared with the historical control group ($P < .001$).

Conclusion.—Staggered radiologist work shifts that include an early-morning shift can improve the timeliness of reporting urgent findings on overnight portable chest radiography of hospitalized patients.

▶ This is an article no radiologist really wants to read. It addresses a relatively common clinical problem that may be a patient safety issue. Specifically, what is the potential harm that may come to a patient who has a portable chest radiograph in the middle of the night, reviewed as unremarkable by a nonradiologist clinician but which contains an urgent radiologic finding not reported until the next morning? Because of the patterns and time delay between usual radiological morning shifts and work, there is the potential that critical findings could go unobserved for 12 hours or more.

The authors reviewed this experience at a large Harvard teaching hospital. They concluded that about 5% of overnight portable chest radiographic studies contained urgent findings requiring immediate communication, most often for tube or line malposition, pneumothorax, or lung collapse. By institution of a 3 AM to 11 AM radiology shift (vs the standard shift that begins at 8 AM), the median time for reporting such abnormalities was reduced from 457 to 350 minutes. Whether there will be many radiologists lining up as volunteers for the 3 AM shift remains to be seen.

A. D. Elster, MD

Lung Nodule Computer-Aided Detection as a Second Reader: Influence on Radiology Residents
Teague SD, Trilikis G, Dharaiya E (Indiana Univ School of Medicine, Indianapolis; Philips Healthcare, Cleveland, OH)
J Comput Assist Tomogr 34:35-39, 2010

Objective.—The purpose of this study was to evaluate the use of a computed tomographic lung nodule computer-aided detection (CAD) software as a second reader for radiology residents.

Methods.—The study involved 110 cases from 4 sites. Three expert radiologists identified nodules that were 4 to 30 mm in maximum diameter to form the ground truth. These cases were then interpreted by 6 board-certified radiologists and 6 radiology residents. The residents read each case without and then with a CAD software (Lung Nodule Assesment, Extended Brilliance Workspace; Philips Healthcare, Highlands Heights, OH) to identify nodules that were 4 to 30 mm in maximum diameter.

Results.—The experts identified 91 nodules as the ground truth for the study. The mean sensitivity of the 6 board-certified radiologists was 89%. The mean sensitivity of the residents was 85% without the CAD and 90% ($P < 0.05$) with the CAD as a second reader.

Conclusions.—The CAD software can help improve the sensitivity of residents in the detection of pulmonary nodules on computed tomography, making them comparable with board-certified radiologists.

▶ A number of studies have shown that the use of computer-aided detection (CAD) software as a second reader can improve the sensitivity of radiologists in detecting small nodules on chest CT.[1,2] This study is an interesting twist on this theme, using radiology residents to analyze chest CTs with and without CAD software as a second reader on a large series of cases collected from multiple sites. The sensitivity of the residents was then compared with the sensitivity of board-certified radiologists at various experience levels. Typically, the sensitivity of inexperienced and experienced readers for the detection of pulmonary nodules differs by about 5%.

The lung nodule CAD software proved to be a very effective second reader. It improved the sensitivity of the second-, third-, and fourth-year residents in detecting lung nodules to levels comparable with board-certified radiologists.

A. D. Elster, MD

References

1. Rubin GD, Lyo JK, Paik DS, et al. Pulmonary nodule on multiYdetector row CT scans: performance comparison of radiologists and computer-aided detection. *Radiology.* 2005;234:274-283.
2. Peldschus K, Herzog P, Wood S, Cheema JI, Costello P, Schoepf UJ. Computer-aided diagnosis as a second reader: spectrum of findings in CT studies if chest interpreted as normal. *Chest.* 2005;123:1517-1523.

Incidental Findings Are Frequent in Young Healthy Individuals Undergoing Magnetic Resonance Imaging in Brain Research Imaging Studies: A Prospective Single-Center Study
Hartwigsen G, Siebner HR, Deuschl G, et al (Christian-Albrechts-Univ, Kiel, Germany; et al)
J Comput Assist Tomogr 34:596-600, 2010

Objective.—There is an ongoing debate about how to handle incidental findings (IF) detected in healthy individuals who participate in research-driven magnetic resonance imaging (MRI) studies. There are currently no established guidelines regarding their management.

Methods.—We prospectively assessed the frequency of IF in 206 young healthy volunteers who additionally underwent structural MRIs of the whole brain as part of a scientific MRI protocol.

Results.—Assessment of the structural MRI by 2 board-certified neuro-radiologists revealed IF in 19% of the subjects (n = 39). In approximately half of these subjects (n = 21), these findings were of potential clinical relevance (eg, arteriovenous malformations, cavernomas, pituitary abnormalities) and required further diagnostic investigations. None of these potentially relevant IF prompted immediate active medical treatment.

Conclusions.—Incidental findings are very frequent in young healthy volunteers. Because many of the IF require further diagnostic workup, standardized procedures for MRI and the handling of these images are mandatory to ensure competent clinical management.

▶ Whenever research imaging studies are conducted in normal volunteers, a perplexing problem commonly arises: the detection of an incidental but potentially clinically significant lesion that may adversely impact the volunteer's future health unless noted and addressed. This article adds to the existing literature and controversy.

A number of previous articles have looked at such incidental lesions, especially in the brain.[1-4] In the aggregate, such studies have found incidental lesions in about 2% to 8% of subjects. This study found a much higher number (19%) that may represent sampling error but may also relate to the fact that their study used fluid attenuated inversion recovery imaging, which is known to be more sensitive than conventional T2-weighted images for the detection of white matter disease and other abnormalities.

A good discussion follows concerning the ethical responsibility that supervising imaging scientists have for reviewing scans in these subjects and notifying them and their health care provider of the abnormalities detected.

A. D. Elster, MD

References

1. Illes J, Kirschen MP, Edwards E, et al. Ethics. Incidental findings in brain imaging research. *Science.* 2006;311:783-784.
2. Vernooij MW, Ikram MA, Tanghe HL, et al. Incidental findings on brain MRI in the general population. *N Engl J Med.* 2007;357:1821-1828.
3. Yue NC, Longstreth WT Jr, Elster AD, Jungreis CA, O'Leary DH, Poirier VC. Clinically serious abnormalities found incidentally at MR imaging of the brain: data from the Cardiovascular Health Study. *Radiology.* 1997;202:41-46.
4. Morris Z, Whiteley WN, Longstreth WT Jr, et al. Incidental findings on brain magnetic resonance imaging: systematic review and meta-analysis. *BMJ.* 2009; 339:b3016.

Revised RECIST Guideline Version 1.1: What Oncologists Want to Know and What Radiologists Need to Know

Nishino M, Jagannathan JP, Ramaiya NH, et al (Dana-Farber Cancer Inst, Boston, MA)
AJR Am J Roentgenol 195:281-289, 2010

Objective.—The objectives of this article are to review the new Response Evaluation Criteria in Solid Tumors (RECIST) guideline, version 1.1, highlighting the major changes in the new version compared with the original RECIST guideline (version 1.0), and to present case examples with representative imaging.

Conclusion.—Familiarity with the revised RECIST is essential in day-to-day oncologic imaging practice to provide up-to-date service to oncologists and their patients. Some of the changes in the revised RECIST affect how radiologists select, measure, and report target lesions.

▶ If you don't know what RECIST is, you should. The acronym stands for Response Evaluation Criteria in Solid Tumors and was introduced in 2000 by an international working party to standardize and simplify tumor response criteria.[1]

Key features of the system included definitions of the minimum size of measurable lesions, instructions about how many lesions to follow and the use of unidimensional measures for evaluation of overall tumor burden. RECIST has been widely accepted as a standardized measure of tumor response, particularly in oncologic clinical trials worldwide. The original system has now been supplanted by a modified version, RECIST 1.1, published in 2009.[2]

Major changes in RECIST 1.1 pertaining to imaging include: (1) the number of target lesions, reduced from 5 to 2 per organ (Fig 7 in the original article); (2) detailed instructions about how to measure and assess lymph nodes; (3) clarification of disease progression; (4) clarification of unequivocal progression of nontarget lesions; and (5) inclusion of [^{18}F]-fluorodeoxyglucose positron emission tomography in the detection of new lesions.

In summary, if you are involved with imaging cancer patients, you probably need to be familiar with the RECIST 1.1 system.

A. D. Elster, MD

References

1. Therasse P, Arbuck SG, Eisenhauer EA, et al. New guidelines to evaluate the response to treatment in solid tumors. European Organization for Research and Treatment of Cancer, National Cancer Institute of the United States, National Cancer Institute of Canada. *J Natl Cancer Inst.* 2000;92:205-216.
2. Eisenhauer EA, Therasse P, Bogaerts J, et al. New response evaluation criteria in solid tumours: revised RECIST guideline (version 1.1). *Eur J Cancer.* 2009;45:228-247.

Impact of new technologies on dose reduction in CT
Lee T-Y, Chhem RK (Robarts Res Inst, London, Ontario, Canada; International Atomic Energy Agency, Vienna, Austria)
Eur J Radiol 76:28-35, 2010

The introduction of slip ring technology enables helical CT scanning in the late 1980's and has rejuvenated CT's role in diagnostic imaging. Helical CT scanning has made possible whole body scanning in a single breath hold and computed tomography angiography (CTA) which has replaced invasive catheter based angiography in many cases because of its ease of operation and lesser risk to patients. However, a series of recent articles and accidents have heightened the concern of radiation risk from CT scanning. Undoubtedly, the radiation dose from CT studies, in particular, CCTA studies, are among the highest dose studies in diagnostic imaging. Nevertheless, CT has remained the workhorse of diagnostic imaging in emergent and non-emergent situations because of their ubiquitous presence in medical facilities from large academic to small regional hospitals and their round the clock accessibility due to their ease of use for both staff and patients as compared to MR scanners. The legitimate concern of radiation dose has sparked discussions on the risk vs benefit of CT scanning. It is recognized that newer CT applications, like CCTA and perfusion, will be severely curtailed unless radiation dose is reduced. This paper discusses the various hardware and software techniques developed to reduce radiation dose to patients in CT scanning. The current average effective dose of a CT study is ∼ 10 mSv, with the implementation of dose reduction techniques discussed herein; it is realistic to expect that the average effective dose may be decreased by 2−3 fold.

▶ This is the best modern review article I have found that covers all the currently available methods to reduce patient dose on computed tomography (CT). Only 8-pages long including references, nearly everything is covered here: automatic exposure control in the axial, z-axis, and 3D modes; electrocardiographic current-modulated and gating techniques; dual-source and 256-slice scanner characteristics; and iterative reconstruction methods. The only technical item missing is a discussion of cone-beam CT systems, which are currently mostly a niche market for dentists and head and neck surgeons. A brief section on reducing patient exposures by reducing the kilovolt (peak) is also included.

In summary, this is a great review that provides a highly understandable discussion of all major topics in dose reduction with abundant references and without dumbing down the presentation to layperson levels. This is a must-read for every radiologist.

A. D. Elster, MD

Medical Malpractice

Stability and Infrequency of Radiologic Technologist Malpractice Payments: An Analysis of the National Practitioner Data Bank
Duszak R Jr, Berlin L, Ellenbogen PH (Mid-South Imaging and Therapeutics, Memphis, TN; NorthShore Univ Health System, Skokie, IL; Texas Health Presbyterian Hosp of Dallas)
J Am Coll Radiol 7:705-710, 2010

Purpose.—The aim of this study was to describe characteristics and trends of radiologic technologist (RT) malpractice payments.

Methods.—National Practitioner Data Bank data files were analyzed for details of RT malpractice payments from 1991 through 2008. Payment amounts, sources, and allegations were all identified and summarized, along with geographic and demographic data.

Results.—Between 1991 and 2008, a total of 155 RT malpractice payments were reported nationally, ranging from $750 to $11.5 million (median, $57,500; mean, $293,655 ± $1,305,091), with 153 (99%) <$1 million. Adjusting for outliers and inflation, payments changed little over the 18-year interval. More than half of all cases originated in 8 states, with per capita payments most common in Louisiana and New Jersey. Alleged errors in diagnosis accounted for one third of all cases.

Conclusion.—Malpractice payments on behalf of RTs are very infrequent (on average, <9 nationally each year) and usually relatively small (almost half <$50,000). Frequency and mean adjusted payment have remained stable over nearly two decades, likely related in part to "deep pocket" shielding by hospitals and radiologists.

▶ Although considerable interest has been directed to medical malpractice issues of radiologist physicians, little or no attention has been given to the liability issues of radiological technologists (RTs). Over the last 17 years, about 115 malpractice payments were made on behalf of RTs, and this article reviews this experience.

Compared with cases against physicians and hospitals, the number of cases (only about 7-9 per year) against RTs is very small, and the payouts are likewise modest (median = $57 500). The rate and levels of payments have been relatively constant over the period. More than half of the cases came from 8 states, the worst being New Jersey, Louisiana, Texas, and California. Allegations of malpractice included failure to diagnose (24%) and improper technique (15%).

This small database shows that even shallow pockets (RTs) are from time to time subjected to malpractice actions and may be held responsible for suboptimal care resulting in patient injury.

A. D. Elster, MD

Objective Determination of Standard of Care: Use of Blind Readings by External Radiologists
Semelka RC, Ryan AF, Yonkers S, et al (Univ of North Carolina at Chapel Hill; et al)
AJR Am J Roentgenol 195:429-431, 2010

Objective.—The purpose of this study was to determine whether specific findings determined to be critical and standard of care by expert witnesses in a legal case are identifiable by radiologists blinded to clinical outcome and litigation.

Subjects and Methods.—Images from six CT studies were sent to radiologists for interpretation. Two studies were performed for screening after major trauma, one of the cases being the subject of a settled legal action; three were randomly selected from studies performed in the evaluation of emergency department patients; and one was the control. The cases were selected to simulate a typical emergency department caseload.

In the medicolegal case, four plaintiff expert witness radiologists had identified three findings in the CT study that were not described by the radiologist of record (primary reader). One of these findings was considered critical and was the basis for the legal case.

Results.—Thirty-one radiologists participated in the study. The three findings made by the expert witnesses—T3 and T10 vertebral body fractures and 1-mm symmetric widening of the facet joints at T10—were made by none, 19 (61.3%), and none of the 31 radiologists in this study.

Conclusion.—Thirty-one radiologists who had no knowledge of the clinical outcome or litigation did not confirm the expert witness interpretation. This finding prompts questions about the current method of determining standard of care in legal cases, that is, use of paid medical expert witnesses. Our findings suggest that use of radiologists blinded to clinical outcome may be a more objective method of evaluating legal cases.

▶ From time to time, radiologists may be subject to a medical malpractice lawsuit in which it is alleged that they failed to make an observation or render a diagnosis that others would have made. The legal question asked is, "Did the radiologist fall below the standard of care in his/her interpretation of the study?" While the precise definition of standard of care may vary somewhat among jurisdictions, a common definition is what a reasonably competent physician would do under like or similar circumstances. Obviously this definition is unclear, and there is wide latitude in deciding how reasonably competent one needs to be and how similar the circumstances of a given case are to others.

In litigation, both plaintiff and defense hire expert radiology witnesses who opine as to whether a breach in the standard of care has occurred. While I have never been a defendant in a malpractice action, I have served as an expert witness on several occasions over the years and had to make this determination. I have always tried to be fair and keep an open mind to both sides, yet when an attorney calls and asks you to review some films, your suspicion is naturally heightened toward finding an abnormality, and it is difficult to assume the position of the original first reader of the study in the setting of the radiology reading room.

It has also been my experience that occasionally attorneys will (intentionally or unintentionally) present such cases to their experts with additional information that may potentially bias the expert toward a certain opinion. Such confounding information may be relatively subtle and relate to outcome, such as, "This child became paralyzed the next day. Tell me if you see anything on the first CT." Sometimes even more blatant bias is introduced, "Please look at this scan and tell me if you see any sign of lung cancer."

So the study by Semelka et al shows how such biases may occur in the system and the superiority of using independent readers who are blinded to all history. I have always believed such a blinded panel method would be a much better way of establishing standard of care for radiologists, but I am afraid it may take a long time for the US legal system to accept such a radical change to its procedures.

A. D. Elster, MD

6 Interventional Radiology

Introduction

Investigators continue to develop and enhance innovative and sometimes controversial image-guided therapies. One of the strengths of interventional radiology has always been the drive to constantly seek new ways of treating diseases and other medical states using more optimal yet less-invasive methods. Often in doing so, accepted treatment algorithms are questioned and sometimes are ultimately abandoned. This is one of the hallmarks of medical progress and scientific advancement, and the interventional radiology community continues to have a leadership role in this regard.

The current economic climate and the ever-increasing costs of providing accessible high-quality health care have raised serious questions regarding imaging utilization by physicians and patients, along with additional concerns regarding cumulative radiation exposure. Minimally invasive image-guided interventions sometimes represent far more expensive alternatives to more traditional treatments. Despite these constraints, however, therapeutic options continue to evolve, and when new therapies prove superior to existing ones, they are embraced, as they should be. Reporting such medical advances through unbiased peer-reviewed medical journals is crucial to improving the quality of care that we can offer to our patients.

In this year's selections for the YEAR BOOK OF DIAGNOSTIC RADIOLOGY, I have selected some innovative and occasionally controversial topics that have been recently published. In all instances, the investigators seek to expand the armamentarium that we have available for dealing with various medical issues, while hopefully also allowing us to improve patient outcomes in a less-invasive manner.

I hope that the readers will enjoy the articles that I have chosen this year.

T. Gregory Walker, MD

Balloon Angioplasty/Stents

A 5-Year Evaluation Using the Talent Endovascular Graft for Endovascular Aneurysm Repair in Short Aortic Necks

Jim J, Sanchez LA, Rubin BG, et al (Washington Univ School of Medicine, St Louis, MO; et al)
Ann Vasc Surg 24:851-858, 2010

Background.—Although endovascular aneurysm repair has been shown to be an effective way to treat abdominal aortic aneurysm (AAA), certain anatomic characteristics such as a short aortic neck, limit its applicability. Initially, commercially available devices were approved only for the treatment of AAA with an aortic neck length ≥15 mm. The purpose of this study was to evaluate the outcomes of the recently approved Talent endograft for AAAs with a short aortic neck length (10-15 mm).

Method.—Data were obtained from the prospective, nonrandomized, multicenter Talent enhanced Low Profile Stent Graft System trial which enrolled patients between February 2002 and April 2003. A total of 154 patients with adequate preoperative imaging were identified for this study. Subgroup analyses were performed for AAA with 10-15 mm aortic neck and those with >15 mm neck. Safety and effectiveness endpoints were evaluated at 30 days, 1 year, and 5 years postprocedure.

Results.—Patients treated with aortic neck lengths of 10-15 mm ($n = 35$) and those with >15 mm ($n = 102$) had similar age, gender, and risk factor profile. Both groups had similar preoperative aneurysm morphology in terms of maximum aneurysm size, degree of neck angulation, or proximal neck diameter. There were no statistically significant differences in freedom from major adverse events and mortality rates at 30 and 365 days. Similarly, there was no difference in the effectiveness endpoints at 12 months. At 5 years, there was no difference in migration rate, endoleaks, or change in aneurysm diameter from baseline. In addition, there is no difference in freedom from aneurysm-related mortality (94% vs. 99%).

Conclusions.—AAAs with short aortic necks (10-15 mm) and otherwise suitable anatomy for endovascular repair can be safely and effectively treated with the Talent endograft with excellent 1 and 5 year outcomes (Tables 1 and 2).

▶ Endovascular abdominal aortic aneurysm (AAA) repair has become widely accepted for treating aneurysms located in the infrarenal portion of the aorta. Currently in the United States, over 50% of all AAAs are repaired using this technique. Multiple clinical trials comparing endovascular aneurysm repair (EVAR) with traditional open surgical repair have confirmed the perioperative benefits of EVAR. In particular, 2 randomized trials, the EVAR 1 and the Dutch Randomized Endovascular Aneurysm Repair, demonstrated significantly lower perioperative mortality, operative time, transfusion requirements, and length of hospital stay with EVAR. Despite its benefits, EVAR is indicated

TABLE 1.—Patient Characteristics

	Group 1 (neck 10-15 mm)	Group 2 (neck >15 mm)	p Value
Number of patients	35	102	—
Aged—mean (range)	73.5 (51-86)	74.6 (53-89)	0.455
Male	32 (91.4%)	95 (93.1%)	0.715
Comorbid conditions (%)			
Angina	25.7% (9/35)	14.7% (15/102)	0.196
Arrhythmia	45.7% (16/35)	42.2% (43/102)	0.843
Coronary artery bypass graft (CABG)	25.7% (9/35)	27.5% (28/102)	>0.999
Coronary artery disease (CAD)	62.9% (22/35)	54.9% (56/102)	0.436
Cancer	31.4% (11/35)	30.4% (31/102)	>0.999
Congestive heart failure (CHF)	45.7% (16/35)	24.5% (25/102)	0.031
Chronic obstructive pulmonary disease (COPD)	45.7% (16/35)	30.4% (31/102)	0.105
Cerebral vascular accident (CVA)	22.9% (8/35)	22.5% (23/102)	>0.999
Diabetes	17.1% (6/35)	14.7% (15/102)	0.787
Hypertension	82.9% (29/35)	86.3% (88/102)	0.590
Myocardial infarction (MI)	31.4% (11/35)	38.2% (39/102)	0.545
Percutaneous transluminal coronary angioplasty (PTCA)	20.0% (7/35)	14.7% (15/102)	0.438
Peripheral vascular disease	48.6% (17/35)	48.0% (49/102)	>0.999
Renal insufficiency	54.3% (19/35)	56.9% (58/102)	0.843
Tobacco use	94.3% (33/35)	79.4% (81/102)	0.064
SVS classification (%)			
SVS 0 (none/low)	5.7% (2/35)	6.9% (7/102)	>0.999
SVS 1 (mild)	34.3% (12/35)	52.0% (53/102)	0.080
SVS 2 (moderate)	51.4% (18/35)	39.2% (40/102)	0.237
SVS 3 (high/severe)	8.6% (3/35)	2.0% (2/102)	0.105

TABLE 2.—Baseline AAA Morphology—Mean, Median (Range), n

	Group 1 (Neck, 10-15 mm)	Group 2 (Neck >15 mm)	p Value
Proximal neck length (mm)	12.9, 12.0 (10-15), 35	29.0, 25.5 (16-75), 102	NA
Proximal neck diameter (mm)	26.4, 27.0 (17-32), 35	25.3, 26.0 (16-31), 102	0.105
Proximal neck angle (°)	28.6, 28.0 (5-51), 25	30.5, 30.0 (0-72), 87	0.617
Maximum aneurysm diameter (mm)	56.3, 55.0 (40-82), 35	54.2, 52.0 (38-85), 102	0.228

only in select patients who have a favorable aortic anatomy. Certain anatomic characteristics, such as severe angulation, a large-diameter neck, or a short aortic neck, may preclude the applicability of EVAR. Currently, the indications for use (IFU) for most commercially available devices require an aortic neck length of at least 15 mm. However, the Talent endograft (Medtronic Vascular, Santa Rosa, CA) is the only device that is approved in the United States for the treatment of aneurysms with short aortic necks between 10 and 15 mm on the basis of their IFU. The current article evaluates the outcomes of EVAR using Talent endograft for aneurysms with a short aortic neck length (10-15 mm).

The Medtronic Talent eLPS study was originally initiated as a short-term, nonrandomized, multicenter, prospective, Investigational Device Exemption trial to confirm that design enhancements of the original Talent LPS would have a favorable effect on patient safety and device performance. During the 2002 to 2003 study period, 137 patients at various study sites throughout the United States received the Talent device for EVAR. Patients included in the trial were suitable candidates for elective surgical repair of nonruptured AAAs and aortoiliac aneurysms, who were at low to moderate risk for open surgical repair. Further inclusion criteria were aneurysms that were ≥4.0 cm in diameter, 1.5 times the diameter of the native aorta, or symptomatic and a proximal AAA neck ≥5 mm in length and ≥14 to ≤32 mm in diameter, with ≤60°, a distance of ≥9 cm between the renal arteries and the aortic bifurcation, a distal iliac neck length of ≥15 mm, and distal iliac diameters ≥8 and ≤18 mm. They were excluded from the trial if they were deemed at high risk for elective surgical repair (Society for Vascular Surgery/International Society for Cardiovascular Surgery score 3). Additional exclusion criteria were circumferential mural thrombus at the proximal neck; an aneurysm involving both internal iliac arteries; no distal vascular bed (≥1 vessel runoff was required); a known allergy to the fabric or metal components of the stent graft device; an untreated bleeding diathesis or a hypercoagulable state; a history of congenital degenerative collagen disorders; a systemic infection; a history of contraindications to contrast agents; and an episode of myocardial infarction, cerebral vascular accident, or major surgery within 3 months.

All patients underwent conventional angiography with a calibrated catheter and spiral computed tomography (CT), with minimum 3-mm slices. All patients underwent EVAR with the Talent device. Composition of the interventional team varied across sites, with only surgeons at some sites and with combinations of surgeons, radiologists, and cardiologists at other sites. Before discharge from the hospital, all patients underwent a physical examination, clinical laboratory tests, a 2-view (anteroposterior and lateral) plain abdominal radiography, and a spiral CT to evaluate device placement, graft patency, aneurysm size, renal artery patency, and presence or absence of endoleak. The recommendations for CT follow-up included contrast and noncontrast phases, performed at a minimum of 3-mm sections. The same studies were repeated at 1, 6, and 12 months and annually thereafter. All films, both preoperative and postoperative, were reviewed locally at each investigational site. In addition, all imaging were to be reviewed by the independent core laboratory during the first year of follow-up. However, sites were encouraged, but not required, to submit additional imaging to the core laboratory for analysis after the first year.

The study was designed to compare the acute and 1-year safety and efficacy outcomes of EVAR using the Talent endograft for low-risk AAA with conventional open surgical repair and to evaluate long-term safety and efficacy outcomes of the device through 5 years of follow-up. The primary safety end point was freedom from major adverse events (MAE) at 30 days. MAE were defined as all-cause mortality, myocardial infarction, renal failure, respiratory failure, paraplegia, stroke, bowel ischemia, and procedural blood loss ≥ 1000 mL. Additional safety end points were freedom from MAE at 1 year and freedom from all-cause and aneurysm-related mortality (ARM) at 30 days, 1 year, and 5 years; aneurysm rupture at 1 and 5 years; and conversion to surgery at 1 and 5 years. ARM was defined as death that occurred within 1 month of the index procedure to treat the AAA or death that was caused by

AAA rupture and a conversion to open or any other secondary procedure intended to treat the AAA. The primary effectiveness end point was successful aneurysm treatment at 1 year based on composite achievement of all 3 outcome states: technical success, absence of aneurysm expansion through 1 year, and absence of reintervention for type I and III endoleaks through 1 year. Technical success was defined as successful deployment without endoleak at completion angiography; deployment success was defined as ability to gain endovascular access and deliver the stent graft to the intended site in the aorta. Additional end points were related to procedural events such as blood transfusion requirements and duration of operation.

Two groups of patients were identified: those treated with aortic neck lengths of 10 to 15 mm (n = 35) and those with > 15 mm (n = 102). Both groups had similar age, gender, and risk factor profiles and both groups had similar preoperative aneurysm morphology in terms of maximum aneurysm size, degree of neck angulation, or proximal neck diameter. The patient characteristics and baseline AAA morphologies are summarized in Tables 1 and 2.

Both groups had a similar successful aneurysm treatment rate (88.0% vs 93.7%, $P > .39$). Technical failure occurred in 2 patients in group 2, and these were related to access issues secondary to diseased and calcified vessels. There was no device malfunction. Both groups had a similar rate of freedom from secondary endovascular intervention (84.8% vs 91.2%, $P > .32$), with no need for conversion to open surgical repair in either group. Combining the end points of successful aneurysm treatment and freedom from secondary endovascular intervention also showed no difference between the 2 groups. There were no cases of aneurysm rupture in the entire study. There was no difference in the effectiveness endpoints at 12 months.

At 5 years, there was no difference in migration rate, endoleaks, or change in aneurysm diameter from baseline. In addition, there was no difference in freedom from ARM (94% vs 99%).

The authors conclude that although AAAs with short aortic necks have traditionally been much more difficult to treat with EVAR, this study demonstrates the effective use of the Talent endograft in aneurysms with a short aortic neck length of 10 to 15 mm. They performed similarly when compared with aneurysms with a traditional neck length of > 15 mm.

T. G. Walker, MD

Drug-eluting Tibial Stents: Objective Patency Determination
McMillan WD, Leville CD, Long TD, et al (Minneapolis Vascular Physicians and Minneapolis Vascular Res Foundation, Plymouth)
J Vasc Interv Radiol 21:1825-1829, 2010

Purpose.—Endovascular management of limb-threatening ischemia often requires treatment of tibial occlusive disease. This study was preformed to examine the patency of drug-eluting tibial stents.

Materials and Methods.—The medical records of all patients undergoing drug-eluting tibial stent placement for limb-threatening ischemia from June 2004 to June 2008 were retrospectively reviewed. Postprocedural antiplatelet therapy included clopidogrel and aspirin. Patients were followed with serial arterial duplex ultrasonography and had selective subsequent angiographic evaluation based on noninvasive findings. Primary patency of the target lesion, limb salvage, and survival rates were reported.

Results.—A total of 240 patients underwent 283 tibial angioplasty procedures to treat limb-threatening ischemia during the 4-year period. Fifty-two patients (22%) had a suboptimal balloon result and were treated with a drug-eluting tibial stent. Balloon-expandable paclitaxel-eluting stents were used in all patients (1.2 stents per patient; range, 1–3; median diameter, 2.75 mm; range, 2.5–3.5 mm; median length, 24 mm; range, 20–32 mm). Forty-eight of those 52 patients (92%) had simultaneous endovascular treatment of proximal lesions. Mean follow-up was 14.3 months (range, 1–48 months). Target lesion patency of the drug-eluting tibial stent was 73% at 24 months (SE < 10%). Limb salvage rate in patients treated with drug-eluting tibial stents was 86% at 26 months (SE < 10%), and the survival rate was 65% at 24 months (SE < 10%).

Conclusions.—Drug-eluting tibial stents are a viable option for the endovascular management of limb-threatening ischemia and have acceptable patency rates. The majority of patients require multilevel endovascular treatment, and close surveillance is required for limb salvage (Figs 1 and 2, Tables 1, 2 and 3).

▶ Although the use of drug-eluting stents to inhibit restenosis has revolutionized the treatment of coronary atherosclerosis, the role of these agents in the

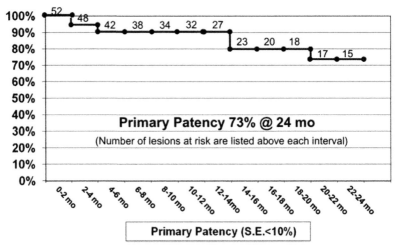

FIGURE 1.—Primary patency of target lesions. (Reprinted from McMillan WD, Leville CD, Long TD, et al. Drug-eluting tibial stents: objective patency determination. *J Vasc Interv Radiol.* 2010;21:1825-1829.)

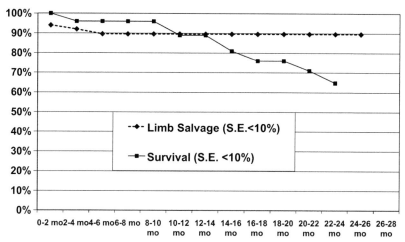

FIGURE 2.—Limb salvage and survival outcomes. (Reprinted from McMillan WD, Leville CD, Long TD, et al. Drug-eluting tibial stents: objective patency determination. *J Vasc Interv Radiol.* 2010;21:1825-1829.)

TABLE 1.—Patient Characteristics

Characteristic	Value
Mean (range) age (y)	73 (46–92)
Diabetic	32 (62)
Smokers	25 (48)
Dialysis	10 (20)
Male	34 (65)
Hypertensive	45 (87)
Hyperlipidemia	42 (80)

Note.—Values in parentheses are percentages unless specified otherwise.

TABLE 2.—Lesion Types

Lesion Treated	Number
Tibioperoneal trunk	12 (24)
Peroneal	16 (31)
Posterior tibial	17 (32)
Anterior tibial	7 (13)

Note.—Values in parentheses are percentages.

treatment of peripheral vascular disease remains undefined. Several trials have examined the potential application of these agents in the superficial femoral artery, with varying results. There are few data regarding the potential role of drug-eluting stents for the treatment of tibial occlusive disease. Endovascular

TABLE 3.—Target Lesion Primary Patency Rates (SE < 10%)

Interval (mo)	Target Lesions Patent At Interval Start	At Interval End	Cumulative Patency (%)	SE (%)
0–2	52	48	94.2	3.1
2–4	48	42	90.1	4.1
4–6	42	34	85.5	5.3
8–10	34	32	85.5	5.6
10–12	32	27	85.5	5.8
12–14	27	23	85.5	6.3
14–16	23	20	77.5	7.7
16–18	20	18	77.5	8.2
18–20	18	17	77.5	8.7
20–22	17	15	72.7	9.2
22–24	15	10	72.7	9.8
24–26	10	10	72.7	>10

treatment options for tibial occlusive disease are limited to balloon angioplasty, atherectomy, and tibial stent placement. Published patency data for each option are disappointing. Contemporary series of tibial angioplasty report 12-month patency rates between 51% and 63%, while reported patency rates for tibial atherectomy range between 58% and 42% at 18 months. Only a few studies have examined the patency of bare metal tibial stents, with reported patency rates ranging between 60% and 75% at 6 months. Drug-eluting coronary stents are an appealing option for the treatment of short-segment tibial occlusive disease, as the size of the vessels are similar and the patency rates of these stents in the coronary circulation are well documented. However, few published studies report the extended patency of drug-eluting stents in the tibial arteries. The purpose of the current retrospective study was to determine the objective patency rates for tibial paclitaxel-eluting stents placed for suboptimal angioplasty result at a single institution.

The authors retrospectively examined the records of 240 consecutive patients undergoing 283 consecutive tibial interventions for limb salvage in a 4-year period in their institution. Interventions consisted of primary angioplasty with drug-eluting tibial stent placement for a suboptimal balloon result (ie, flow-limiting dissection or residual stenosis of > 50%). Fifty-two consecutive patients (22% of all patients with tibial lesions treated) had 52 vessels treated with 62 Taxus stents (Boston Scientific, Natick, Massachusetts) for suboptimal balloon results. All patients received 300 mg clopidogrel at least 1 hour preprocedurally and 75 mg daily for at least 6 months after stent placement. Patients with sensitivity to clopidogrel were treated with ticlopidine. During the study period, all patients undergoing endovascular treatment of tibial lesions, including those undergoing simultaneous proximal intervention, were included in the study group. No patients were treated with bare metal tibial stents or other forms of tibial endovascular intervention (ie, atherectomy, cryoplasty). Taxus stents were used exclusively.

All patients had limb-threatening ischemia at the time of treatment (ie, Rutherford class 4-6). All patients were followed with duplex ultrasonography (US) at 1 month, 3 months, 6 months, and then yearly. The 1-month US study was used as the baseline for follow-up studies. Angiography was performed for US findings, including a decrease of greater than 0.2 in ankle-brachial index or an increase in peak systolic velocity across a stent-implanted segment exceeding 200 cm/s.

Forty-two percent of patients presented with gangrene, 40% with ulceration, and 18% with rest pain. (During the course of the study, patients with rest pain were offered tibial intervention only if they had an ankle-brachial index less than 0.4, if obtainable, and at least 2 levels of arterial occlusive disease.) Follow-up was achieved in all patients. Tables 1 and 2 respectively show the patient demographics and lesion distributions.

Only 1 tibial vessel in each patient was treated to restore inline flow to the foot. An average of 1.2 stents (range, 1-3) was used per vessel treated, with a mean lesion length of 28 mm (range, 20-32 mm). The mean stent diameter was 2.75 mm (range, 2.5-3.5 mm). Forty-eight of the 52 patients (92%) had simultaneous intervention on more proximal disease. Thirty-two patients had treatment of lesions in superficial femoral or popliteal arteries, 8 had iliac stents placed, and 8 had the iliac and superficial femoral or popliteal artery treated at the time of tibial intervention. The 4 patients who had isolated tibial intervention were all treated for gangrene or nonhealing ulcers. Primary stent patency, or target lesion patency, rates are shown in Fig 1 and Table 3. Paclitaxel tibial stents placed for suboptimal balloon results had a 24-month patency rate of 72%. The corresponding limb salvage and survival rates are shown in Fig 2. The overall limb salvage rate was 87% at 26 months and the survival rate for the cohort was 65% at 24 months.

This series adds to the existing data that suggest reasonable patency rates for drug-eluting tibial stents and provides the longest follow-up data available for their use in the treatment of tibial occlusive disease.

The authors add a caveat to this technique: they note early limb loss in a subset of their treated patients. In all, almost 80% of the limb loss occurred within 1 month of treatment. In each case of early limb loss, amputation was necessary despite a patent stent. Better patient selection could have avoided treatment for nonviable limbs. In most cases, endovascular intervention was undertaken as a "last-ditch" effort and, in retrospect, should have been avoided, with primary amputation chosen as the single best option.

The allure of minimally invasive endovascular therapy still needs to be tempered by the futility of intervention in limbs that are not salvageable.

The present study demonstrates that paclitaxel-eluting tibial stents used to treat short-segment tibial disease after failed balloon angioplasty have reasonable patency. Close surveillance and aggressive follow-up of all treated segments are needed to ensure limb salvage.

T. G. Walker, MD

Endovascular and open surgery for acute occlusion of the superior mesenteric artery

Block TA, Acosta S, Björck M (St Göran Hosp, Stockholm, Sweden; Malmö Univ Hosp, Sweden; Uppsala Univ, Sweden)
J Vasc Surg 52:959-966, 2010

Background.—Acute thromboembolic occlusion of the superior mesenteric artery (SMA) is associated with high mortality. Recent advances in diagnostics and surgical techniques may affect outcome.

Methods.—Through the Swedish Vascular Registry (Swedvasc), 121 open and 42 endovascular revascularizations of the SMA at 28 hospitals during 1999 to 2006 were identified. Patient medical records were retrieved, and survival was analyzed with multivariate Cox-regression analysis.

Results.—The number of revascularizations of the SMA increased over time with 41 operations in 2006, compared to 10 in 1999. Endovascular approach increased sixfold by 2006 as compared to 1999. The endovascular group had thrombotic occlusion $(P < .001)$ and history of abdominal angina $(P = .042)$ more often, the open group had atrial fibrillation more frequently $(P = .031)$. All the patients in the endovascular group, but only 34% after open surgery, underwent completion control of the vascular reconstruction $(P < .001)$. Bowel resection $(P < .001)$ and short bowel syndrome (SBS; $P = .009$) occurred more frequently in the open group. SBS (hazard ratio [HR], 2.6; 95% confidence interval [CI], 1.3-5.0) and age (HR, 1.03/year; 95% CI, 1.00-1.06) were independently associated with increased long-term mortality. Thirty-day and 1-year mortality rates were 42% vs 28% $(P = .03)$ and 58% vs 39% $(P = .02)$, for open and endovascular surgery, respectively. Long-term survival after endovascular treatment was better than after open surgery (log-rank, $P = .02$).

Conclusion.—The results after endovascular and open surgical revascularization of acute SMA occlusion were favorable, in particular among the endovascularly treated patients. Group differences need to be confirmed in a randomized trial.

▶ Acute thromboembolic occlusion of the superior mesenteric artery (SMA) is associated with poor prognosis. With the advancement of radiologic imaging, early detection is feasible and may result in a more planned technique for achieving intestinal revascularization. Hence, it is likely that more patients may be treated in present times and that the development of endovascular options offers a possibility to improve clinical outcome. However, prospective studies are difficult to carry out because of the low incidence and emergency presentation of these patients. Data from the Swedish vascular registry (Swedvasc, a nationwide registry for open and endovascular vascular surgery with high reported validity) from 1999 to 2006 were analyzed to study the outcome in patients undergoing intestinal revascularization and to assess the influence of radiologic imaging and endovascular treatment in a large patient cohort. The purpose of the present study was to analyze time trends and patient-related and management-related factors for outcome after open and endovascular intestinal revascularization for acute SMA occlusion.

The authors identified 174 revascularizations performed on the indication of acute intestinal ischemia during the period 1999 to 2006. Registry data were supplemented by retrospective analysis of patient medical records from 28 surgical departments. Long-term mortality data were obtained by crossmatching with the national population registry in September 2009 using the personal identity codes. Patients with symptoms of previous chronic mesenteric ischemia were included if they presented with an acute onset of intestinal ischemia. Eleven patients were excluded because of misclassification. The remaining 163 procedures and 161 patients were included in this study.

The onset of abdominal pain was divided into sudden (instantaneous, within minutes), acute (within 1 hour), or insidious (more than 1 hour). The clinical triad of acute embolic occlusion of the SMA was defined as pain out of proportion to abdominal signs, possible source of embolus (such as atrial fibrillation), and bowel emptying (diarrhea and/or vomiting). Chronic mesenteric ischemia was defined as postprandial abdominal pain with weight loss and/or chronic diarrhea. Patient's delay was defined as the time delay from onset of symptoms to hospital admission, and doctor's delay was defined as the time from hospital admission to start of the operation. Total delay was patient's + doctor's delay. Short bowel syndrome was defined as the need of parenteral nutrition or anti-diarrheal medication at discharge. The distinction between open and endovascular surgery was based on the primary vascular reconstruction. As a consequence, patients undergoing laparotomy with exposure of the SMA and retrograde open mesenteric stenting of the SMA through an open abdomen were considered part of the endovascular group. A second-look operation was defined as a planned control of bowel viability after endovascular or open surgery. If a laparotomy was performed as an immediate procedure in conjunction with an endovascular revascularization, it was not considered a second-look procedure but a part of the primary procedure. If, however, a laparotomy was performed later after an endovascular procedure at a defined time interval, it was considered a second-look despite the fact that it was indeed the first laparotomy performed. A reoperation was defined as being performed for deterioration or unexpected surgical complications. Completion control refers to any method used to objectively assess the patency of the vascular reconstruction at the end of open or endovascular surgery.

The procedures performed for embolic occlusion ($n = 99$) were open SMA embolectomy ($n = 85$), local SMA thrombolysis ($n = 9$), and endovascular aspiration SMA embolectomy from the groin ($n = 3$). Two failed SMA embolectomies resulted in 2 aorto-SMA bypasses. The procedures performed for thrombotic occlusion ($n = 54$) were antegrade stenting of the SMA ($n = 18$), thromboendarterectomy ($n = 10$), aorto-SMA bypass ($n = 15$), retrograde open mesenteric stenting ($n = 4$), local SMA thrombolysis ($n = 4$), thromboendarterectomy with a balloon catheter ($n = 2$), and reimplantation of the SMA into the aorta ($n = 1$).

Revascularization due to acute SMA dissection was performed in 5 patients with the following procedures: aorto-SMA bypass ($n = 2$), stenting ($n = 1$), fenestration ($n = 1$), and embolectomy ($n = 1$).

One patient had an acute thrombotic occlusion of a previously inserted stent within the SMA for chronic mesenteric ischemia, which was treated with recanalization and stenting. In 4 patients, the pathophysiology could not be determined. They were treated with bypass ($n = 1$) and embolectomy ($n = 3$).

This study indicated that the delay from onset of symptoms to revascularization was not significantly correlated with survival. This is probably explained by patient selection. Patients with severe symptoms are more easily diagnosed but also suffer from a more severe intestinal ischemia. Time delay to intervention is important, but the study results imply that revascularization may still be considered as a treatment option in cases with a significant delay to surgery. This finding has been reported previously and could be explained by the rich collateral mesenteric blood flow in some patients. Patients with a verified acute SMA occlusion at a nonvascular center could benefit from transport to an emergency vascular service with the possibility of both open and endovascular surgery. Such a strategy might offer a higher chance of proper intervention and survival. Insidious onset was, on the other hand, both associated with a longer delay to intervention and a higher mortality rate, which could reflect a lower diagnostic activity.

Computed tomographic angiography (CTA) is readily available in virtually every modern surgical department and was the most frequent preoperative diagnostic method in this study. A previous study showed a trend toward a higher rate of correct diagnosis by CTA if the referral letter included a suspicion of intestinal ischemia and/or SMA occlusion. In this study, clinical suspicion in the referral letter resulted in a higher proportion of correct diagnosis by CTA, and correct diagnosis after CTA was associated with an improved early survival rate. This is an important observation; the clinician should guide the radiologist by expressing his or her suspicion.

The endovascular group had a more favorable outcome compared with those treated with open surgery, both in the short term and long term. There were no significant differences between the 2 groups regarding age or gender. The endovascular group had a higher frequency of thrombotic occlusion and abdominal angina, whereas the group treated with open surgery had a higher frequency of embolic occlusion, atrial fibrillation, and synchronous embolism. There was a trend toward a higher frequency of previous vascular surgery in the endovascular group and previous cerebrovascular disease in the group treated with open surgery. Previous studies have reported that both thrombotic occlusion and previous vascular surgery are factors associated with adverse outcome. The effect of disease severity in patients receiving endovascular as opposed to open surgery could only be addressed in a randomized trial. But such a trial is unlikely to ever be performed because of the low frequency of SMA revascularization in most centers.

Completion control by angiography was more often performed in the endovascular group, which may have implications on outcome. Doppler scan measurement was used in a large proportion of patients in the open group, and this method should be considered inaccurate, whereas blood flow measurement with ultrasonic transit-time flow meter is more accurate, but inferior to angiography. No patient in the open group underwent angiography as completion control. It must be emphasized that angiography is superior for controlling the result after vascular intervention and provides accurate imaging and flow dynamics of the mesenteric vascular tree. Any insufficient revascularization can be visualized and small peripheral emboli can be detected. The information at completion control could be considered to have prognostic implications. It seems advisable to validate the revascularization with angiography whenever possible. Blood flow measurement of the main stem of the SMA should preferably be performed in the abdomen before and after open surgery revascularization.

In previous discussions on the advantages and shortcomings of open and endovascular therapy, the advantages of open surgery including completion control and inspection of the bowel have been evaluated. The results of this study imply that better completion control of the vascular reconstruction, being an integrated part of endovascular therapy, may be equally important. Second-look operation was more frequent in the open group compared to the endovascular group but was not associated with increased survival. This finding may be a result of selection bias. Patients with the most favorable prognosis, not experiencing any bowel symptoms after revascularization, are not likely to undergo a second-look procedure. This, however, is also the case for those with poor prognosis who are not considered candidates for further operative treatment because of advanced age or multiple comorbidities.

The authors conclude that endovascular therapy hypothetically offers many advantages over open surgery, in particular when only endovascular therapy without subsequent laparotomy for evaluation of the intestines is performed. It gives immediate and complete visualization of the vascular tree before and after intervention, and the patient can be treated without the inherent risks of general anesthesia. With the endovascular technique, the surgical trauma can be minimized and thus reduce infection, inflammatory response, postoperative ileus, opioid medication, and immobilization. All of the above could affect the clinical outcome in this group of usually elderly patients with multiple comorbidities. The authors demonstrated that the results after endovascular and open surgical revascularization of acute SMA occlusion were favorable, in particular among the endovascularly treated patients. Group differences need to be confirmed in a randomized trial.

T. G. Walker, MD

Iliofemoral stenting for venous occlusive disease
Titus JM, Moise MA, Bena J, et al (Cleveland Clinic Foundation, OH)
J Vasc Surg 2010 [Epub ahead of print]

Background.—Venous hypertension is a significant cause of patient morbidity and decreased quality of life. Common etiologies of venous hypertension include deep venous thrombosis (DVT) or congenital abnormalities resulting in chronic outflow obstruction. We have implemented an aggressive endovascular approach for the treatment of iliac venous occlusion with angioplasty and stenting. The purpose of this study was to determine the patency rates with this approach at a large tertiary care center.

Materials/Methods.—All patients undergoing iliofemoral venous angio-plasty and stenting over a 4-year period were identified from a vascular surgical registry. Charts were reviewed retrospectively for patient demographics, the extent of venous system involvement, the time course of the venous pathology, and any underlying cause. Technical aspects of the procedure including previous angioplasty or stenting attempts, and presence of collaterals on completion venogram were then recorded. Patency upon follow-up was determined using primarily ultrasound scans; other imaging methods were used if patency was not clear using an ultrasound scan.

Results.—A total of 36 patients (40 limbs) were stented from January 2005 through December 2008. Of these patients, 27 were women (75%). Both lower extremities were involved in 4 patients. Thrombolysis was performed in 19 patients (52.8%). Thrombosis was considered acute (<30 days) in 13 patients (38%). The majority of patients who had a recognized underlying etiology were diagnosed with May-Thurner syndrome (15 patients; 42%). In 9 patients, an etiology was not determined (25%). The mean follow-up time period in the study population was 10.5 months. One stent in the study occluded acutely and required restenting. Primary patency rates at 6, 12, and 24 months were 88% (75.2-100), 78.3% (61.1-95.4), and 78.3% (61.1-95.4), respectively. Secondary patency rates for the same time frames were 100% (100.0, 100.0), 95% (85.4, 100.0), and 95% (85.4, 100.0). Better outcomes were seen in stenting for May-Thurner syndrome and idiopathic causes, whereas external compression and thrombophilia seemed to portend less favorable outcomes ($P < .001$). Symptomatic improvement was reported in 24 of 29 patients (83%) contacted by telephone follow-up.

Conclusion.—Iliofemoral venous stenting provides a safe and effective option for the treatment of iliac venous occlusive disease. Acceptable patency rates can be expected through short-term follow-up, especially in the case of May-Thurner syndrome. Further experience with this approach and longer-term follow-up is necessary. Thrombophilia workup should be pursued aggressively in this population, and further studies should be undertaken to determine the optimal length of anticoagulation therapy after stent placement.

▶ Venous outflow obstruction can lead to ambulatory venous hypertension and chronic venous insufficiency. The symptoms of chronic venous insufficiency, including ulcerations, chronic pain, and/or swelling, are a significant cause of morbidity and decreased quality of life for patients. Common causes of outflow obstruction include acute deep venous thrombosis (DVT) and extrinsic compression of the iliac vein.

Chronic outflow obstruction after an episode of acute DVT manifests itself as a constellation of symptoms known as the postthrombotic syndrome (PTS). This includes symptoms of persistent pain, swelling, skin changes, and ulceration. Up to 29% to 82% of patients will develop PTS after an episode of DVT. These symptoms are thought to result from the chronic outflow obstruction after thrombosis and occlusion of the venous lumen. During this process, inflammatory changes take place that can result in vein wall fibrosis, leading to valve dysfunction, reflux, and insufficiency. Studies have shown that early thrombus removal and decreasing the incidence of recurrent thrombotic events can reduce the likelihood of developing PTS.

Chronic outflow obstruction can also result from extrinsic forces compressing the iliac vein. These include entities such as May-Thurner syndrome (compression of the left iliac vein from an overriding right common iliac artery) or pelvic tumors, fluid collections, or fibrosis. Catheter-based treatment of outflow obstruction in the form of angioplasty and stenting has been shown to relieve symptoms and improve quality of life. It has also been found to have comparable if not better patency rates than the currently available open surgical alternatives (bypass). This article evaluates the iliofemoral venous stenting experience in a single institution and reviews different technical and clinical factors in an effort to clarify risk factors for stent thrombosis.

Thirty-six patients were treated with venous stenting for symptomatic iliofemoral occlusive disease. Both patients who presented acutely and those whose disease was chronic were included in this study. In addition, patients who had their initial stent placed at another hospital and subsequently presented to the authors' institution after stent thrombosis for further care were included, provided that they required additional stenting. Those who did not require further stenting were not included.

Extent of the thrombosis was judged according to preoperative ultrasound scans and intraoperative venography findings. Clinical factors included clinical severity and time course of symptoms. Clinical severity was documented according to the clinical, etiologic, anatomic, pathophysiologic (CEAP) classification before the procedure. Etiology of the patient's DVT was determined based on patient history, findings in the preoperative workup, and intraoperative data. These were divided into 4 classes: May-Thurner syndrome, external compression from another source, thrombophilia, and idiopathic/unknown DVT. The disease was considered acute if symptoms had been present for < 30 days.

Popliteal vein access was used for intervention in most of the patients (20 patients), femoral access was used in 13 patients, and 3 patients had a combined femoral/jugular approach. Venography was performed to determine the extent of the thrombosis or obstruction. In all patients, balloon angioplasty was attempted before stents were placed. After angioplasty, the presence of recoil or persistent obstruction prompted the use of stents. A variety of nitinol self-expanding stents were used in most patients, and size was based on the vessel in which it was deployed. Two patients had steel self-expanding stents placed. Median stent diameter was 14 mm (range, 9-28 mm). Completion venography was then obtained to identify the presence of persistent collaterals or the need for further stenting. Inferior vena cava (IVC) filter placement was used selectively in patients who were felt to be at a very high risk for pulmonary embolus based on individual surgeon assessment. In these cases, retrievable filters were used. Postoperatively, all patients were started or continued on anticoagulation therapy with warfarin (goal-international normalized ratio, 2-3) or Lovenox for at least 6 months. Follow-up imaging was primarily done with duplex ultrasound scan. A small number of patients were reimaged with computed tomography, magnetic resonance imaging, and/or repeat venography because of difficulty in obtaining adequate imaging of the stents by ultrasound scan alone. No follow-up data were available for 3 patients.

Forty limbs were stented in the 36 patients who underwent lower extremity venous stenting for occlusive disease, as 4 patients (11%) had bilateral lower extremity involvement. The occlusion was considered acute in 14 of the patients (39%) presenting for treatment. In the categories of defined etiology of the occlusion, 15 patients (41.7%) had May-Thurner syndrome, 9 patients (25%) had an idiopathic/unknown cause, 7 patients had external compression (19.4%), and 5 patients (13.9%) had a known underlying thrombophilia.

Clot burden was isolated to the left side in 24 patients (66.7%), the right side in 7 patients (19.4%), and bilateral in 4 patients (11%). IVC involvement was noted in 12 patients (33%), femoral veins were occluded in 26 patients (19 left, 6 right, and 1 bilateral), and the clot extended down to the popliteal vein in 14 patients (38.9%). Initial thrombolysis was done in 19 patients (52.8%), which took place for 12 to 72 hours. Three of the 19 patients had residual clot present at the cessation of thrombolysis. In all, 73 stents were placed in 40 limbs.

Postoperatively, 1 stent had early thrombosis and required acute reoperation. Otherwise, there were no complications associated with the stenting; no incidences of pulmonary embolus were recorded and no bleeding complications were noted. Primary patency rates at 6, 12, and 24 months were 88% (75.2-100), 78.3% (61.1-95.4), and 78.3% (61.1-95.4), respectively. Secondary patency rates for the same time frames were 100% (100.0, 100.0), 95% (85.4, 100.0), and 95% (85.4, 100.0), respectively. Mean follow-up time was 10.5 months with a range of 0 to 38 months. At follow-up, mean CEAP clinical severity score had decreased to 1.97. One patient in this study had venous ulceration preoperatively; upon follow-up, this had healed.

Results from this small retrospective study show that excellent patency rates and symptomatic improvement can be obtained with stenting for venous outflow occlusion. The primary and secondary patency rates at 2 years of 78% and 95%, respectively, are comparable to those found by previous studies. Primary patency was lost in 5 patients at mean follow-up of 10 months, all but one of these stents was able to be reopened. In the last patient, another operation was refused by the patient and actually not recommended by the surgeon, as the patient's symptoms of edema, claudication, and skin changes were improving.

Other studies have divided the etiologies into thrombotic and nonthrombotic disease, but no study has looked at the different causes of thrombotic disease to discern its effect on stent outcome. This study showed a worse outcome with etiologic factors of diagnosed thrombophilia and external compression as opposed to May-Thurner syndrome or idiopathic causes. Of the stents that lost primary patency, 2 patients had diagnosed thrombophilia and 3 had external compression as the underlying etiologies. Two of the patients in the external compression group occluded their stents within a month of being taken off their anticoagulation. One of the 2 patients was subsequently found to have an underlying thrombophilia. Once anticoagulation was restarted, there were no further problems. This brings forward the question of how long to continue anticoagulation in people with venous stents and whether to pursue a hypercoagulable workup more frequently in this patient population.

In summary, the results of this study indicate that venous stenting for iliofemoral occlusive disease is a safe and effective method of treatment. It can be done with excellent patency rates expected in cases of idiopathic occlusion and May-Thurner syndrome. However, in cases in which external compression or inherent thrombophilia is the cause of the underlying occlusion, poorer outcomes can be expected. In addition, perhaps a more aggressive approach toward hypercoagulability assessment should be pursued in this patient population, and studies to determine the optimal duration of anticoagulation therapy after venous stenting are needed.

T. G. Walker, MD

Management of Transjugular Intrahepatic Portosystemic Shunt (TIPS)-associated Refractory Hepatic Encephalopathy by Shunt Reduction Using the Parallel Technique: Outcomes of a Retrospective Case Series
Cookson DT, Zaman Z, Gordon-Smith J, et al (Royal Infirmary, Edinburgh, Scotland, UK)
Cardiovasc Intervent Radiol 34:92-99, 2011

Purpose.—To investigate the reproducibility and technical and clinical success of the parallel technique of transjugular intrahepatic portosystemic shunt (TIPS) reduction in the management of refractory hepatic encephalopathy (HE).

Materials and Methods.—A 10-mm-diameter self-expanding stent graft and a 5–6-mm-diameter balloon-expandable stent were placed in parallel inside the existing TIPS in 8 patients via a dual unilateral transjugular approach. Changes in portosystemic pressure gradient and HE grade were used as primary end points.

Results.—TIPS reduction was technically successful in all patients. Mean ± standard deviation portosystemic pressure gradient before and after shunt reduction was 4.9 ± 3.6 mmHg (range, 0–12 mmHg) and 10.5 ± 3.9 mmHg (range, 6–18 mmHg). Duration of follow-up was 137 ± 117.8 days (range, 18–326 days). Clinical improvement of HE occurred in 5 patients (62.5%) with resolution of HE in 4 patients (50%). Single episodes of recurrent gastrointestinal hemorrhage occurred in 3 patients (37.5%). These were self-limiting in 2 cases and successfully managed in 1 case by correction of coagulopathy and blood transfusion. Two of these patients (25%) died, one each of renal failure and hepatorenal failure.

Conclusion.—The parallel technique of TIPS reduction is reproducible and has a high technical success rate. A dual unilateral transjugular approach is advantageous when performing this procedure. The parallel technique allows repeat bidirectional TIPS adjustment and may be of significant clinical benefit in the management of refractory HE (Figs 3, 5 and 6).

▶ Hepatic encephalopathy (HE) is a common complication of transjugular intrahepatic portosystemic shunt (TIPS) procedures, with reported incidences of 5% to 35%. TIPS-associated HE refractory to medical therapy occurs in 3% to 7% of patients. Treatment options in this setting include liver transplant, TIPS reduction or occlusion, and embolization of splenorenal portosystemic shunts.

Multiple TIPS-directed procedures have been described and are associated with different advantages and disadvantages in terms of their potential reversibility and risk of adverse outcomes. TIPS reduction by parallel placement of

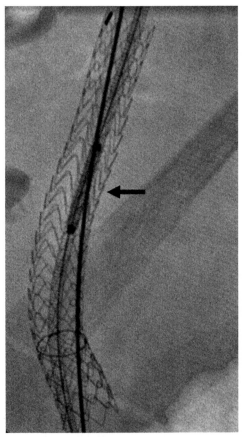

FIGURE 3.—Undeployed balloon-expandable stent (*arrow*) within 6F sheath at the midpoint of the covered portion of TIPS. (Reprinted from Cookson DT, Zaman Z, Gordon-Smith J, et al. Management of transjugular intrahepatic portosystemic shunt (tips)-associated refractory hepatic encephalopathy by shunt reduction using the parallel technique: outcomes of a retrospective case series. *Cardiovasc Intervent Radiol*. 2011;34:92-99, with permission from Springer Science+Business Media, LLC and the Cardiovascular and Interventional Radiological Society of Europe (CIRSE).)

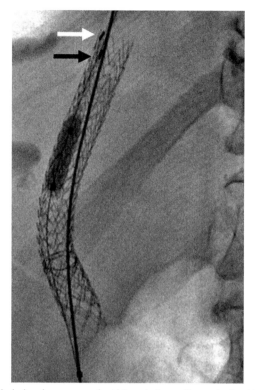

FIGURE 5.—Fully deployed new stent graft with lateral release of its proximal end (*black arrow*) toward the inner wall of the old stent graft (*white arrow*). (Reprinted from Cookson DT, Zaman Z, Gordon-Smith J, et al. Management of transjugular intrahepatic portosystemic shunt (tips)-associated refractory hepatic encephalopathy by shunt reduction using the parallel technique: outcomes of a retrospective case series. *Cardiovasc Intervent Radiol.* 2011;34:92-99, with permission from Springer Science+Business Media, LLC and the Cardiovascular and Interventional Radiological Society of Europe (CIRSE).)

a self-expanding stent graft and a balloon-expandable stent inside an existing TIPS allows bidirectional adjustment of shunt diameter and portosystemic pressure gradient (PSPG), thereby optimizing control of TIPS configuration and flow. Repeat bidirectional TIPS adjustment is also feasible using this method. These advantages are not conferred by alternative TIPS reduction procedures. The published data experience of the parallel technique is, however, limited to a small number of case reports and case series. This study is the second largest to date of the parallel technique and comprises the largest reported experience of its accomplishment via a solely transjugular approach. The reproducibility of this procedure and its technical and clinical success were investigated by means of changes in PSPG and HE grade as primary end points.

Eight patients underwent TIPS reduction using the parallel technique. The median interval from TIPS creation to TIPS reduction was 509.6 days. TIPS creation was performed in a total of 61 patients during the study period. All patients were referred after hepatology assessment by a specialist. Child-Pugh scores at the time of initial patient referral were B (n = 3; 37.5%) and C

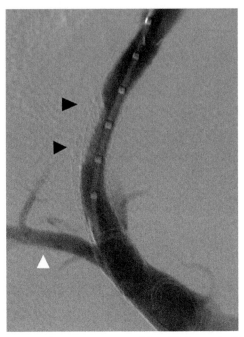

FIGURE 6.—TIPS angiogram demonstrating narrowed shunt (*black arrowheads*) and increased intrahepatic portal vein opacification (*white arrowhead*). (Reprinted from Cookson DT, Zaman Z, Gordon-Smith J, et al. Management of transjugular intrahepatic portosystemic shunt (tips)-associated refractory hepatic encephalopathy by shunt reduction using the parallel technique: outcomes of a retrospective case series. *Cardiovasc Intervent Radiol.* 2011;34:92-99, with permission from Springer Science+Business Media, LLC and the Cardiovascular and Interventional Radiological Society of Europe (CIRSE).)

(n = 5; 62.5%). The indication for TIPS reduction was HE refractory to medical treatment. HE at the time of initial patient referral was classified as grade I (n = 1; 12.5%), grade II (n = 3; 37.5%), grade III (n = 2; 25%), and grade IV (n = 2; 25%). Medical treatment of HE included regular oral administration of lactulose (n = 8; 100%) and neomycin (n = 4; 50%) supplemented in one patient with the administration of phosphate enemas as appropriate. Upper gastrointestinal endoscopy was performed during the admission period in all patients with a history of variceal hemorrhage (n = 6; 75%). Prophylactic treatment by banding was also carried out at this time if required.

TIPS creation was performed with 10-mm-diameter self-expanding polytetra-fluoroethylene-covered nitinol Viatorr stent grafts (W. L. Gore & Associates, Flagstaff, AZ) that were postdilated to 10 mm in all patients. The mean PSPG before and after TIPS creation was 20.2 ± 8.6 mm Hg and 4.5 ± 3.4 mm Hg, respectively. The decrease in PSPG was 15.8 ± 6.6 mm Hg (range, 5-27 mm Hg).

TIPS reduction was performed according to the technique described by Holden et al via the right (n = 7) or left (n = 1) internal jugular vein. The procedure was carried out in an angiography suite using local anesthesia in all patients and moderate sedation as required. Systemic venous pressure was recorded with a 40-cm 10F sheath placed within the right atrium. The TIPS was then accessed through the 10F sheath with standard catheters and wires. TIPS angiography and portal venous pressure measurement were performed with a pigtail catheter, and the initial PSPG was recorded. The 10F sheath was then advanced through the TIPS into the portal vein. A 45-cm 6F Destination sheath was subsequently advanced through the TIPS into the portal vein via a second puncture of the ipsilateral internal jugular vein. A short 5-mm-diameter (n = 5) or 6-mm-diameter (n = 3) balloon-expandable uncovered stent was then introduced through the 6F sheath and positioned at the midpoint of the covered portion of the in situ Viatorr stent graft (Fig 3). A new 10-mm-diameter Viatorr stent graft was then introduced through the 10F sheath over a stiff guide wire and advanced until the radiopaque ring marking the junction of its covered and uncovered portions was level with the marker ring of the in situ stent graft. The 6F sheath was then withdrawn into the right atrium to allow deployment of the balloon-expandable stent. The uncovered portion of the new stent graft was deployed by withdrawal of the 10F sheath into the right atrium, maintaining superimposition of the ring markers of both stent grafts. The balloon-expandable stent was then dilated to its nominal diameter, and the covered portion of the new stent graft was subsequently deployed with the angioplasty balloon still inflated (Fig 5).

The new stent graft was thereby focally narrowed at its midpoint by extrinsic compression from the balloon-expandable stent. Postreduction TIPS angiography was then performed to confirm patency of the narrowed shunt (Fig 6), and the postreduction PSPG was recorded. The angioplasty balloon was subsequently deflated and removed. Hemostasis was achieved by manual compression of both puncture sites after sheath and guide wire removal.

Clinical follow-up was performed by the same hepatologists responsible for initial patient referral.

Study end points were the technical and clinical success of the procedure. Technical success was defined as an increase in PSPG associated with correct placement of the stent graft and balloon-expandable stent in the absence of any immediate complications. Note was also made of any increase in intrahepatic portal perfusion immediately after performing TIPS reduction. This was determined by the presence of antegrade angiographic opacification of a greater length and/or number of intrahepatic portal vein branches in comparison with the preliminary angiogram. TIPS reduction was considered to be clinically successful if the worst HE grade at follow-up was better than that at the time of referral. Recurrence of gastrointestinal hemorrhage and any other adverse clinical events after TIPS reduction were also recorded.

TIPS reduction was technically successful in all patients. The mean PSPG before and after shunt reduction was 4.9 ± 3.6 mm Hg and 10.5 ± 3.9 mm Hg, respectively. The increase in PSPG was 5.6 ± 2.1 mm Hg (range, 2-8 mm Hg). Intrahepatic portal vein perfusion increased in 3 patients (37.5%). There was no clear correlation between changes in PSPG or intrahepatic portal vein perfusion and changes in HE grade. Opacification of portosystemic varices was noted in 1 patient (12.5%) with a final PSPG of 6 mm Hg. Variceal opacification was present before TIPS reduction in this case and did not significantly increase. Prophylactic embolization was not concurrently performed in this or any other patient.

Mean ± SD duration of follow-up was 137 ± 117.8 days (range, 18-326 days). Follow-up was performed to the end of the study period (n = 5), death (n = 2), or liver transplant (n = 1). Mean encephalopathy grade improved from 2.6 to 1.5. Clinical improvement of HE occurred in 5 patients (62.5%), with resolution of HE in 4 patients (50%) and partial improvement in 1 patient (12.5%). No adverse clinical events occurred in patients in whom HE grade improved. HE grade failed to improve in 3 patients (37.5%). Single episodes of recurrent gastrointestinal hemorrhage occurred in these 3 cases.

The findings of this study confirm the reproducibility and high technical success rate of the parallel technique. A dual unilateral transjugular approach was successful in all cases and allowed accurate and reliable positioning of the stent graft and stent. A combined transjugular and transfemoral approach is an alternative, but TIPS catheterization via the transfemoral route is less anatomically favorable and may not be possible. Dual unilateral access via the right internal jugular vein is straightforward and is suggested as the first-line approach to this procedure. A left-sided transjugular approach is also feasible if required. TIPS reduction was beneficial in most patients, with clinical improvement (62.5%) and resolution (50%) of HE, comparable with previous results that used the parallel technique. Overall clinical outcomes were not, however, universally favorable. In accordance with previous findings, the occurrence of persistently severe or progressive postprocedural encephalopathy was associated with significant morbidity and mortality. An increased risk of complications of portal hypertension is also expected after TIPS reduction. Routine periprocedural endoscopy is, therefore, recommended in all patients with a history of varices to minimize the incidence of recurrent gastrointestinal hemorrhage. The 3 patients (37.5%) in this study with recurrent hemorrhage were successfully treated by conservative management and were not referred for TIPS reevaluation.

The optimal procedural end point of TIPS reduction is uncertain and may vary between patients. An increase in PSPG was used as the end point in this study and was achieved in all patients.

The authors conclude that the parallel technique is a reproducible method of TIPS reduction and has a high technical success rate. A dual unilateral transjugular approach is advantageous when performing this procedure. The parallel technique allows repeat bidirectional TIPS adjustment and may be of significant clinical benefit in the management of refractory HE. Additional investigation is required to further define the end points of TIPS reduction associated with optimum clinical outcome.

T. G. Walker, MD

The Carotid Revascularization Endarterectomy Versus Stenting Trial (CREST): Stenting Versus Carotid Endarterectomy for Carotid Disease

Mantese VA, for the CREST Investigators (St John's Mercy Med Ctr/St Louis Vascular Ctr, St Louis, MO; et al)
Stroke 41:S31-S34, 2010

Background and Purpose.—Carotid artery stenosis causes up to 10% of all ischemic strokes. Carotid endarterectomy (CEA) was introduced as a treatment to prevent stroke in the early 1950s. Carotid stenting (CAS) was introduced as a treatment to prevent stroke in 1994.

Methods.—The Carotid Revascularization Endarterectomy versus Stenting Trial (CREST) is a randomized trial with blinded end point adjudication. Symptomatic and asymptomatic patients were randomized to CAS or CEA. The primary end point was the composite of any stroke, myocardial infarction, or death during the periprocedural period and ipsilateral stroke thereafter, up to 4 years.

Results.—There was no significant difference in the rates of the primary end point between CAS and CEA (7.2% versus 6.8%; hazard ratio, 1.11; 95% CI, 0.81 to 1.51; $P=0.51$). Symptomatic status and sex did not modify the treatment effect, but an interaction with age and treatment was detected ($P=0.02$). Outcomes were slightly better after CAS for patients aged <70 years and better after CEA for patients aged >70 years. The periprocedural end point did not differ for CAS and CEA, but there were differences in the components, CAS versus CEA (stroke 4.1% versus 2.3%, $P=0.012$; and myocardial infarction 1.1% versus 2.3%, $P=0.032$).

Conclusions.—In CREST, CAS and CEA had similar short- and longer-term outcomes. During the periprocedural period, there was higher risk of stroke with CAS and higher risk of myocardial infarction with CEA.

Clinical Trial Registration.—www.clinicaltrials.gov. Unique identifier: NCT00004732 (Tables 1 and 2).

▶ Carotid endarterectomy (CEA) has been shown to be effective as a preventive treatment for symptomatic and asymptomatic cervical carotid arterial stenotic disease, while carotid artery stenting (CAS) provides another option for treatment. However, results of randomized trials comparing CAS with CEA for symptomatic participants have varied. The Carotid Revascularization Endarterectomy Versus Stenting Trial (CREST) prospectively compared CAS with CEA in both symptomatic and asymptomatic patients.

Table 1 details that in the 2052 participants, there was no significant difference in the primary end point between CAS and CEA (7.2% vs 6.8%).

Trial enrollment was carried out at 117 CREST centers, and participants could not be randomized until operators had been selected at each site through a validated selection process for CEA or a training and credentialing program for CAS. To be eligible, symptomatic patients had to have had a transient ischemic attack, amaurosis fugax, or minor nondisabling stroke in the distribution of the study artery within 180 days of randomization and had to have carotid artery stenosis ≥50% by angiography, ≥70% by ultrasound, or ≥70% by CT

TABLE 1.—Selected Characteristics of the Study Cohort by Treatment Group*

Characteristic	CAS (N=1262)	CEA (N=1240)
Age, years*	68.9±9.0	69.2±8.7
Male sex, % of patients	63.9	66.4
Asymptomatic arteries, % of patients	47.1	47.3
Risk factors, % of patients		
Hypertension	85.8	86.1
Diabetes	30.6	30.4
Dyslipidemia†	82.9	85.8
Current smoker	26.4	26.1
Percent stenosis at randomization		
Severe (≥70%)	86.9	85.1
Median time from randomization to treatment (no. of days)	6	7

*Means ± SD.
†P=0.05 for the difference in the baseline rate of dyslipidemia between the 2 groups.

TABLE 2.—Composite Primary End Point and Components of the Primary End Point

	4-Year Study Period (Including Periprocedural Period*) No. of Patients (%±SE)		Absolute Treatment Effect of CAS Versus CEA (95% CI) Percentage Points	P†
	CAS (N=1262)	CEA (N=1240)		
Stroke				
Any stroke	105 (10.2±1.1)	75 (7.9±1.0)	2.3 (−0.6 to 5.2)	0.03
Major ipsilateral	16 (1.4±0.3)	6 (0.5±0.2)	0.8 (0.1 to 1.6)	0.05
Minor ipsilateral	52 (4.5±0.6)	36 (3.5±0.6)	1.0 (−0.7 to 2.7)	0.10
Primary end point (any periprocedural stroke, myocardial infarction, or death or post procedural ipsilateral stroke)	85 (7.2±0.8)	76 (6.8±0.8)	0.4 (−1.7 to 2.6)	0.51

Editor's Note: Please refer to original journal article for full references.
*For patients who received the assigned procedure within 30 days after randomization, the periprocedural period was defined as the 30-day period after the procedure. For patients who did not receive the assigned procedure within 30 days after randomization, the periprocedural period was defined as the 36-day period after randomization.
†P values were calculated based on significance of the hazard ratios.[7]

angiography or MR angiography if ultrasound was 50% to 69%. Asymptomatic patients had to have carotid artery stenosis of ≥60% by angiography, ≥70% by ultrasound, or ≥80% by CT angiography or MR angiography if ultrasound was 50% to 69%. Patients were not eligible if they had a previous disabling stroke or chronic atrial fibrillation.

CAS was performed with the use of the RX Acculink stent; the RX Accunet embolic protection device was required except when not technically feasible. For both CAS and CEA, antiplatelet therapy was required before and after the procedure. The National Institutes of Health Stroke Scale, modified Rankin Scale, Transient Ischemic Attack Stroke Questionnaire, cardiac enzymes, electrocardiogram, and carotid ultrasound were performed at baseline. Cardiac enzymes were obtained 6 to 8 hours postprocedure; repeat neurological evaluation, the National Institutes of Health Stroke Scale, and the Transient Ischemic Attack Stroke Questionnaire were performed at 18 to 54 hours; and an electrocardiogram was obtained at 6 to 48 hours and at 1 month. The National Institutes of Health Stroke Scale, the modified Rankin Scale, and the carotid ultrasound were also performed at 1, 6, and 12 months and annually thereafter. A telephone follow-up call was performed at 3 months and every 6 months thereafter. The Medical Outcomes Study 36-item Short Form Instrument was obtained at baseline, 2 weeks, and 1 month postprocedure and 1 year after randomization.

The primary end point was the occurrence of any stroke, myocardial infarction (MI), or death during the periprocedural period or ipsilateral stroke thereafter up to 4 years. Stroke was defined as an acute neurological event with focal symptoms and signs lasting for ≥24 hours consistent with focal cerebral ischemia. MI was defined as an elevation of cardiac enzymes (CK-MB or troponin) to a value twice or greater than the upper limit of normal for the local center laboratory plus the occurrence of either chest pain or equivalent symptoms consistent with myocardial ischemia or electrocardiogram evidence of ischemia, including new ST segment depression or elevation >1 mm in ≥2 contiguous leads (as determined by the centralized core laboratory). Analysis was intention to treat. Proportional hazards analysis adjusting for age, sex, and symptomatic status was used to test for treatment differences.

Table 1 details that in the 2052 participants, there was no significant difference in the primary end point between CAS and CEA (7.2% vs 6.8%). During the periprocedural period, the incidence of the primary end point was similar for CAS and CEA, but there were differences in the end point components (stroke, 4.1% vs 2.3%; MI, 1.1% vs 2.3%; and death, 0.7% vs 0.3%). Thereafter, ipsilateral stroke was infrequent for both CAS and CEA (2.0% vs 2.4). Neither symptomatic status nor sex showed an effect on treatment difference per preplanned effect modification analyses. Patient age did interact with treatment efficacy. Outcomes were slightly better after CAS for patients younger than 70 years and better after CEA for patients older than 70 years.

During the periprocedural period, the occurrence of the primary end point components (stroke, MI, or death) for CAS and CEA was not different for symptomatic (6.7% vs 5.4%) or asymptomatic subjects (3.5% vs 3.6%). The risk of stroke and death was significantly higher for CAS in symptomatic patients (6.0% vs 3.2%) but not for asymptomatic patients (2.5% vs1.4%); however, a smaller total number of events occurred in the asymptomatic strata, resulting in lower statistical power to detect treatment differences. Cranial nerve palsies were less frequent for CAS (0.3% vs 4.7%). Table 2 details the composite primary end point and components of the primary end point.

The authors noted that CAS and CEA had similar net outcomes for symptomatic and asymptomatic men and women. However, there was a lower incidence of MI immediately after CAS and a lower incidence of stroke immediately after CEA. CAS, when done by experienced and skilled interventionists, has patient outcomes similar to those of CEA done by experienced and skilled surgeons. During the perioperative period, more strokes occur after CAS and more MIs occur after CEA. Younger patients have slightly better outcomes with CAS and older patients have better outcomes with CEA. For the future, both CEA and CAS appear to be useful tools for preventing stroke.

This was a well-designed and thorough trial that gives very important comparative data regarding carotid artery revascularization methodologies.

T. G. Walker, MD

Embolization

Does Size Really Matter? Analysis of the Effect of Large Fibroids and Uterine Volumes on Complication Rates of Uterine Artery Embolisation
Parthipun AA, Taylor J, Manyonda I, et al (St George's Hosp, London, UK)
Cardiovasc Intervent Radiol 33:955-959, 2010

The purpose of this study was to determine whether there is a correlation between large uterine fibroid diameter, uterine volume, number of vials of embolic agent used and risk of complications from uterine artery embolisation (UAE). This was a prospective study involving 121 patients undergoing UAE embolisation for symptomatic uterine fibroids at a single institution. Patients were grouped according to diameter of largest fibroid and uterine volume. Results were also stratified according to the number of vials of embolic agent used and rate of complications. No statistical difference in complication rate was demonstrated between the two groups according to diameter of the largest fibroid (large fibroids were classified as ≥ 10 cm; Fisher's exact test $P = 1.00$), and no statistical difference in complication rate was demonstrated according to uterine volume (large uterine volume was defined as ≥ 750 cm^3; Fisher's exact test $P = 0.70$). 84 of the 121 patients had documentation of the number of vials used during the procedure. Patients were divided into two groups, with ≥ 4 used defined as a large number of embolic agent. There was no statistical difference between these two groups and no associated increased risk of developing complications. This study showed no increased incidence of complications in women with large-diameter fibroids or uterine volumes as defined. In addition, there was no evidence of increased complications according to quantity of embolic material used. Therefore, UAE should be offered to women with large fibroids and uterine volumes (Tables 1 and 2).

▶ Uterine artery embolization (UAE) has been established as a safe and effective treatment for symptomatic fibroids. However, reports have suggested that large fibroids may be a relative contraindication to UAE because of increased incidence of complications, such as infection, sepsis, uterine necrosis, and death, and it has been suggested that UAE should not be performed for large fibroids (≥ 10 cm in diameter) or uteri with > 100 cm^3 volume. Some investigators have excluded patients on the basis of uterine volume, for example, uterus with > 24-week pregnancy volume, > 1000 cm^3. Other studies have refuted this and found no increased risk of complications associated with large fibroids or large uterus volume.

TABLE 1.—Relationship Between Fibroid Size and Complications

Presence of Complications	≥10 cm (group A)	<10 cm (group B)	Total
Complication	1	5	6
No complication	29	86	115
Totals	30	91	121

TABLE 2.—Relationship Between Uterine Volume and Complications

Presence of Complications	≥750 ml (group C)	<750 ml (group D)	Total
Complication	2	4	6
No complication	50	65	115
Totals	52	69	121

In view of the conflicting results in the literature, the authors sought to determine whether dominant uterine fibroid diameter ≥10 cm is associated with increased complication rate, whether uterine volume ≥750 cm^3 is associated with increased complication rate, and whether there is an association between the number of vials of embolic agent used and the complication rate.

The current study prospectively registered 121 consecutive nonrandomized patients in a single institution treated with uterine fibroid embolization from 2004 to 2008. All patients (100%) had full registry documentation of uterine volume, diameter of largest fibroid, and follow-up information for a minimum 6 months, including complications, documented in the registry, with review of the clinical notes where necessary. Of the 121 patients, 112 (93%) had 12 months of follow-up documented in the registry. All patients were premenopausal and symptomatic and had undergone ultrasound assessment of their fibroids before UAE. The number of vials of embolic material was recorded routinely in the registry. Results were analyzed using a cutoff point as follows: a large fibroid was defined as ≥10 cm and a large uterine volume was defined as ≥750 cm^3.

UAE was performed using a standard technique with single or bilateral common femoral arterial punctures and bilateral catheterization of the uterine arteries with 4F catheters. Embolization was performed using nonspherical polyvinyl alcohol (PVA) particles 355 to 500 μm in diameter or tris-acryl gelatin microspheres 500 to 900 μm in diameter (Embosphere; Biosphere Medical, Louvres, France). The angiographic end point for embolization was defined as almost complete stasis of contrast in the uterine arteries when using nonspherical PVA or a pruned tree for embospheres. Manual compression was applied to the puncture site at the end of the procedure. Each patient was reviewed in the outpatient gynecology clinic at 6 weeks and in the radiology clinic at 6 months and again at 1 year to assess the outcome of the procedure and to ascertain whether there had been any complications. Statistical analysis of the relationship between (1) fibroid diameter and complications and (2) uterine volume and complications was performed using Fisher exact test. In addition, statistical analysis of the correlation between the number of embolic vials used and incidence of complications was also performed using Fisher exact test.

Tables 1 and 2 respectively show the relationship between fibroid size and complications related to embolization and the relationship between uterine volume and complications. No statistical difference was present between the 2 groups in either circumstance. The overall complication rate was 5%.

The authors conclude that there is no correlation between the numbers of vials of embolic agent used, size of the fibroid, and risk of developing complications. On the basis of these findings, they feel that continuing to offer this service to all women with symptomatic fibroids, with no exclusion based on fibroid or uterine size, is justified.

T. G. Walker, MD

Transcatheter Arterial Chemoembolization for Liver Cancer: Is It Time to Distinguish Conventional from Drug-Eluting Chemoembolization?
Liapi E, Geschwind J-FH (Johns Hopkins Univ School of Medicine, Baltimore, MD)
Cardiovasc Intervent Radiol 34:37-49, 2011

Conventional transcatheter arterial chemoembolization and chemoembolization with drug-eluting beads are increasingly being performed interchangeably in many institutions throughout the world. As both therapies continue to being tested in many phase II and III studies and in combination with other therapies, especially targeted agents, for treatment of primary and metastatic liver cancer, it is imperative to review their current status and evaluate their impact on patient survival. This review critically assesses patient selection, indications, contraindications, techniques, materials, safety, and clinical outcomes of patients treated with conventional chemoembolization and chemoembolization with drug-eluting beads (Table 1).

▶ Transcatheter arterial chemoembolization (TACE) is the mainstay of catheter-based therapies for unresectable primary liver cancer, and its use is expanding for other hepatic metastatic malignancies. Conventional TACE typically involves the injection of chemotherapeutic agents mixed with lipiodol and embolic particles into the branch of the hepatic artery that feeds the tumor. TACE with drug-eluting beads (DEBs) involves the injection of DEBs into the tumor-feeding artery, offering simultaneous delivery of chemotherapy and embolization with sustained and controlled drug release over time.

Conventional TACE and DEB-TACE are increasingly being performed interchangeably in many institutions throughout the world. As both therapies continue to being tested in many phase II and III studies and in combination with other therapies, especially targeted agents, for treatment of primary and metastatic liver cancer, it is imperative to review their current status and

TABLE 1.—Exclusion Criteria for TACE and DEB-TACE

Characteristic	DEB-TACE	TACE
Liver disease	• Child-Pugh class C (except with isolated tumor feeder) • Active gastrointestinal bleeding • Encephalopathy • Mild or severe ascites • Bilirubin levels >3 mg/dl • Albumin <2.5 g/dl • ALT and AST >5 times upper limit of normal	• Child-Pugh class >C11 • Active gastrointestinal bleeding
Tumor status	• Tumor resectability • BCLC class C (vascular invasion including segmental portal obstruction, extrahepatic spread) • BCLC class D • Main PVT or portal vein occlusion • Extensive tumor involvement (>50% of the liver) • Extrahepatic metastases	• Tumor resectability • BCLC class D
Patient performance status	• ECOG >3	• ECOG >3
Doxorubicin related	• WBC <3000 cells/mm^3 Neutrophils <1500 cells/mm^3 • LV ejection fraction <50%	• WBC <3000 cells/mm^3 Neutrophils <1500 cells/mm^3 • LV ejection fraction <50%
Procedural	• Portosystemic shunt • Hepatofugal blood flow • Platelet count <50,000/mm^3 • Prothrombin activity <50%) • Renal insufficiency/failure • Serum creatinine >2 mg/dl (177 μmol/l)	• Renal insufficiency/failure • Serum creatinine >2 mg/dl (177 μmol/l) • Uncorrectable bleeding disorder

ALT alanine aminotransferase, *AST* aspartate aminotransferase, *WBC* white blood cell count, *LV* left ventricle.

evaluate their impact on patient survival. This review critically assesses patient selection, indications, contraindications, techniques, materials, safety, and clinical outcomes of patients treated with conventional TACE and DEB-TACE.

Conventional TACE is used for palliative treatment of unresectable hepatocellular carcinoma (HCC), as well as an adjunctive therapy to liver resection, as a bridge to liver transplantation, and before or after radiofrequency ablation. TACE is also used for palliative treatment of unresectable cholangiocarcinoma, hepatic metastatic neuroendocrine tumors, metastatic sarcomas to the liver, breast hepatic metastases, and hepatic colorectal metastases. Similarly, DEB-TACE has been performed for patients with unresectable HCC, cholangiocarcinoma, neuroendocrine tumors, and hepatic colorectal metastases.

Contraindications to both techniques are similar. Current absolute contraindications to conventional TACE include tumor resectability, intractable systemic infection, an uncorrectable bleeding disorder, uncorrectable contrast allergy, leukopenia (white blood cell count < 1000/μL), cardiac or renal insufficiency hepatic encephalopathy, or East Coast Oncology Group (ECOG) performance status > 2. Contraindications, such as the absence of hepatopetal blood flow and presence of encephalopathy and biliary obstruction, have been recently reclassified as relative ones. Portal vein thrombosis (PVT) should not be considered a contraindication to TACE. A study by Georgiades et al reported that TACE is safe to perform in patients with PVT and identified that the key prognostic factor to survival was the Child-Pugh numerical disease stage. In the presence of PVT, a highly selective approach and adjustment of the chemotherapeutic dosage may minimize liver damage.

Relative contraindications to conventional TACE include a variety of other factors, including, but not limited to, serum bilirubin > 3 mg/dL, lactate dehydrogenase > 425 U/L, aspartate aminotransferase more than 5 times the upper limit of normal, tumor burden involving > 50% of the liver, presence of extrahepatic metastases, poor performance status, cardiac or renal insufficiency, ascites, recent variceal bleeding, significant thrombocytopenia, intractable arteriovenous fistula, surgical portocaval anastomosis, severe portal vein thrombosis, and tumor invasion to the inferior vena cava (IVC) and right atrium.

Because DEB-TACE is still relatively new and thus clinical data have not been collected for as long as for conventional TACE, the list of exclusion criteria is more extensive for DEB-TACE. Currently, most investigators will not treat patients with Child-Pugh class C, diffuse tumors, or portal vein thrombosis. Table 1 summarizes the list of exclusion criteria for conventional TACE and DEB-TACE.

In conventional TACE, the most widely used single chemotherapeutic agent is doxorubicin, and the combination of cisplatin, doxorubicin, and mitomycin C is the most common drug combination used in the United States. Although none of these agents is extracted by the liver during the first pass, their pharmacokinetic profile is modified when they are combined with lipiodol. The emulsion allows prolonged transit of the drugs within the tumor bed, leading to greater contact time between the cancer cells and the chemotherapeutic agents. As a result, favorable tumor drug concentration with concurrent low systematic drug load can be achieved. The oily medium of lipiodol is a key ingredient to the chemoembolization procedure because of its unique combination of properties as a drug-carrying, tumor-seeking, and embolizing agent. Lipiodol localizes in hepatic tumors when administered via the hepatic artery, and it is typically retained by HCC for months, even up to a year, while it is cleared from normal or cirrhotic liver within 4 weeks. Several embolic agents have been used in conjunction with conventional TACE. The intended purpose of embolization is 2-fold: to prevent washout of the drug at the site of tumor and to induce ischemic necrosis. These agents may produce different effects on vasculature, resulting in permanent or transient obstruction, by acting at different levels in the arterial system. Usually the injection of embolic agents follows the injection of the chemotherapeutic mixture. Embolic materials for conventional TACE can be spherical or nonspherical agents.

Drug-eluting microspheres commercially available for DEB-TACE include DC Bead, Precision Bead microspheres, and Paragon Bead microspheres (Biocompatibles, UK), and Superabsorbent polymer Quadrasphere (Hepasphere for Europe). The microspheres are loaded with various chemotherapeutic agents (eg, doxorubicin, irinotecan, cisplatin), which then elute from the microspheres in vivo.

In 2002, 2 landmark studies showed that TACE provided a statistically significant survival advantage over that of best supportive care in selected patients with well-preserved liver function. The first of these studies, by Llovet et al, prospectively evaluated the survival outcomes in patients treated with fixed interval chemoembolization, embolization, and supportive measures. This trial ended when a survival benefit of patients treated with chemoembolization compared with those treated conservatively was shown. In the second randomized controlled trial, Lo et al reported on a select group of patients with unresectable HCC treated with TACE or supportive care, demonstrating that TACE significantly improved survival over supportive care. In this trial, the most common complications of patients treated with TACE were fever 33%, abdominal pain 26%, vomiting 16.7%, ascites 5.2%, and gastrointestinal bleeding 4.2%.

The largest case series ever reported (8510 patients) on patients treated with TACE comes from Japan. Median survival in this series was 34 months.

In regards to metastatic disease, for metastatic neuroendocrine hepatic metastases, TACE has been shown to be effective in controlling hormonal symptoms and tumor growth. Investigators have concluded that TACE is effective in prolonging survival in metastatic cholangiocarcinoma and for colorectal disease metastatic to liver. Metastatic breast cancer and other metastatic disease may show similar benefit.

The results from the Prospective Randomised Study of Doxorubicin in the Treatment of Hepatocellular Carcinoma by Drug-Eluting Bead Embolisation trial, which is the only prospective, controlled, randomized study involving the efficacy of DEB-TACE, were recently published.

In this trial, a total of 212 patients were enrolled and received TACE with either doxorubicin or doxorubicin-loaded microspheres. DEB-TACE with doxorubicin showed a higher rate of complete response, objective response, and disease control compared with conventional TACE (27 vs 22%, 52 vs 44%, and 63 vs 52%, respectively). Patients with Child-Pugh class B, ECOG score 1, bilobar disease, and recurrence after curative treatment benefited more from the DEB-TACE procedure than they did from conventional TACE, as demonstrated by a significant increase in objective response ($P = .038$). There was a marked reduction in serious liver toxicity in patients treated with DEB-TACE. The rate of doxorubicin-related side effects were significantly lower ($P = .0001$) in the DEB group than in the conventional TACE one. Results about the survival benefits of each therapy will be reported within the next 2 years. There is also ongoing investigation into the role of DEB-TACE in metastatic disease to the liver, with early encouraging results.

Both TACE and DEB-TACE are potent palliative options for the treatment of primary and metastatic liver cancer. Initial results in patients with unresectable HCC, including a randomized phase II study, have shown that DEB-TACE is superior to TACE in terms of local tumor response, liver toxicity, and systemic toxicity. Results regarding the potential survival benefits of DEB-TACE in patients with HCC are to be reported within the next 2 years. Results regarding the potential survival benefit of patients with hepatic metastases treated with DEB-TACE should also become available in the near future.

T. G. Walker, MD

Embolization of Acute Nonvariceal Upper Gastrointestinal Hemorrhage Resistant to Endoscopic Treatment: Results and Predictors of Recurrent Bleeding
Loffroy R, Rao P, Ota S, et al (The Johns Hopkins Univ School of Medicine, Baltimore, MD)
Cardiovasc Intervent Radiol 33:1088-1100, 2010

Acute nonvariceal upper gastrointestinal (UGI) hemorrhage is a frequent complication associated with significant morbidity and mortality. The most common cause of UGI bleeding is peptic ulcer disease, but the differential diagnosis is diverse and includes tumors; ischemia; gastritis; arteriovenous malformations, such as Dieulafoy lesions; Mallory-Weiss tears; trauma; and iatrogenic causes. Aggressive treatment with early endoscopic hemostasis is essential for a favorable outcome. However, severe bleeding despite conservative medical treatment or endoscopic intervention occurs in 5–10% of patients, requiring surgery or transcatheter arterial embolization. Surgical intervention is usually an expeditious and gratifying endeavor, but it can be associated with high operative mortality rates. Endovascular management using superselective catheterization of the culprit vessel, « sandwich» occlusion, or blind embolization has emerged as an alternative to emergent operative intervention for high-risk patients and is now considered the first-line therapy for massive UGI bleeding refractory to endoscopic treatment. Indeed, many published studies have confirmed the feasibility of this approach and its high technical and clinical success rates, which range from 69 to 100% and from 63 to 97%, respectively, even if the choice of the best embolic agent among coils, cyanoacrylate glue, gelatin sponge, or calibrated particles remains a matter of debate. However, factors influencing clinical outcome, especially predictors of early rebleeding, are poorly understood, and few studies have addressed this issue. This review of the literature will attempt to define the role of embolotherapy for acute nonvariceal UGI hemorrhage that fails to respond to endoscopic hemostasis and to summarize data on factors predicting angiographic and embolization failure (Tables 1-3).

▶ Nonvariceal upper gastrointestinal (UGI) bleeding is usually caused by peptic ulcer disease, although there are many other causes, including benign and malignant tumors; ischemia; gastritis; arteriovenous malformations, such as Dieulafoy lesions; Mallory-Weiss tears; trauma; and iatrogenic injury. Effective treatment requires an accurate diagnosis (location and etiology), and unlike lower gastrointestinal bleeds, most patients have undergone endoscopic examination and treatment before their referral to interventional radiology. Surgery is typically reserved for those patients whose bleeding failed to respond to all previous treatments. Increasingly, transcatheter arterial embolotherapy (TAE) is employed in patients who have failed medical and endoscopic management. Although TAE has been performed for at least 3 decades and has been shown to be effective at controlling hemorrhage and decreasing mortality, there are few published series that have analyzed factors predicting angiographic and

TABLE 1.—Published Series of Angiographic Embolization for Acute Nonvariceal UGI Bleeding that Included >20 Patients During a 17-Year Period

Reference	Patients (*n*)	Mean Age (y)	Previous Endoscopy (%)	Active Extravasation (%)	Technical Success (%)
Lang [18]	57	52	NA	100	91
Encarnacion [7]	29	55	NA	NA	62
Toyoda [40]	30	62	100	NA	100
Walsh [23]	50	64	100	50	92
Schenker [27]	163	58	90	37	95
Defreyne [29]	20	54	NA	60	95
Aina [25]	75	62	100	61	99
De Wispelaere [36]	28	69	100	39	89
Ripoll [50]	31	75	100	NA	100
Holme [10]	40	70	100	30	100
Loffroy [52]	35	71	100	66	94
Larssen [53]	36	80	100	42	92
Poultsides [28]	57	65	100	61	93
Loffroy [26]	60	69	100	63	95
Padia [34]	108	66	93	33	NA
All studies	819	65	99	54	93

The number of patients per study, mean patient age, number of patients who underwent endoscopy before embolization, proportion of the patients who were found to have active extravasation on initial angiography, and technical success rate of embolization are presented.
NA not available.
Editor's Note: Please refer to original journal article for full references.

TABLE 2.—Outcomes in Selected Case Series

Reference	Clinical Success (%)	Rebleeding Rate (%)	Need for Surgery (%)	Complication Rate (%)	30-Day Mortality (%)
Lang [18]	86	56	2	16	4
Encarnacion [7]	62	11	17	17	45
Toyoda [40]	80	23	13	NA	23
Walsh [23]	52	52	37	4	40
Schenker [27]	58	29	NA	10	33
Defreyne [29]	60	37	26	20	30
Aina [25]	73	23	16	5	35
De Wispelaere [36]	64	36	21	0	46
Ripoll [50]	71	29	16	0	26
Holme [10]	65	28	35	0	25
Loffroy [52]	94	17	14	6	21
Larssen [53]	72	9	30	8	17
Poultsides [28]	51	47	21	26	21
Loffroy [26]	72	28	12	10	27
Padia [34]	44	66	21	5	20
All studies	67	33	20	9	28

The rates of clinical success, recurrent bleeding after a technically successful embolization, need for operative intervention to control bleeding, complications, and periprocedural mortality are presented.
NA not available.
Editor's Note: Please refer to original journal article for full references.

embolization failure. In this review, the authors summarize data on outcomes and factors that may influence the outcome of patients who have undergone embolization procedures for acute nonvariceal UGI hemorrhage.

TABLE 3.—Predictors of Rebleeding Within 30 Days of Embolization in the Series Under Review

Reference	Patients (n)	Factors Associated with Rebleeding in Univariate Analysis ($P < 0.05$)	Factors Associated with Rebleeding in Multivariate Analysis ($P < 0.05$)
Encarnacion [7]	29	Coagulopathy[a]	Coagulopathy[b]
Walsh [23]	50	Longer time to angiography	Longer time to angiography
		Greater number of total PRBCs	Greater number of total PRBCs
		Previous surgery	Previous surgery
Schenker [27]	163	NA	Multiorgan system failure[c]
			Coagulopathy[d]
			Bleeding subsequent to trauma or invasive procedures
Defreyne [29]	20	Blood loss (hemoglobin level <80 g l^{-1})	NA
		Hypovolemic shock	
		Corticosteroid use	
		Greater number of PRBCs transfused before angiography	
		Greater number of fresh frozen plasma transfused before angiography	
Aina [25]	75	Coagulation disorders[e]	Coagulation disorders[f]
		Presence of cirrhosis	Use of coils as the only embolic agent
Poultsides [28]	57	>6 units of PRBCs before the procedure	>6 units of PRBCs before the procedure
			Previous suture-ligated duodenal ulcer
Loffroy [26]	60	Coagulopathy[g]	Coagulopathy[h]
		≥2 comorbidities	Use of coils as the only embolic agent
		Longer time from shock onset to angiography	
		Larger number of PRBCs transfused before angiography	
		Use of coils as the only embolic agent	

NA not available.
Editor's Note: Please refer to original journal article for full references.
[a,b,d]Prothrombin ratio >1.3, partial thromboplastin time >40 s, or platelet count <80,000 µl^{-1}.
[c]Defined as at least three of the following underlying conditions: serious cardiovascular compromise (myocardial infarction, cardiac ischemia, heart failure, hypotension, or hypovolemic shock), dialysis-dependent renal failure, steroid-dependent chronic obstructive pulmonary disease, ventilator-dependent lung disease, cirrhosis, or sepsis.
[e,f,g,h]International normalized ratio >1.5, partial thromboplastin time >45 s, or platelet count <80,000 µl^{-1}.

The authors identified case series on embolization for acute nonvariceal UGI bleeding from 1992 to 2009 using PubMed queries, adding further bibliography by manual searches of reference lists. Studies that included 20 or more subjects were selected for review when they had well-defined indications for intervention and offered a detailed description of outcomes, including technical and clinical success rates, rebleeding and reintervention rates, the need for surgery to control bleeding, and morbidity and mortality rates. This article reviews 15 studies (819 patients, mean age 65 years) on endovascular management of intractable nonvariceal UGI bleeding (Tables 1 and 2). Among them, only 7 studies identified factors affecting the success of embolotherapy using statistical analysis (Table 3). Endoscopy had been performed and failed in 99% of patients.

As detailed in Table 1, TAE was successful technically in 762 (93%) patients. The causes for endovascular technique failure were as follows: difficult vascular anatomy, arterial dissection, vasospasm, false-negatively read angiogram, multiple bleedings, and tumoral bleeding. A variety of embolic materials, including coils, polyvinyl alcohol particles, blood clot, Gelfoam, and cyanoacrylate glue were used. The sandwich technique, with placement of embolic material at both sides of the bleeding vessel, was used in most series to minimize the chance of recurrent bleeding caused by rich collaterals. Active extravasation was present at the time of embolization in only 442 (54%) patients. Consequently, 46% of patients underwent blind embolization guided by the findings on endoscopy or placement of clips around the area of the bleeding vessel.

In most cases, gelatin sponge or coils were then used for embolization. From the subgroup that underwent technically successful embolization, 549 (67%) patients responded well clinically and had cessation of bleeding (Table 2). Thirty-three percent of patients continued to bleed, but almost half of them responded to repeat embolization. Major and minor embolization-related complications developed in 9% (74) of patients, and the overall 30-day mortality rate was 28% (229 patients). Although the mortality rate appears to be as high as in some surgical series for emergent open repair of UGI bleeding, one should keep in mind that the patients treated with embolotherapy had been, on most occasions, turned down for open repair because of significant comorbidities and advanced age.

Although conclusions from all retrospective studies must be drawn with caution, some investigators have identified several clinical and technical factors that may influence the embolization outcome (Table 3). Although coagulopathy has been shown to adversely affect the success rate for embolotherapy, investigators reported successful TAE control approaching 50% in coagulopathic patients. Consequently, although every effort should be made to correct coagulopathy before, during, and after intervention, patients with coagulopathy should by no means be excluded from angiographic treatment for emergent arterial UGI hemorrhage. As summarized in Table 3, other clinical variables have been identified as predictors of early rebleeding after embolization.

The authors note that although blind embolization is controversial, because massive bleeding is often intermittent, most groups have adopted a policy to embolize on the basis of endoscopic findings even in situations where no extravasation is seen angiographically. As a useful technique to guide endovascular treatment in patients with failed endoscopic control, the endoscopists marked the site of bleed with clips placed at the junction of the ulcer and the adjacent normal mucosa so that this can serve as a reference at the time of angiography.

The influence of the type of embolic agent on the clinical outcome remains controversial. It is generally accepted that embolic therapy is superior to vasopressin infusion for the treatment of UGI hemorrhage from gastroduodenal ulcers. The choice of the best embolic agent is still debatable.

The authors conclude that the safety and efficacy of transcatheter embolization for the treatment of life-threatening acute nonvariceal UGI bleeding is now widely accepted and is considered the gold standard for endoscopy-refractory patients. Embolization may be effective for even the most gravely ill patients for whom surgery is not a viable option, even when extravasation is not visualized by angiography. As described in this review, several clinical and technical factors must be known by interventional radiologists since they may influence the clinical outcome of embolotherapy in such a setting. Specifically, every effort should be made to perform embolization early after bleeding onset and to correct coagulations disorders. In addition, it seems that careful selection of the embolic agents according to the bleeding vessel may play a role in a successful outcome.

T. G. Walker, MD

Hepatic Intra-Arterial Injection of Drug-Eluting Bead, Irinotecan (DEBIRI) in Unresectable Colorectal Liver Metastases Refractory to Systemic Chemotherapy: Results of Multi-Institutional Study
Martin RCG, Joshi J, Robbins K, et al (Univ of Louisville School of Medicine, KY; Baptist Health, Little Rock, AR; et al)
Ann Surg Oncol 18:192-198, 2011

Introduction.—Response rates and overall outcome for patients who have failed first-line and in some cases second-line chemotherapy are as low as 12% and 7 months, respectively. The aim of this study is to evaluate the efficacy of hepatic arterial sulfonate hydrogel microsphere (drug-eluting beads), irinotecan preloaded therapy (DEBIRI) in metastatic colorectal cancer refractory to systemic chemotherapy.

Methods.—This was a multicenter multinational single-arm study of metastatic colorectal cancer patients who received DEBIRI after failing systemic chemotherapy from 10/2006 to 8/2008. Primary endpoints were safety, tolerance, tumor response rates, and overall survival.

Results.—Fifty-five patients who had received prior systemic chemotherapy and who underwent a total of 99 DEBIRI treatments were reviewed. The median number of DEBIRI treatments was 2 (range 1—5), median treatment dose was 100 mg (range 100—200 mg), with total hepatic treatment of 200 mg (range 200—650 mg), with 86% of treatments performed as lobar infusion and 30% of patients treated with concurrent simultaneous chemotherapy. Adverse events occurred in 28% of patients with median grade of 2 (range 1—3) with no deaths at 30 days post procedure. Response rates were 66% at 6 months and 75% at 12 months. Overall survival in these patients was 19 months, with progression-free survival of 11 months.

Conclusions.—Hepatic arterial drug-eluting bead, irinotecan (DEBIRI) was safe and effective in treatment of metastatic colorectal cancer (MCC) refractory to multiple lines of systemic chemotherapy. DEBIRI is an acceptable therapy for treatment of metastatic colorectal cancer to the liver (Tables 1-5).

▶ Systemic chemotherapy for unresectable metastatic colorectal cancer (MCC) is the standard initial management. After a patient has failed first-line chemotherapy and in some cases second-line chemotherapy, the response rates to

TABLE 1.—Clinical and Chemotherapy Characteristics of DEBIRI-Treated Patients

Characteristic	N = 55
Age (years) (median, range)	60 (34−82)
Gender (M/F)	32/23
Performance status	
0	27
1	12
2	16
Colon/rectal primary	40/15
Synchronous/metachronous	17/38
Prior liver surgery	
Hepatic resection (lobectomy)	11
Ablation	5
Liver involvement	
<25%	30
26−50%	18
>50%	17
Number of liver tumors (median, range)	4 (1−20)
1	11
2	10
≥3	33
Total sum of all target lesion(s) size (median, range)[a]	9 cm (5.5−28 cm)
Prior systemic chemotherapy regimes	
FOLFOX + Avastin	17
FOLFOX + Avastin and FOLFIRI + Erbitux	14
FOLFOX + Avastin and FOLFIRI + Eribitux and Xelox + Vectibex or other	24

[a]Up to five target lesions are used for the total sum.

TABLE 2.—DEBIRI Technical Outcomes

	N = 99 Total DEBIRI Treatments
Number of bead courses	2 (range 1−5)
1	5
2	34
3	3
4	3
5	1
Technical success	100%
Bead size	
100−300 μm	54
300−500 μm	6
100−300 and 300−500 μm	10
300−500 and 500−700 μm	29
Dose delivered (median, range)	100 mg (50−200 mg)
Total hepatic dose exposure	185 (150−650)
Adverse events (%)	28 (28%)
Extrahepatic infusion	1 (1%)

further systemic chemotherapy fall to as low as 12%. Approximately 60% of patients with new colorectal cancer will develop liver metastasis during the course of their disease in the United States. In approximately 30% of these patients who develop liver metastasis, the metastatic disease will remain confined to the liver. For the 70% to 75% of patients with colorectal liver

TABLE 3.—DEBIRI Treatment-Related Morbidity

Side-Effect ($n = 99$)	All Grades, No. of Events (%)	Severe Grade,[a] No. of Events (%)
Nausea	6 (6%)	0%
Vomiting	4 (4%)	0%
Hypertension	4 (4%)	0%
Liver dysfunction/failure	6 (6%)	3 (3%)[b]
Anorexia	3 (3%)	1 (1%)
Pain	2 (2%)	0%
Cholecystitis	1 (1%)	1 (1%)
Gastritis	1 (1%)	1 (1%)
Myocardial infarction	1 (1%)	1 (1%)[b]

[a]Defined as grade 3 or higher
[b]Defined as cause of death in one patient

TABLE 4.—Response Rates for All 55 Patients Evaluated

Response ($n = 55$)	3 Months	6 Months	12 Months
Complete response	7 (12%)	7 (12%)	8 (15%)
Partial response	28 (53%)	21 (38%)	14 (25%)
Stable disease	15 (30%)	19 (34%)	23 (42%)
Progression of disease	3 (5%)	8 (15%)	10 (18%)
Dead of disease	0	5	9
Death of other cause	2	0	0

TABLE 5.—Progression-Free, Hepatic-Specific, and Overall Survival

Survival	Median (Months)	At 1 Year (%)
PFS	11	55
Hepatic	15	75
Extrahepatic	13	45
Overall survival	19	75

PFS progression-free survival.

metastasis not suitable for hepatic resection or similarly ablative therapy with curative intent, the short-term prognosis is relatively poor since optimal palliative chemotherapy has been able to produce overall survival of approximately 22.4 months.

In patients with liver-dominant metastatic colorectal cancer to the liver, direct arterial infusion of the chemotherapeutic agent is another treatment option. In these patients in whom the majority of their disease is confined to the liver, colorectal liver metastases are preferentially perfused (nearly 90%-95%) by the hepatic arterial network, whereas nontumoral liver parenchyma is preferentially perfused by the portal vein. These colorectal liver metastases can be exposed to high concentrations by using direct arterial infusion of the chemotherapy agent, avoiding the liver first-pass effect, thus reducing overall systemic side effects. However, given the past response rates of hepatic arterial infusion through hepatic arterial infusion pump, yttrium-90, or drug-eluting bead chemotherapy, there have been limited randomized controlled trials clearly demonstrating improvement in overall survival, and a majority of studies have only been able to demonstrate increased response rates. However, the invasiveness of pump insertion, the significant increased biliary toxicity, and the lack of long-term patency have led to failure to adopt hepatic arterial infusion pumps. The aim of this prospective multi-institutional single-arm treatment registry was to evaluate the efficacy of transcatheter hepatic arterial irinotecan bead therapy in patients with metastatic colorectal cancer (MCC) who have failed first-line and/or second-line or third-line systemic chemotherapy.

Ninety-five patients presenting with liver-dominant (defined as > 50% overall head-to-toe tumor burden confined to the liver) rectal MCC were treated with drug-eluting beads preloaded with irinotecan (DEBIRI) therapy (LC/DC Bead; Biocompatibles, UK Ltd.). Inclusion and exclusion criteria were confirmed diagnosis of liver-dominant MCC, with defined prior chemotherapy treatment and reasons for abandoning that chemotherapy. Standard technique transarterial chemoembolization protocol using DEBIRI was followed for patient treatment; 1 vial of beads was eluted with the desired amount of irinotecan chemotherapy. Treatment was performed in a lobar approach, based on the extent and distribution of the disease, with most treatments being performed in the outpatient setting. The number of treatments was based on the size of lesions, location of lesions (single lobe or bilobar), and the degree of angiographic stasis following each treatment.

DEBIRI was loaded with irinotecan at 50 mg/mL for a total dose of 100 mg per vial. The dose delivered is defined as the single amount of irinotecan that was delivered at 1 DEBIRI administration. Total hepatic exposure was defined as the total sum of irinotecan that was delivered to the patient's entire liver. The primary function of the DEBIRI is to embolize the arteries feeding the tumor site, causing nutrient and oxygen starvation of the tumor, and thereby inducing necrosis in the tumor tissue. The secondary function is to deliver irinotecan in a controlled manner to tumor sites. These functions combine to significantly enhance the cytotoxicity of irinotecan to the tumor and potentially reduce systemic toxicity compared with intravenous chemotherapy.

Follow-up assessments included triphasic CT scan of the liver within at least 1 to 2 months from treatment completion with evaluation of the enhancement pattern of the target lesion and tumor response rates measured according to modified Response Evaluation Criteria in Solid Tumors criteria. Follow-up assessment was then performed at 3-month intervals for the first year and every 6 months for the second year. Hepatic progression-free survival was defined as liver-only progression of disease. Extrahepatic progression-free survival was defined by disease outside of the liver progressing during follow-up.

Fifty-five patients who met the inclusion criteria stated above and had documented liver progression of disease from at least one line of chemotherapy were included in this evaluation. Most patients had good performance status at time of first bead treatment, with the vast majority having colon primaries and presenting with metachronous colorectal metastasis. Liver involvement treated was < 25% in the majority (30 patients), 26% to 50% in 13 patients, and > 50% in 12 patients. The sum of the total lesion sizes that were treated in this study was 9.0 cm with a range of 5.5 to 28.0 cm. Table 1 summarizes the clinical and chemotherapy characteristics of these patients who underwent DEBIRI.

Overall, 99 DEBIRI treatments were performed with a median of 2 (range, 1-5) DEBIRI treatments based on extent of liver involvement, size of the liver lesions to be treated, and the anatomic remaining liver parenchyma since 30% of these patients had already undergone prior hepatectomy. The technical outcomes of the DEBIRI treatments are summarized in Table 2.

Tables 3 and 4 detail the DEBIRI treatment—related morbidity and the response rates for the 55 patients, while Table 5 summarizes the progression-free, hepatic-specific, and overall survival in the group.

This study demonstrated that DEBIRI produced an intention-to-treat overall response rate of 70% and a tumor control rate of 15 months in a heavily pre-treated population of patients with unresectable colorectal liver metastasis.

These results have to be compared with the expected response rate of 10% reported for systemic chemotherapy. DEBIRI treatment also demonstrated hepatic-specific disease progression in which median overall survival of 19 months from DEBIRI treatment was obtained. All patients had previously received and failed a median of 2 lines of systemic chemotherapy with biologic agents, and a majority had failed all potential treatment options for systemic chemotherapy while having ongoing hepatic-specific progression of disease. Considering that this study was performed during the extensive use of all 3 biologic agents that are currently approved in the treatment of colorectal liver metastasis, these results suggest that hepatic arterial infusion with DEBIRI is a viable option in such patients, even after they have failed prior systemic chemotherapy, including oxaliplatin- or irinotecan-based therapy.

The percutaneous nature of this therapy and favorable toxicity profile make this treatment a potential option specifically in the patient with MCC with hepatic-dominant disease. The authors conclude that this promising modality approach should be confirmed in larger populations of chemoresistant patients in conjunction with systemic chemotherapy to optimally demonstrate the timing and use of DEBIRI.

T. G. Walker, MD

Prostatic Arterial Embolization to Treat Benign Prostatic Hyperplasia
Pisco JM, Pinheiro LC, Bilhim T, et al (New Univ of Lisbon, Rua Luz Soriano, Portugal; et al)
J Vasc Interv Radiol 22:11-19, 2011

Purpose.—To evaluate whether prostatic arterial embolization (PAE) might be a feasible procedure to treat lower urinary tract symptoms associated with benign prostatic hyperplasia (BPH).

Materials and Methods.—Fifteen patients (age range, 62—82 years; mean age, 74.1 y) with symptomatic BPH after failure of medical treatment were selected for PAE with nonspherical 200-μm polyvinyl alcohol particles. The procedure was performed by a single femoral approach. Technical success was considered when selective prostatic arterial catheterization and embolization was achieved on at least one pelvic side.

Results.—PAE was technically successful in 14 of the 15 patients (93.3%). There was a mean follow-up of 7.9 months (range, 3−12 months). International Prostate Symptom Score decreased a mean of 6.5 points ($P = .005$), quality of life improved 1.14 points ($P = .065$), International Index of Erectile Function increased 1.7 points ($P = .063$), and peak urinary flow increased 3.85 mL/sec ($P = .015$). There was a mean prostate-specific antigen reduction of 2.27 ng/mL ($P = .072$) and a mean prostate volume decrease of 26.5 mL ($P = .0001$) by ultrasound and 28.9 mL ($P = .008$) by magnetic resonance imaging. There was one major complication (a 1.5-cm^2 ischemic area of the bladder wall) and four clinical failures (28.6%).

Conclusions.—In this small group of patients, PAE was a feasible procedure, with preliminary results and short-term follow-up suggesting good symptom control without sexual dysfunction in suitable candidates, associated with a reduction in prostate volume (Figs 1 and 2).

▶ Benign prostatic hyperplasia (BPH) has a high prevalence rate in men aged 50 to 79 years and is ubiquitous with aging. BPH is a condition often associated with lower urinary tract symptoms, the most frequent of which are decreased urinary stream, greater frequency, and urgency. Prostatectomy by open surgery or transurethral resection of the prostate is still considered the gold standard of treatment. Unfortunately, there are many potential associated surgical complications, such as urinary tract infection, strictures, postoperative pain, incontinence or urinary retention, sexual dysfunction, and blood loss. Alternative options include minimally invasive treatments and prostatic stent placement. Unfortunately, the minimally invasive treatment options have major disadvantages, such as less effective improvement in symptom scores, greater risk of continued catheterization and reoperation, and poorer durability of symptomatic benefit.

Recently, it was suggested that prostatic arterial embolization (PAE) to treat BPH might be analogous to uterine artery embolization for uterine leiomyoma. Animal studies in pigs and dogs have shown that PAE is safe, with no related sexual dysfunction, and can induce prostatic volume reduction. The first report of this technique in the management of BPH in humans was by DeMeritt et al, who reported a single case of BPH with obstructive symptoms and blood loss refractory to other treatments that was successfully managed by PAE with 150- to 250-μm polyvinyl alcohol (PVA) particles. More recently, there has been a report of 2 other patients in similar clinical scenarios who were treated with success with the use of 300- to 500-μm microspheres.

In this prospective study, the authors investigated whether PAE might be a feasible procedure as an alternative treatment option to treat BPH-associated symptoms while preserving sexual function. The study group consisted of 15 patients aged 62 to 82 years who presented with symptomatic BPH refractory to medical treatment for at least 6 months (mean International Prostate

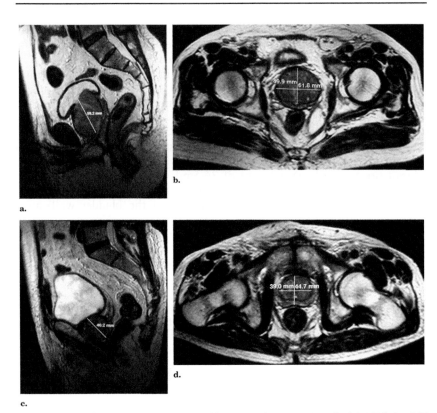

FIGURE 1.—Pelvic MR images in a 78-year-old patient with BPH. (a) Sagittal pelvic MR before PAE shows a prostate cephalocaudal diameter of 59.2 mm and a prostate volume of 95.5 mL. (b) Axial image before PAE shows prostate sagittal and transverse diameters of 49.9 × 61.8 mm and prostate volume of 95.5 mL. (c) Sagittal image 6 months after PAE shows a prostate cephalocaudal diameter of 40.2 mm and prostate volume of 36.6 mL, a decrease of 61.7%. (d) Axial image 6 months after PAE shows prostate sagittal and transverse diameters of 39.0 × 44.7 mm and prostate volume of 36.6 mL, a decrease of 61.7%. (Reprinted from Pisco JM, Pinheiro LC, Bilhim T, et al. Prostatic arterial embolization to treat benign prostatic hyperplasia. *J Vasc Interv Radiol.* 2011;22:11-19, with permission from SIR.)

Symptom Score [IPSS], 21) with a clinical indication for surgery and agreed to undergo PAE. Study criteria included being older than 60 years and having a diagnosis of BPH with moderate to severe lower urinary tract symptoms (ie, IPSS > 18) refractory to medical treatment for at least 6 months, having sexual dysfunction or accepting the risk of developing sexual dysfunction after treatment, and/or having peak urinary flow (Q_{max}) lower than 12 mL/s or acute urinary retention. Malignancy (evaluated by prostate specific antigen [PSA], physical examination, transrectal ultrasound [US], and magnetic resonance [MR] imaging in all patients and by prostatic biopsy in suspicious cases) and advanced atherosclerosis and tortuosity of iliac arteries (based on interventional radiologists' visual evaluation of pelvic MR angiography performed before PAE in all patients) were exclusion criteria. Patients with minimal to moderate lower urinary tract symptoms were also considered for PAE if Q_{max} was lower than

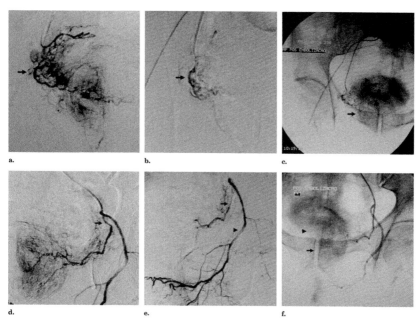

FIGURE 2.—Angiographic findings in a 74-year-old patient with urinary retention with a bladder catheter. Right prostatic arteries before (arrow, **a**) and after (**b**) embolization (arrow). (**c**) After embolization of the right prostatic arteries, in the parenchymal phase of angiography, the prostate is slightly opacified (arrow). The bladder catheter is marked with an arrowhead. Left prostatic arteries before (arrow, **d**) and after (**e**) embolization (arrow). Left internal pudendal artery remains patent (arrowhead). (**f**) After embolization of the left prostatic arteries, in the parenchymal phase of angiography, the prostate is shown with good opacification (arrow). The bladder catheter is marked with an arrowhead. (Reprinted from Pisco JM, Pinheiro LC, Bilhim T, et al. Prostatic arterial embolization to treat benign prostatic hyperplasia. *J Vasc Interv Radiol*. 2011;22:11-19, with permission from SIR.)

12 mL/s if the patients were unsatisfied with the results of medical therapy or had urinary retention. Prostatic biopsy was performed in all cases of suspected prostatic malignancy based on PSA level greater than 4 ng/mL or suspicious focal lesions detected on transrectal US or MR. All cases positive for malignancy were excluded.

All patients were undergoing medical therapy with symptoms that persisted for more than 6 months. Medical therapy was consistent among patients with each receiving 1 α_1-adrenergic receptor antagonist. One patient had a partial prostatectomy 14 years before, and 6 had bladder catheters at the time as a result of acute urinary retention. Pelvic MR angiography with a 1.5-T system was performed before PAE to evaluate the pelvic vessels for tortuosity and atherosclerotic changes of the iliac arteries. All patients were evaluated by clinical observation with measurement of the IPSS and quality of life (QOL)-related symptoms (score from 0 [delighted] to 6 [terrible]), sexual function tests (International Index of Erectile Function; score from 0 to 30), uroflowmetry (Q_{max} and PVR), PSA level, and transrectal US to calculate prostatic volume. Baseline data were obtained before PAE, and the response to treatment was measured at 1, 3, and 6 months after the procedure. The prostate volume was also measured by MR before and 6 months after PAE. Fig 1 shows an example of pre- and post-PAE MR imaging.

In the embolization technique, the patients stopped all prostatic medication 1 week before embolization, and after successful PAE, all prostatic medication was abandoned. Patients started an acid-suppressing drug (omeprazole, 20 mg once daily) and an anti-inflammatory agent (naproxen, 1000 mg twice daily) for 2 days before the procedure and continued to receive them for 10 days after PAE. At the day of PAE, patients received omeprazole, 20 mg, and naproxen, 1000 mg, in the morning before PAE and naproxen, 1000 mg, as post-embolization medication 8 hours after PAE. The patients were admitted to the hospital on the day of the procedure. During embolization, analgesic and anti-inflammatory drugs were given intravenously (ketorolac, 30 mg and metamizole, 2 g).

Embolization was performed under local anesthesia by unilateral approach, usually the right femoral artery. Initially, pelvic angiography was performed to evaluate the iliac and prostatic arteries. Then, a 5F Cobra catheter was introduced into the left hypogastric artery and was positioned in its anterior division. The inferior vesical artery and finally the prostatic vessels were selectively catheterized with a 3F coaxial microcatheter. Repeat angiography was performed to confirm the position of the catheter in the ostium of the prostatic artery before embolization. For embolization, nonspherical 200-μm PVA particles were used. The end point chosen for embolization was slow flow or near stasis in the prostatic vessels with interruption of the arterial flow and prostatic gland opacification. When embolization of the left prostatic arteries was finished, a Waltman loop was formed with the Cobra catheter and the right prostatic arteries were embolized in the same way (Fig 2). The PAE procedure time was measured, as was the fluoroscopy time. Pain assessment was performed during PAE and 6 to 8 hours after PAE by verbal questioning and written questionnaires with a visual analog scale. Patients were asked to rate their pain severity from 0 (sensation of no pain) to 10 (the worst pain imaginable).

Symptoms of postembolization syndrome including pain and fever were not considered complications unless pain and/or fever resulted in prolonged hospitalization or hospital readmission. Postprocedural fever was qualified as a complication when a detailed history, physical examination, and laboratory evaluations confirmed a specific etiology. Complications were categorized as complications of angiography (related to puncture site, contrast agents, or radiation injury), pelvic infection, ischemic complications, sexual dysfunction, nonprostatic embolization, adverse drug reactions, pulmonary embolism, and other. Complications were considered minor if they could be addressed by ambulatory medical treatment and major if they resulted in prolonged hospitalization or hospital readmission and/or need for surgery.

Nine patients underwent prostatic biopsy in view of high PSA levels (> 4 ng/mL) to exclude malignancy. All biopsy findings were negative for neoplasia.

PAE was technically successful in 14 of the 15 patients (93.3%). In 1 patient (6.7%), the procedure was impossible as a result of iliac artery tortuosity and atherosclerosis; surgery was required in this case. We performed PAE bilaterally in 13 patients (technical success rate for bilateral PAE, 86.7%) and unilaterally in 1 patient (patient 11) because of iliac artery tortuosity and atherosclerosis.

The PAE procedure lasted between 25 and 135 minutes (mean, 85 minutes), and fluoroscopy time ranged between 15 and 45 minutes (mean, 35 minutes). Mean follow-up was 7.9 months (range, 3-12 months). Only 1 vial of 200-μm PVA particles was used in each patient.

Six patients had urinary retention with vesical catheters. Only 1 patient (patient 10) felt pain during embolization; no other patients experienced pain during or after the procedure. Twelve patients were discharged from the hospital 6 to 8 hours after the procedure, and the remaining 3 patients were discharged 18 hours after the procedure. Urinary catheters were removed 5 days after the procedure in 4 patients and 10 days after PAE in the remaining 3 patients.

Despite the withdrawal of all prostatic medications after PAE, there was a significant improvement of the IPSS (mean improvement, 6.5 points; range, 2-16 points). QOL improved in all but in 3 patients whose QOL remained stable. The sexual function improved in 5 patients and remained stable in 9 patients. The improvement of erectile function might be explained by the discontinuation of all prostatic medication after PAE, although these results were not statistically significant. There was a tendency for PSA reduction in almost all cases. There were 4 patients with insignificant increases in PSA. There was a significant improvement in Q_{max} (mean improvement, 3.85 mL/s; range, 9.3-1.2 mL/s). There was a significant prostate volume reduction in all patients (mean reduction, 26.5-28.9 mL; range, 7.8%-64.8%, the former reduction in a patient with unilateral PAE). PVR decreased significantly in all patients.

Despite the general improvement in most parameters evaluated, there were 4 clinical failures (28.6%) with persisting severe symptomatology after PAE (ie, IPSS $\geq$ 20 points) or Q_{max} remaining lower than 7 mL/s after PAE. Most of these patients had severe symptoms before PAE despite prostatic medical therapy and had partial relief after PAE without the need for further prostatic medication. Despite the persisting symptoms, 3 patients are currently doing well without the need for prostatic medication or surgery. One patient (patient 10) required surgery for prostatic symptomatic relief and removal of a small area of ischemia at the bladder base.

This study did not compare PAE with placebo, medical therapies, or surgery, so it is not possible to imply if these clinical results after PAE could be comparable to placebo or medical therapy mainly because all patients were receiving prostatic medication and stopped all medication after the procedure, with good outcomes. There is some evidence that other factors besides prostatic volume reduction may account for clinical outcomes after PAE. Further studies are warranted to confirm this hypothesis and to compare PAE with placebo and medical and surgical therapies. Although the results are preliminary, with a small number of patients and a short follow-up period, they are very promising. More studies are needed with greater numbers of patients, different sizes of PVA particles, and longer follow-up period to assess if the procedure can be an effective and a safe alternative in the management of BPH.

T. G. Walker, MD

Transarterial Chemoembolization Can Be Safely Performed in Patients with Hepatocellular Carcinoma Invading the Main Portal Vein and May Improve the Overall Survival

Chung GE, Lee J-H, Kim HY, et al (Seoul Natl Univ Hosp, Yungun-dong, Chongno-gu, Korea; Seoul Natl Univ College of Medicine, Korea)
Radiology 258:627-634, 2011

Purpose.—To determine the efficacy and safety of transarterial chemoembolization (TACE) in patients with hepatocellular carcinoma (HCC) and main portal vein (MPV) invasion.

Materials and Methods.—This study was approved by the institutional review board, and the requirement to obtain informed consent was waived. The authors retrospectively assessed the electronic medical records of patients in whom HCC with MPV invasion was newly diagnosed from January 2004 to December 2007 at a single tertiary medical center. Patients with decompensated hepatic function were excluded. Outcomes of patients treated with TACE were compared with those of patients given supportive care according to Child-Pugh class.

Results.—One hundred twenty-five patients (104 men and 21 women; mean age, 55.7 years; age range, 33.4–83.0 years) were included. The median overall survival was 3.7 months (range, 0.2–33.3 months). Eighty-three of the 125 patients (66.4%) were treated with TACE and 42 (33.6%) received supportive care. Repeated TACE showed significant survival benefits compared with supportive care in patients with Child-Pugh class A (median survival, 7.4 months vs 2.6 months, respectively; $P < .001$) and class B (median survival, 2.8 months vs 1.9 months, respectively; $P = .002$) disease. Results of multivariate analysis showed that treatment with TACE (hazard ratio, 0.263; 95% confidence interval [CI]: 0.164, 0.424; $P < .001$) and Child-Pugh class A status (hazard ratio, 0.550; 95% CI: 0.368, 0.822; $P = .004$) were independent predictive factors of a favorable outcome. There were no procedure-related deaths within 4 weeks after TACE, and patient morbidity was 28.9% (24 of 83 patients).

Conclusion.—TACE can be performed safely and may improve the overall survival of patients with HCC and MPV invasion (Fig 1).

► Hepatocellular carcinoma (HCC) is one of the most common malignant tumors in the world, with an increasing annual incidence. Many HCCs are diagnosed at the intermediate or advanced stages, for which there are no curative therapy and a dismal prognosis. In particular, transarterial chemoembolization (TACE) has been used for palliative treatment in patients with unresectable HCC with invasion of vascular sites other than the main portal vein (MPV) and has been shown to improve survival.

However, TACE has been considered to be contraindicated in patients with HCC and MPV invasion because of the risk of deteriorating hepatic function caused by ischemic liver damage caused by TACE. Instead, the Barcelona Clinic Liver Cancer (BCLC) group recommended treatment with sorafenib, a molecular-targeted agent, as a standard treatment for patients with vascular invasion.

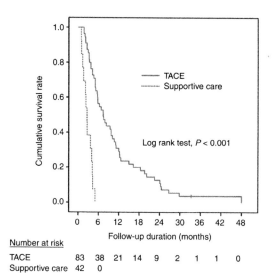

FIGURE 1.—Graph shows cumulative survival rates of patients with HCC and MPV invasion according to treatment. Data were obtained with the Kaplan-Meier method. The median survival of the TACE group (5.6 months) was longer than that for the supportive care group (2.2 months) ($P < .001$, log-rank test). (Reprinted from Chung GE, Lee J-H, Kim HY, et al. Transarterial chemoembolization can be safely performed in patients with hepatocellular carcinoma invading the main portal vein and may improve the overall survival. *Radiology.* 2011;258:627-634, copyright by the Radiological Society of North America.)

However, the Sorafenib Hepatocellular Carcinoma Assessment Randomized Protocol (SHARP) trial, on which the BCLC recommendations are based, included a mixed group of patients with heterogeneous prognoses regarding the presence and degree of vascular invasion and/or extrahepatic metastasis. In fact, while the SHARP trial showed a survival benefit with sorafenib in patients with advanced HCC, macroscopic vascular invasion was confirmed in only 38.5% of the patients. Thus, the results of the SHARP trial may not directly translate into a substantial survival gain with sorafenib treatment in the specific subgroup of patients with HCC and MPV invasion.

It has been recently suggested that TACE could be safely performed even in patients with MPV invasion if the patient has good hepatic function and collateral circulation around the MPV. However, a survival benefit for TACE in patients with HCC and MPV invasion has not been demonstrated. The aim of the current study was to investigate the efficacy and safety of TACE in patients with HCC and MPV invasion.

This was an institutional review board—approved retrospective study in which the electronic medical records of consecutive patients in whom HCC and MPV invasion was newly diagnosed from January 2004 to December 2007 at a university-affiliated hospital. In these patients in whom there was the diagnosis of HCC, the presence of tumor invasion in the MPV was confirmed with the demonstration of a low-attenuation intraluminal mass expanding the portal vein and/or filling defects in the MPV at 3-phase dynamic computed tomography (CT).

If the patient had preserved hepatic function (eg, Child-Pugh class A disease), TACE was recommended as the initial treatment. If the patient had intermediate hepatic function (eg, Child-Pugh class B disease), the treatment strategy, including TACE and supportive care, was determined for each patient on the basis of the attending physician's preference. Patients were excluded from this study if they (1) had decompensated liver function classified as Child-Pugh class C disease; (2) had previously received sorafenib, systemic chemotherapy, or intra-arterial chemoinfusion; (3) had serious medical comorbidities; (4) had or previously had malignant tumors in addition to HCC; and (5) had undergone organ transplantation.

The embolization procedure was performed as selectively as possible through the lobar, segmental, or subsegmental arteries, depending on the tumor distribution and hepatic functional reserve, by using a microcatheter, and doxorubicin hydrochloride was administered into the feeder vessels. The volume of iodized oil ranged from 2 to 12 mL and the amount of doxorubicin ranged from 10 to 60 mg. Gelatin sponge particles were mixed with mitomycin and contrast material and were administered into the arterial feeder vessels until stasis of arterial flow was achieved. Cisplatin was infused into the tumor feeder vessels as a solution with a concentration of 0.5 mg/mL at a rate of 5 to 10 mL/min. The total amount of cisplatin used ranged from 50 to 100 mg depending on the patient's body weight and the level of infusion. In patients with an arterioportal shunt, embolization with gelatin sponge particles was initially performed to occlude the shunt.

This was followed by infusion of a small amount of an iodized oil and doxorubicin hydrochloride emulsion. The extent of chemoembolization was individually adjusted by using a superselective catheterization technique depending on the patient's hepatic functional reserve, similar to that used with surgical hepatectomy.

A noncontrast hepatic CT was performed 3 weeks after TACE to evaluate the liver for traces of iodized oil, and contrast-enhanced 3-phase dynamic CT was performed 1 to 2 weeks before the next TACE session to detect residual viable tumor or recurrent tumor. If the Child-Pugh status remained at class B or higher and there was no evidence of hepatic decompensation (eg, uncontrolled ascites or hepatic encephalopathy), TACE was performed repeatedly over 2 or 3 months until the absence of viable intrahepatic tumor. Complete remission of the intrahepatic tumor was determined by shrinkage of parenchymal and intraportal tumor thrombi without residual enhancing tumor at 3-phase dynamic CT and the lack of tumor staining at follow-up hepatic arteriography. Of the 125 patients, 105 had diffuse HCC, which limited our ability to measure the change in tumor size in response to treatment. In patients in whom serum tumor markers were initially elevated, normalization of those markers along with compatible imaging findings was also required to determine complete tumor response.

One hundred twenty-five patients in whom HCC with MPV invasion was newly diagnosed were included in the study. Of the 125 patients, 83 (66.4%) were treated with TACE and 42 (33.6%) received supportive care. The median interval between diagnosis and initiation of TACE was 13 days. The median number of TACE procedures was 2.7. There were no differences between the

2 groups with respect to patient age, viral cause of underlying liver disease, and tumor stage according to the American Joint Committee on Cancer staging system.

The median overall survival for the 125 patients was 3.7 months. The TACE treatment and a better Child-Pugh class were significant predictive factors of a favorable outcome. The median survival in the TACE group was longer than that in the supportive care group (5.6 months vs 2.2 months, respectively). Fig 1 shows the cumulative survival rates of patients with HCC and MPV invasion according to treatment. Treatment with TACE and Child-Pugh class A status were independent predictive factors associated with better overall survival. In the TACE group, the presence of iodized oil uptake in the MPV after TACE and Child- Pugh class A status were significant favorable prognostic factors. Tumor type (eg, diffuse or nodular) failed to show a significant difference. A greater number of TACE sessions were found to be a favorable prognostic factor. During the follow-up period, 25 adverse clinical events were observed in 24 of the 83 patients (29%) in the TACE group, and 19 adverse events were observed in 19 of the 42 patients (45%) in the supportive care group.

The authors were able to demonstrate a survival benefit of TACE in patients with advanced HCC and MPV invasion. The benefit of TACE on overall survival remained significant after adjusting for baseline liver function. In addition, the results demonstrated that TACE could be performed relatively safely in patients with HCC and MPV invasion; however, patient morbidity was high, at 28.9% (24 of 83 patients).

T. G. Walker, MD

Uterine Artery Embolization in the Treatment of Postpartum Uterine Hemorrhage
Ganguli S, Stecker MS, Pyne D, et al (Brigham and Women's Hosp and Harvard Med School, Boston, MA)
J Vasc Interv Radiol 22:169-176, 2011

Purpose.—To evaluate the clinical effectiveness and safety of uterine artery embolization (UAE) in the treatment of primary postpartum hemorrhage (PPH), secondary PPH, and PPH associated with cesarean section.

Materials and Methods.—All women who underwent UAE for obstetric-related hemorrhage during a 52-month period culminating in April 2009 were included. Clinical success was defined as obviation of hysterectomy. Blood product requirements before and after UAE were calculated. Statistically significant associations between subject characteristics and clinical success were evaluated. The two subgroups of women with uterine artery pseudoaneurysms and women who underwent cesarean section were examined separately as well.

Results.—Sixty-six women (mean age, 33 years; range, 17—47 y) underwent UAE, with an overall clinical success rate of 95% (98% for primary PPH, 88% for secondary PPH, and 94% for PPH associated with cesarean

244 / Diagnostic Radiology

section) and an overall complication rate of 4.5%. Mean pre- and postembolization transfusion requirements were 3.1 U and 0.4 U of packed red blood cells, respectively. The only significant characteristic identified for the cases that necessitated hysterectomy was an increased transfusion requirement after UAE (increase of 1.0 U ± 0.5; $P = .02$). Uterine artery pseudoaneurysms were associated with secondary PPH ($P = .01$) and cesarean section ($P = .03$).

Conclusions.—The threshold for UAE in women with PPH should be low, as it is associated with a high clinical effectiveness rate and a low complication rate. Uterine artery pseudoaneurysms should be suspected in women presenting with secondary PPH after cesarean section.

▶ Obstetric hemorrhage is a leading cause of maternal morbidity and mortality, with an incidence that varies depending on the definition used. Postpartum hemorrhage (PPH), defined as blood loss exceeding 500 mL, is a common entity that complicates as many as 18% of all deliveries. More severe obstetric hemorrhage, defined as blood loss in excess of 1000 mL, may occur in 1%-5% of all deliveries. Obstetric hemorrhage continues to be the single most important cause of maternal mortality worldwide, accounting for 25%-30% of all maternal deaths, and it represents the most common maternal morbidity in the developed world.

Since its introduction as a treatment of PPH, uterine artery embolization (UAE) has been shown to be associated with high technical success rates and good clinical outcomes for the treatment of primary and secondary PPH. However, optimal patient selection and the appropriate position of UAE in the treatment decision tree for PPH remain to be elucidated. Current studies in the literature lack standardization in patient selection as well as embolization techniques, and there is a lack of randomized controlled trials comparing pharmacologic, surgical, and endovascular interventions. As the number and percentage of cesarean deliveries increases in the United States, more data are required in regard to the effectiveness of UAE for PPH in the population of women who have had a cesarean delivery.

The purpose of this retrospective study was to analyze and report the clinical outcomes, including clinical effectiveness and safety of UAE for the treatment of obstetrical uterine hemorrhage at a single tertiary care obstetric hospital in terms of primary and secondary PPH and in the population who had previously undergone a cesarean delivery.

All subjects were referred to the vascular and interventional radiology service for UAE by the obstetric service. UAE for the treatment of PPH was performed only after all usual obstetric maneuvers for the treatment of PPH were used. This usually included intravenous uterotonic agents, aggressive uterine massage, manual extraction of the placenta, examination and repair of genital lacerations, and often balloon tamponade. Those patients with leiomyoma- or tumor-related uterine hemorrhage were excluded. Primary PPH was defined as hemorrhage that occurred within the first 24 hours after delivery. Secondary PPH was defined as hemorrhage occurring more than 24 hours after delivery.

The standard UAE technique was used in treatment of the subjects. As long as a pseudoaneurysm was not visualized with selective uterine angiography, embolization was performed with the use of absorbable gelatin sponge administered in a slurry with saline solution and contrast medium. Embolization was performed until stasis of flow in the uterine artery was achieved. If a pseudoaneurysm was identified, it was embolized with microcoils. Technical success was defined as successful catheterization of both uterine arteries with embolization to stasis, embolization of a nonuterine pelvic vessel giving rise to active contrast agent extravasation, or successful coil embolization of a specific vascular lesion (ie, pseudoaneurysm). Clinical success of UAE was defined as obviation of subsequent hysterectomy. The range and mean requirements for administered blood products before and after UAE were calculated.

A total of 76 women (mean age, 33 years) underwent UAE at our institution for obstetric-related hemorrhage during the study period. The technical success rate was 100%. The mean gravidity of the women was 2.6, and the mean parity of the women was 1.8. Of these 76 women, 6 women underwent UAE for hemorrhage related to an intrauterine ectopic pregnancy and 3 women underwent UAE performed in conjunction with prophylactic placement of internal iliac occlusion balloons for hemorrhage control during elective cesarean delivery associated with known placenta accreta/percreta. Only 1 woman underwent hysterectomy before UAE, in whom embolization was performed for persistent vaginal hemorrhage, and this woman did not require further intervention after UAE. These 10 subjects were excluded from the analysis. Of the remaining 66 women, only 3 went on to subsequent hysterectomy, indicating a clinical success rate of UAE of 95% and a hysterectomy rate of 5% (3 of 66). The reasons for subsequent hysterectomy in the 3 women included persistent PPH in 2 women and endometritis in 1 woman (2 weeks after UAE). In addition to these 3 clinical failures, there were 3 complications potentially related to the UAE procedure, including 1 woman who developed a left lower extremity deep vein thrombosis, 1 woman who developed postprocedural pancreatitis, and 1 woman who was readmitted for intravenous antibiotic treatment for presumed endometritis and underwent UAE as well as dilation and curettage. No women in the study had a repeat UAE procedure.

Of the 66 women included in the study, 50 (76%) underwent UAE for primary PPH and 16 (24%) for secondary PPH. Forty-eight women (73%) underwent UAE following vaginal deliveries, and 18 (27%) had cesarean deliveries. The mean pre-embolization transfusion requirement was 3.1 U (range, 0-12 U) of packed red blood cells (PRBCs) and the mean postembolization transfusion requirement was 0.4 U of PRBCs. The mean hospital stay after UAE was 3.5 days.

Nine pregnancies were identified after UAE in 9 women. Of these 9 pregnancies, there were 2 spontaneous abortions and 7 viable gestations, 6 of which had standard vaginal deliveries and 1 was cesarean delivery. Therefore, 7 of 66 women had a subsequent viable pregnancy (10.6%). An area of interest to clinicians and women regarding UAE is its effect on subsequent fertility, and the data in the literature regarding this topic are limited. The transient subischemic conditions induced by UAE on the uterus raise the important question of long-term effect on future fertility. Previous investigators have concluded that UAE offers a safe and conservative alternative to surgical interventions for PPH in women who desire to preserve future fertility. In this series, the documentation of 9 pregnancies that were identified after UAE in 9 women appear to coincide with those found in other series, but the numbers are relatively low. There are not enough data to make definitive recommendations in this area, but the data suggest that the endometrium is not impaired by UAE. A careful discussion with women considering UAE who desire future fertility is warranted. However, the fact that UAE preserves the uterus and can preclude hysterectomy is vital in this regard.

The authors conclude that UAE for obstetric-related hemorrhage has a high clinical effectiveness for primary PPH (98%), secondary PPH (88%), and PPH related to cesarean delivery (94%). This was associated with an overall complication rate of 4.5%, although some complications may have been related to hemorrhage-related comorbidities and other contemporaneous procedures. Blood product requirements after UAE were low, and the surgical risks and absolute loss of fertility associated with hysterectomy were avoided. Interventional radiology and UAE should be included in multidisciplinary algorithms and rapid-response team plans to optimize outcomes of women with PPH, and given the relatively low incidence of complications, the authors propose that embolization of the uterus should be considered early in the algorithm of PPH management.

T. G. Walker, MD

Endografts

Detection of Type II Endoleak After Endovascular Aortic Repair: Comparison Between Magnetic Resonance Angiography and Blood-Pool Contrast Agent and Dual-Phase Computed Tomography Angiography
Wieners G, Meyer F, Halloul Z, et al (Univ Hosp, Magdeburg, Germany)
Cardiovasc Intervent Radiol 33:1135-1142, 2010

Purpose.—This prospective study was designed to assess the diagnostic value of magnetic resonance angiography (MRA) with blood-pool contrast agent (gadofosveset) in the detection of type-II endoleak after endovascular aortic repair (EVAR).

Methods.—Thirty-two patients with aortic aneurysms who had undergone EVAR were included in this study. All patients were examined by dual-phase computed tomography angiography (CTA) as well as MRA with gadofosveset in the first-pass and steady-state phases. Two independent readers evaluated the images of CTA and MRA in terms of endoleak type II, feeding vessel, and image quality.

Results.—Median follow-up-time after EVAR was 22 months (range 4 to 59). Endoleak type II was detected by CTA in 12 of 32 patients (37.5%); MRA detected endoleak in all of these patients as well as in another 9 patients ($n = 21$, 65.6%), of whom the endoleaks in 6 patients showed an increasing diameter. Most endoleaks were detected in the steady-state phase ($n = 14$). The decrease in diameter of the aneurysmal sac was significantly greater in the patients without a visible endoleak that was visible on MRA ($P = 0.004$). In the overall estimation of diagnostic accuracy, MRA was judged superior to CTA in 66% of all examinations.

Conclusion.—MRA with gadofosveset appeared superior to CTA, and has higher diagnostic accuracy, in the detection of endoleak after EVAR (Figs 1 and 2).

▶ Endovascular aneurysm repair (EVAR) is now a mainstay of treatment of aortic aneurysms. This minimally invasive endovascular treatment, in which a stent graft is inserted into the affected part of the aorta, has become increasingly popular because it is associated with fewer perioperative risks, a lower rate of short-term complications, and shorter hospitalization stay compared with conventional open surgery. Following EVAR, diagnostic surveillance imaging must be periodically performed to evaluate possible complications, such as endoleak, which can lead to recurrent high pressure in the aneurysmal sac, thus causing enlargement and risk of rupture. The second reason for long-term follow-up is to ensure that the device is structurally intact and that the stent graft has not migrated.

Imaging techniques used for post-EVAR surveillance include ultrasound, computed tomography (CT), and magnetic resonance imaging. New contrast agents have improved the sensitivity of ultrasound, but this technique is extremely dependent on the experience of the investigator. Helical CT angiography (CTA) in arterial and venous phases is currently the reference standard.

The aim of this prospective study was to investigate the diagnostic value of magnetic resonance angiography (MRA) with the new blood pool magnetic resonance (MR) contrast agent gadofosveset (Vasovist; Bayer Schering Health Care, Germany) for the detection of postoperative endoleak after EVAR for aneurysms. Gadofosveset is a blood pool MR contrast agent that binds to albumin and has a half-life of approximately 15 hours. The relaxivity of gadofosveset is approximately 5 to 7 times higher than that of gadopentetate dimeglumine with 1.5-T scanners. The authors compared the MRA technique with

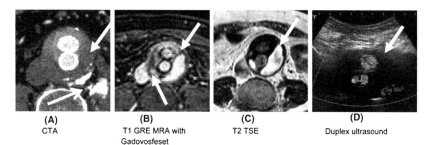

(A)	(B)	(C)	(D)
CTA	T1 GRE MRA with Gadovosfeset	T2 TSE	Duplex ultrasound

FIGURE 1.—(A) CTA of EVAR and postpuncturing of endoleak with application of an embolic agent (Ethibloc) (*open arrow*) 6 months after EVAR. No further endoleak is detectable. (B) T1 GRE MRA with gadovosfeset shows endoleak in the steady-state phase (*arrow*). (C) T2 TSE with hyperintense signal in the region of the endoleak. (D) In the duplex ultrasound, no endoleak is detectable. (Reprinted from Wieners G, Meyer F, Halloul Z, et al. Detection of type II endoleak after endovascular aortic repair: comparison between magnetic resonance angiography and blood-pool contrast agent and dual-phase computed tomography angiography. *Cardiovasc Intervent Radiol.* 2010;33:1135-1142, with permission from Springer Science+Business Media, LLC and the Cardiovascular and Interventional Radiological Society of Europe (CIRSE).)

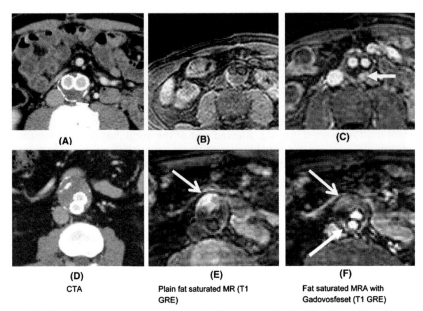

(A) (B) (C)

(D) (E) (F)
CTA Plain fat saturated MR (T1 Fat saturated MRA with
     GRE)   Gadovosfeset (T1 GRE)

FIGURE 2.—Example of two patients (no. 1 [A–C] and no. 2. [D–F) without detectable endoleak in the CTA (A, D). Fat saturated T1 GRE with gadovosfeset demonstrates new contrastation in the aneurysmatic sac compared to the plain fat-saturated T1 GRE (*closed arrow*). Susceptibility artefacts in the aneurysmatic sac (*open arrow*). (Reprinted from Wieners G, Meyer F, Halloul Z, et al. Detection of type II endoleak after endovascular aortic repair: comparison between magnetic resonance angiography and blood-pool contrast agent and dual-phase computed tomography angiography. *Cardiovasc Intervent Radiol.* 2010;33:1135-1142, with permission from Springer Science+Business Media, LLC and the Cardiovascular and Interventional Radiological Society of Europe (CIRSE).)

an improved dual-phase (ie, arterial and venous phases) CTA scan in 32 consecutive patients who were undergoing follow-up examination to exclude endoleak type II after previous implantation of nitinol aortic stent grafts for infrarenal aneurysms as follows: 25 Excluder AAA Endoprosthesis (Gore Medical, Newark, Delaware), 4 Talent Stent Graft (Medtronic, Germany), and 3 Anaconda endovascular device (Vascutek, Germany). All patients were examined by dual-phase CTA during routine follow-up after EVAR, twice in the first year (after 1, 3, and 6 months) and then once a year. MRA was performed as a single additional examination, irrespective of the date of EVAR, between October 2007 and October 2008. The time between CTA and MRA was not to be more than 1 month.

The CTA protocol comprised a dual-phase technique with a slice thickness of 1 mm, KV 120, and modulated milliampere. Iodinated contrast agent (80-100 mL) was injected at a speed of 4 mL/s and followed by 30 mL saline solution. The CT images were reconstructed additionally in the coronal and sagittal orientations. MRA was performed with a 1.5-T scanner. Before the administration of contrast agent, a plain T1 gradient echo sequence and a T2–turbo spin echo sequence were performed. The MRA protocol included a first-pass examination after administration of the blood pool contrast agent gadofosveset with a 3-dimensional reconstruction and a breath-triggered isovoxel steady-state examination 5 minutes after administration of the contrast agent. The examination was completed with an axial fat-saturated T1 gradient echo sequence. Gadofosveset (0.03 mmol/kg body weight) was injected at a flow rate of 1 mL/s; at the concentration supplied, this required a bolus of approximately 10 mL (administration during approximately 10 seconds). Gadofosveset reaches an equilibrium phase in arterial and venous blood vessels within 5 minutes of administration.

The CTA and MRA images were evaluated by 2 experienced readers, in a blinded fashion, with a final consensus reading of the images according to the criteria for detection of endoleak, feeding vessel, hyperintense signal on T2-weighted (T2W) images, and image quality. An endoleak in MRA was defined as new hyperintense signal inside the aneurysmal sac around the nitinol stent graft on the steady-state or the postcontrast T1-weighted (T1W) gradient echo sequence compared with plain T1W gradient echo imaging with identical parameters. The image quality was rated on a scale of 1 (excellent) to 5 (very poor), and possible artifacts were included in the evaluation of image quality. The hyperintense signal in T2W images was considered equivalent to the fluid phase in the aneurysmal sac using a 4-point scale from 0 (none) through 1 (mild), 2 (moderate), and 3 (strong) hyperintense signals, with the signal from the liquor in the spinal canal as reference. All diameters of the aneurysmal sac in each patient were measured by CTA during the follow-up period.

In 12 patients (37.5%), type II endoleak was detected on CTA; of these endoleaks, 67% (n = 8) were seen in the arterial phase and 33% (n = 4) were seen only in the delayed venous phase. The inflow or outflow vessels detected on CTA were in 3 cases lumbar arteries (73%) and in 3 cases the inferior mesenteric and lumbar arteries (27%). It was not possible to identify which vessel is the inflow or outflow vessel on CTA or MRA because no dynamic study or sequences, such as phase contrast, was performed. Image quality for the CT scans was rated as excellent in 94% (n = 30) and good in 6% (n = 2) of the examinations.

All 12 patients displaying a type II endoleak on CTA were also found by MRA to have a type II endoleak. Nine patients who had negative results on CTA showed regions of pathologic contrast on contrast-enhanced MRA, compared with plain (unenhanced) T1W gradient echo sequence, that were classified as type II endoleak. This means that in 66% of patients (n = 21) (Table 3 in the original article) after EVAR, type II endoleak was detected on MRA. Of these type II endoleaks detected on MRA, 33% were seen in the first-pass (n = 7) and 67% in the steady-state phase (n = 14). In 6 of these 9 patients undetected by CTA, there was an increase in the aneurysm sac diameter (median 0.6 cm; range 0.2-1.0). Figs 1 and 2 illustrate patients in whom CTA was negative for type II endoleak, whereas the MR examination was positive.

It is generally accepted that CTA allows the easy detection of relatively large endoleaks. However, the detection of small endoleaks (especially those close to high-attenuation components, such as metallic portions of the stent graft and calcifications) or low-flow endoleaks can be difficult, requiring thorough analysis of CT images. Determining the source of an endoleak and the direction of flow are necessary for proper classification; however, although CTA has high sensitivity and specificity for detecting endoleak, it is limited in its ability to show direction of flow.

The results of this study suggest that the sensitivity of MRA with gadofosveset in the detection of endoleak may be superior to that of CTA. Even given the small population studied, the sensitivity of MRA (assuming CTA as the reference standard) was found to be 100% with a lower 95% confidence limit of approximately 76%. All 21 cases definitively showed endoleaks on MRA, which was defined as new hyperintense signal inside the residual aneurysm sac around the nitinol stent graft that had not previously been seen on plain T1W gradient echo imaging. The authors therefore conclude that artifacts can be excluded as possible reasons for these endoleaks. Future studies should address the question of whether MRA with gadofosveset is superior to dual-phase CTA.

T. G. Walker, MD

Patient Care

A Comparison of Transjugular and Plugged-Percutaneous Liver Biopsy in Patients with Contraindications to Ordinary Percutaneous Liver Biopsy and an "In-House" Protocol for Selecting the Procedure of Choice

Atar E, Ben Ari Z, Bachar GN, et al (Hasharon Hosp, Petach Tikva, Israel; Beilinson Hosp, Petach Tikva, Israel; et al)
Cardiovasc Intervent Radiol 33:560-564, 2010

The purpose of this study was to evaluate the effectiveness and safety of transjugular liver biopsy (TJLB) and plugged-percutaneous liver biopsy (PB) in consecutive patients with severe liver disease associated with impaired coagulation, ascites, or both and to verify the in-house protocol used to select the appropriate procedure. In 2000–2006, 329 patients (208 male [62.8%] and 121 female [37.2%]), aged 1 month to 81 years (mean, 46.8 years), underwent 150 TJLBs (39.1%) or 233 PBs (60.9%) procedures at a major tertiary center, as determined by an in-house protocol. The groups were compared for specimen characteristics, technical success, and complications. Technical success rates were 97.4% for TJLB (146/150) and 99.1% for PB (231/233). TJLB was associated with a lower average core length (1.29 vs. 1.43 cm) and lower average number of specimens obtained (2.44 vs. 2.8), but both methods yielded sufficient tissue for a definitive diagnosis. There were no major complications in either group. TJLB and PB can be safely and effectively performed for the diagnosis of hepatic disease in patients with contraindications for standard percutaneous liver biopsy. When both are technically available, we suggest PB as the procedure of choice, especially in transplanted livers.

▶ Liver biopsy is widely used in the diagnostic workup for mortality (0.01%) and morbidity (0.2%). The most common serious complication is severe hemorrhage due to damage to the arterial or portal tree or to the intercostal arteries. McGill et al found that among 9212 liver biopsies, 0.24% were complicated by nonfatal hemorrhage and 0.11% by fatal hemorrhage.

The optimal diagnostic method in patients with coagulopathy or ascites, which preclude standard percutaneous liver biopsy, is still controversial. Transjugular liver biopsy (TJLB) has been found to have a low major morbidity and mortality. Although TJLB specimens were initially considered inferior to percutaneous liver biopsy specimens owing to their smaller size and excessive fragmentation, this disadvantage was largely eliminated with the introduction of the thinner Tru-cut needles. Currently, a liver specimen > 15-mm long is considered sufficient for diagnosis of diffuse liver disease.

Percutaneous liver biopsy in which the needle tract is plugged with absorbable foam (PB) is a well-known procedure for the diagnosis of coagulation disorders. It is easy to perform, requires no intravenous cannulation, and is less time consuming than TJLB. A previous report suggested that PB might also be more effective than TJLB for obtaining adequate liver tissue, and it is not generally associated with an increased incidence of bleeding. Others, however, found a slightly higher incidence of bleeding episodes in patients with impaired coagulation undergoing PB compared with TJLB. The aims of this study were to evaluate the effectiveness and safety of TJLB and PB in consecutive patients with severe liver disease associated with impaired coagulation, ascites, or both and to verify the in-house protocol used to select the appropriate procedure in this setting.

This retrospective study included 329 consecutive patients who underwent 383 TJLB or PB procedures at a tertiary, university-affiliated facility between January 2000 and December 2006. Data on routine demographic, clinical, and laboratory parameters were collected from the medical files. In all cases, TJLB or PB was performed because of contraindications to standard percutaneous liver biopsy. Selection of TJLB or PB in each case was based on the authors' in-house protocol. TJLB was indicated in patients with ascites, a platelet count of $< 60\,000/mm^3$, or an INR of ≥ 2; PB was indicated in patients with an INR of 1.4 to 2 and a platelet count of $60\,000$ to $100\,000/mm^3$. In young children with ascites for whom the TJLB set was too large, we performed complete peritoneal percutaneous paracentesis with ultrasound verification of the evacuation of the ascitic fluids, followed by PB. In adult patients, after whole-liver transplantation, PB was performed when possible because of the various venous anastomoses between the donor and the recipient hepatic veins.

TJLB was performed in the interventional radiology suite according to previously reported techniques, under local anesthesia (adults) or intravenous or general sedation (children). A 20-guage Cook TJLB set (Cook, Bloomington, IN, USA) was used in all cases. Before taking the biopsy, the wedge and hepatic vein pressures were recorded. Three or 4 quick-core needle passes were usually needed to obtain sufficient liver tissue (at least 2 long tissue cores). TJLB was considered technically unsuccessful if it was impossible to obtain a liver sample for any reason. Major complications (ie, supraventricular tachycardia, capsular perforation, or intraperitoneal hemorrhage) were recorded. Day cases were followed in hospital for up to 12 hours; inpatients were followed for 24 hours.

PB was also performed in the interventional radiology suite, using previously reported techniques, under local anesthesia (adults) or intravenous sedation using a laryngeal mask airway (children). An 18- or 20-guage (according to patient size) coaxial quick-core firing needle set (Cook) was used. The preferred biopsy site was the left liver lobe or segment 4 in the subxyphoid region. Three or 4 core needle specimens were obtained under ultrasound guidance prior to tract embolization using gel-foam pledgets, followed by ultrasound examination of the puncture site and the liver capsule. Day patients were followed in hospital for up to 6 hours. Inpatients were followed for 24 hours and then discharged home if there were no symptoms and no change in serum hemoglobin level.

A total of 150 TJLB procedures were performed in 97 male patients and 53 female patients. The indications for TJLB were ascites in 57 patients (38%), liver cirrhosis in 32 (21.3%), and after liver transplantation in 13 (8.6%). The maximum number of repeated TJLB procedures in individual patients was 4, in 1 patient. A total of 233 PB procedures were performed in 38 male patients (59.2%) and 95 female patients (40.8%); 25 patients were children. The indications for PB were ascites in 23 children (9.9%), liver cirrhosis in 14 patients (6.1%), and after liver transplantation in 125 patients (53.7%). The 3 patients who had 5 or more PB procedures were all young children after split-liver transplantations.

One to 6 needle passes were required per patient (average, 2.44 cores) in the TJLB group, with a technical success rate of 97.4% (146/150). Two of the technical failures were attributed to acute angulation of the right hepatic vein relative to the intravenous catheter caused by cranial displacement of the liver by severe ascites. In the remaining failures, the liver tissue obtained was inadequate for a definitive diagnosis (fragmented in one, too small a specimen in the other).

Thirteen TJLB procedures were performed in adults after whole-liver transplantation. In all cases, the anastomoses between the recipient and the host catheters or hepatic veins were verified first.

One to 6 cores were obtained (average, 2.8 cores per patient) in the PB group, with a technical success rate of 99.1% (231/233 procedures). In 2 cases, the liver specimen was too small for a definitive diagnosis. No major or minor complications were recorded. In the PB procedures performed for ascites during the later study period (initially, TJLB was preferred), the fluid was drained first.

Although the specimens obtained with TJLB were significantly smaller and fewer than those obtained with PB, they were not less adequate for histological evaluation. There was no statistically significant difference between the groups in technical success rate or complication rate. Both techniques were associated with high success.

In liver biopsy, adequate specimens are crucial for accurate histological interpretation, elimination of sampling error, and minimization of intraobserver or interobserver variability. Although Vibhakorn et al concluded that at least 4 passes should be performed in TJLB procedures when liver specimens are needed for grading and staging, the current data do not show a better diagnostic yield with a larger number of passes. The technical failure rate (2.8%) was also close to that reported by others for 7649 biopsies summarizing 64 series (3.2%), and the total complication rate was considerably lower (0.9% vs 7.1% in the earlier study).

The reported rate for major complications of TJLB, usually life-threatening intraperitoneal bleeding, was 0.6% and the mortality rate 0.09%. Further studies are needed to determine the minimal number of passes required to obtain enough tissue for diagnosis. Since the study by Riley et al in 1984, percutaneous liver biopsy with plugging of the needle track has been considered a feasible alternative method for obtaining liver tissue in patients with clotting disorders. It is easier and quicker to perform than TJLB. Major complications include major bleeding and death, and minor complications are mainly hemorrhage but also arterioportal fistulas, biliary fistulas, bile leak, and infections. Embolization of the needle tract makes it possible to use wider biopsy needles. The authors used 18-guage needles and 16-guage coaxial needles in adults and 20-guage biopsy needles and 18-guage outer needles in children. No major complications occurred during the study period.

There is only 1 published study comparing TJLB and PB. The sample included 100 consecutive patients presenting with liver disease and moderately severe coagulation defects. The biopsy specimens obtained by the transjugular method were on average smaller than those obtained with PB. Hemorrhage occurred in 3.5% of the patients who underwent PB, treated by transfusion in all cases, and in none of the patients after TJLB. The success rate was higher in the PB group (91% vs 84% for TJLB).

The authors believe that because of its simplicity, lower cost, high success rate, and very low complication rate, PB is the procedure of choice (according to the coagulation data), especially in liver transplant recipients. PB can be performed even in patients with ascites following paracentesis. In patients with severe impairment on coagulation tests and ascites because of the reduced risk of blood extravasation through the liver capsule, TJLB is preferred and is as safe as PB.

T. G. Walker, MD

Endovascular Treatment of Complications of Femoral Arterial Access
Tsetis D (Univ Hosp of Heraklion, Crete, Greece)
Cardiovasc Intervent Radiol 33:457-468, 2010

Endovascular repair of femoral arterial access complications is nowadays the treatment of choice in a group of patients who cannot tolerate vascular reconstruction and bleeding due to advanced cardiovascular disease. Endovascular procedures can be performed under local anesthesia, are well tolerated by the patient, and are associated with a short hospitalization time. Ninitinol stent technology allows for safe stent and stent-graft extension at the common femoral artery (CFA) level, due to increased resistance to external compression and bending stress. Active pelvic bleeding can be insidious, and prompt placement of a stent-graft at the site of leakage is a lifesaving procedure. Percutaneous thrombin injection under US guidance is the treatment of choice for femoral pseudoaneurysms (PAs); this can theoretically be safer with simultaneous balloon occlusion across the entry site of a PA without a neck or with a short and wide neck. In a few cases with thrombin failure due to a large arterial defect or accompanying arteriovenous fistula (AVF), a stent-graft can be deployed. The vast majority of catheter-induced AVFs can be treated effectively with stent-graft implantation even if they are located very close to the femoral bifurcation. Obstructive dissection flaps localized in the CFA are usually treated with prolonged balloon inflation; however, in more extensive dissections involving iliac arteries, selfexpanding stents should be deployed. Iliofemoral thrombosis can be treated effectively with catheter-directed thrombolysis (CDT) followed by prolonged balloon inflation or stent placement. Balloon angioplasty and CDT can occasionally be used to treat stenoses and occlusions complicating the use of percutaneous closure devices.

▶ The number of percutaneous endovascular interventions performed worldwide has been growing rapidly due to important technological advances, improved long-term clinical outcomes, and, also the lower morbidity associated with these procedures compared with traditional surgical treatment methods. The common femoral artery (CFA) is the most common access site for endovascular procedures, and it is therefore essential for interventionists to know how to recognize and manage the complications associated with this type of access. Table 1 in the original article outlines the most frequent complications that occur with femoral arterial access; these include hematoma, uncontrollable groin and/or retroperitoneal bleeding, pseudoaneurysm, arteriovenous fistula (AVF), and in situ arterial dissection with or without associated thrombosis. Less frequent complications include distal embolization, nerve damage, abscess, and lymphocele. This review examines the risk factors for complications that may occur in association with femoral arterial access, compares the endovascular versus the surgical treatment of iatrogenic femoral arterial access complications, and details the endovascular treatment options for various specific types of complications that are seen with this route of access.

The authors note that although the success of surgical repair of iatrogenic femoral access lesions is nearly 100%, this treatment is associated with a postoperative morbidity of up to 25% and a postoperative mortality that may approach 3.5% if there are significant comorbidities of the treated patients. As a result, when appropriate, endovascular repair of femoral arterial access complications may be the treatment of choice, and as such, interventionists must be familiar with these complications and the endovascular treatment options.

The most common significant complication is either hematoma or uncontrollable bleeding, requiring either transfusion or invasive treatment. This occurs in < 1% of endovascular procedures and almost always occurs during the attempt to achieve postprocedural hemostasis. While groin-expanding hematomas are readily evident, a massive retroperitoneal hematoma can develop without any external sign of bleeding. It is vital to recognize the clinical signs of pelvic bleeding while the patient is still on the angiographic table and thus can be treated on the spot; these include hypotension, tachycardia, loss of ipsilateral distal pulses, faintness, confusion, agitation, and abdominal pain. It is not unusual for an occult pelvic bleeding to occur several hours after the procedure, and in this context, unexplained tachycardia may be the first sign of this complication. As soon as there is suspicion of intra-abdominal bleeding, an abdominal computed tomographic scan should be obtained to confirm or rule out the diagnosis. If positive, diagnostic angiography should be performed in order to identify and treat the possible site of extravasation. This is typically performed through a contralateral retrograde femoral approach. Treatment with covered stent placement may be appropriate, depending upon the location of the vascular injury.

Another relatively common complication is postcatheterization pseudoaneurysm (PSA), with a reported incidence ranging from 2% to 8%. Symptoms and signs of PSA are pain, swelling, and severe bruising at the site of recent arterial puncture, and clinical examination may reveal a palpable thrill or pulsatile mass. The most serious complication of PSA is rupture, which is related mainly to the size of the PSA sac; other complications include persistent pain and swelling around the affected area, distal embolization, local skin ischemia and necrosis, infection, and compression of adjacent vessels or nerves. Diagnosis is confirmed with ultrasound evaluation, and thrombin injection under ultrasound guidance is now the treatment of choice for uncomplicated femoral artery PSAs with a distinct neck. In some circumstances, PSAs that do not respond to thrombin injection may benefit from covered stent placement. This may be useful in high-risk surgical patients, but the typical location of a PSA in the femoral artery may pose a problem for covered stent placement in the majority of patients.

AVFs may also be treated with covered stents, with the same caveats regarding the location of the lesion in the femoral artery. In some instances, embolotherapy of the AVF may be appropriate.

Arterial occlusion related to thrombosis or dissection at the access site is seen in < 0.5% of cases. An obstructive dissection may sometimes be effectively treated with prolonged inflation of an angioplasty balloon, but often an intravascular stent is required. Once more, the femoral artery location may be problematic. Thrombosis may require catheter-directed thrombolysis for the restoration of patency.

There may also be complications associated with closure devices, usually resulting in arterial occlusion. Once again, intravascular stent placement may be appropriate in selected cases.

The author concludes that endovascular repair is a less invasive treatment option than surgery for the treatment of various types of iatrogenic femoral access complications. Stent grafts are safe, effective, and durable devices for the treatment of uncontrollable bleeding, AVFs, and occasionally PSAs not amenable to treatment with percutaneous thrombin injection. New designs of currently available covered stents may allow for safe placement in the CFA in selected cases.

T. G. Walker, MD

Occupational Radiation Protection in Interventional Radiology: A Joint Guideline of the Cardiovascular and Interventional Radiology Society of Europe and the Society of Interventional Radiology

Miller DL, Vañó E, Bartal G, et al (Uniformed Services Univ of the Health Sciences, Bethesda, MD; San Carlos Univ Hosp and Complutense Univ, Madrid, Spain; Meir Med Ctr, Kfar Saba, Israel; et al)
J Vasc Interv Radiol 21:607-615, 2010

Background.—Fluoroscopically guided interventional procedures are increasingly being performed because they offer extensive benefits to patients. However, these procedures also have the potential to expose workers to radiation doses high enough to cause adverse effects and concerns. The Cardiovascular and Interventional Society of Europe (CIRSE) and the Society of Interventional Radiology (SIR) Safety and Health Committee have produced guidelines for providing occupational radiation protection for workers in interventional radiology settings. These guidelines are based on evidence-based data, critical review of peer-reviewed articles, and regulatory documents.

Exposure Issues.—Radiation dose limits are expressed in terms of equivalent dose in an organ or tissue for exposure of the body part and effective dose (E) for whole body exposures. The unit used is the sievert (Sv). Equivalent dose and E cannot be measured directly, but are instead calculated from more readily measured quantities. Personal dosimeters are worn to measure the dose equivalent of soft tissue at 0.07 mm and 10 mm below the surface of the body where the dosimeter is located. The dose delivered to the surface of the unshielded skin and to the lens of the eye is represented by the dosimeter worn at the collar over protective garments. Some uncertainties arise in occupational dosimetry, so for safety reasons, most formulas for estimating an individual's E produce overestimates. Personal dosimeters in interventional laboratories measure radiation field exposures from x-rays that irradiate the dosimeter directly and from radiation scattered back from the wearer's body. Two dosimeters are worn: one under the apron and the other at collar level above the lead apron.

The relatively high occupational exposures occurring in interventional laboratories require the use of more stringent monitoring programs than for areas with lower radiation exposures. The dose limit for E is 20 mSv/year averaged over 5 years. E may not exceed 50 mSv in any year. The lifetime limit is 10 mSv multiplied by the person's age in years. For pregnant women, the standard of protection should ensure that the embryo/fetus does not receive more than 1 mSv during the course of the pregnancy, or a 0.5-mSv equivalent dose monthly. Dosimeters are checked monthly; the "internal" dosimeter is worn at waist level. The current limit for exposure of the lens of the eye is less than 150 mSv annually, but evidence suggests that this is too high and it is being reviewed. The collar dosimeter readings are used to indicate exposure of the lens. Annual limits for the hands and feet are 500 mSv. A ring badge is recommended for hand dose estimates. Busy interventional radiologists who take all precautions will most likely have an E of 2 to 4 mSv/year.

Personal dosimetry data are evaluated monthly, noting E and information on the equivalent dose to the lens of the eye and the hand. If the records exceed the recommendations, investigation should check to see that the dosimeter reading is accurate, note any change in procedures, and observe the worker in action to monitor equipment settings, the worker's proximity to the patient, and the use of equipment-mounted shields and personal protective equipment. Suggestions are then made about how to keep the worker's dose as low as reasonably achievable (ALARA).

Protective Tools.—Controlling patient dose also reduces scatter and limits the amount of radiation to which the operator is exposed. Chronic radiation exposure requires that protective tools be used to limit occupation radiation dose. Three types of shielding can be used: architectural (built into the walls), equipment-mounted, and personal protective devices. Protective drapes suspended from the table and ceiling substantially reduce operator doses and should be used whenever possible. Personal protective devices include aprons, thyroid shields, eyewear, and gloves. All are advised to limit exposure. Leaded gloves do not provide protection when the hands are in the primary radiation beam, and it is recommended that operators stay out of the primary beam.

Specific suggestions for safe practice include minimizing fluoroscopy time, minimizing the number of fluoroscopic images, using available patient dose reduction strategies, employing good imaging-chain geometry, using collimation, using all available information to plan the procedure, positioning yourself in an area of low scatter, using protective shielding, using the right fluoroscopic imaging equipment, undergoing appropriate training, and wearing the dosimeters and knowing what your dose is.

Management Responsibilities.—To ensure that the radiation dose remains controlled, management should provide the right level of resources, including staff, facilities, and equipment. Quality assurance is essential to the monitoring program, with each department analyzing occupational radiation doses. Protective gear should be inspected each year but visually assessed daily or weekly for defects or damage. Because there is a wide range of attenuation values for aprons, standardized methods for acceptance testing of protective gear should be used. Training should be provided for all personnel appropriate to their job, including management.

▶ Fluoroscopically guided interventional procedures are performed in large numbers in Europe and in the United States, and the volume has increased over the past 20 years. Many of these procedures, while indisputably beneficial, have the potential to produce patient radiation doses high enough to cause radiation effects and occupational doses to interventional radiologists high enough to cause concern. A joint Society of Interventional Radiology-Cardiovascular and Interventional Society of Europe guideline on patient radiation management has addressed patient issues. This guideline is intended to serve as a companion to that document and provides guidance to help minimize occupational radiation dose.

The radiation dose received by interventional radiologists can vary by more than an order of magnitude for the same type of procedure and for similar patient dose. Recently, there has been particular concern regarding occupational dose to the lens of the eye in interventional radiologists. New data from exposed human populations suggest that cataracts occur at doses far lower than those previously believed to cause cataracts. Statistical analysis of the available data suggests absence of a threshold dose, although if one does exist, it is possible that it is less than 0.1 gray. Additionally, it appears that the latency period for radiation cataract formation is inversely related to radiation dose.

Occupational radiation protection is a necessity whenever radiation is used in the practice of medicine; it requires both appropriate education and training for the interventional radiologist and the availability of appropriate protection tools and equipment. Occupational dose limits are expressed in terms of equivalent dose in an organ or tissue for exposure of part of the body and effective dose for whole body exposure. The unit for both quantities is the sievert (Sv). Radiation workers are monitored to determine their level of exposure. To allow adequate time for identification of practices leading to high personal dose and implementation of work habit changes, monthly monitor replacement is recommended for operators conducting interventional procedures.

Occupational dose limits recommended by the International Commission on Radiological Protection (ICRP) have been adopted by most of the countries in the world including the European Union and the United States, with slightly differing limits in various nations. In the United States, individual state governments set occupational dose limits, but in most cases, the recommendations developed by the National Council on Radiation Protection and Measurements are used. These recommendations include an occupational limit of 50 mSv in 1 year and a lifetime limit of 10 mSv multiplied by the individual age in years. The current limit for the annual equivalent dose to the lens of the eye is 150 mSv. This limit is under review by an ICRP Task Group, as there is evidence that it is too high. The annual limit for the hands and feet is 500 mSv. The dose received by specific tissues such as the lens of the eye can be estimated by placing a dosimeter on or near the tissue of interest. The collar badge is commonly used to estimate eye dose in interventional laboratories. This method is usually acceptable if the X-ray tube is mounted below the patient. It is not possible to accurately estimate an operator hand dose using a body or wrist dosimeter because of the proximity of the hands to the X-ray beam. A ring badge is recommended to estimate hand dose.

The facility Radiation Safety section or Medical Physics Service should review the personal dose records of individual workers regularly to ensure that dose limits are not exceeded. The World Health Organization recommends investigation when monthly exposure reaches 0.5 mSv for the effective dose, 5 mSv for dose to the lens of the eye, or 15 mSv to the hands or extremities. The Radiation Safety officer or a qualified medical physicist should contact the worker directly to determine the cause of the unusual dose and to make suggestions about how to keep the worker dose as low as reasonably achievable. Badge readings for interventionalists can be expected to be higher than for most other hospital workers, and any investigation should reflect this difference, in order to avoid unnecessary investigations. Investigation of a high personal dose value begins with a check of the validity of the dosimeter reading. Potential sources of invalid dosimeter readings include wearing designated under- and overprotective apron dosimeters in the wrong location, wearing of the dosimeter of a different worker, and dosimeter storage in a location where it is exposed to radiation. If an invalid reading is suspected, the reading for the next monitoring period of an individual should be reviewed to ensure the problem has been corrected. Additionally, the worker should be asked if there was a change in work habits that could explain the increase in radiation exposure, and sometimes an explanation for a temporary cause is identified. If the cause is not thought to be temporary, or if no cause can be identified, the individual working habits should be observed during a series of representative procedures. The observer could be a qualified medical or health physicist or a physician colleague with knowledge of radiation protection principles and the operation of the specific imaging equipment being used.

The greatest source of staff radiation exposure is scatter from the patient. Generally, controlling patient dose also reduces scatter and limits operator dose. However, chronic radiation exposure in the workplace mandates using protective tools to limit occupational radiation dose to an acceptable level and to improve operator and staff safety without impeding the procedure or jeopardizing patient safety. Decreasing patient dose will result in a proportional decrease in scatter dose to the operator. Therefore, techniques that reduce patient dose will generally also reduce occupational dose. This is a win-win situation; the operator and the patient both benefit. Available patient dose reduction technologies include low fluoroscopy dose rate settings, low frame rate pulsed fluoroscopy, removal of the antiscatter grid, spectral beam filtration, and use of increased X-ray beam energy. The patient should be positioned as far as possible from the X-ray tube and the image receptor placed as close as possible to the patient. Collimators should be tightly adjusted to the area of interest, as tight collimation reduces patient dose and improves image quality by reducing scatter. The operator should stay as far away from the X-ray beam as possible. Remember the inverse square law. Tubing extensions or needle holders should be used so that the hands are away from the exposed field; the hands should never be placed in the X-ray beam. Power injectors should be used for contrast material injections when feasible, and the staff should step out of the procedure room during fluorographic acquisitions or digital subtraction angiography. When using angulated or lateral projections, the highest intensity of scattered radiation is located on the X-ray beam entrance side of the patient. When using these projections, the X-ray tube should be on the side opposite to the operator whenever possible.

A personal protective apron and a thyroid shield should be worn during all fluoroscopic procedures. Ceiling suspended shields can provide significant additional dose reduction, especially to unprotected areas of the head and neck. Leaded eyewear is recommended if ceiling suspended shields cannot be used continuously during the entire procedure. Under table lead drapes reduce lower extremity dose substantially and should be used whenever possible. Protective aprons should be examined fluoroscopically on an annual basis and inspected visually on a daily or weekly basis for damage and defects. Standardized methods for acceptance testing of protective aprons are needed because of the wide variation in actual attenuation values of aprons.

Adequate and relevant training programs should be provided for all levels of staff within the organization, including management, to develop a commitment to radiologic protection and in order that all concerned can contribute to the reduction and control of exposures.

T. G. Walker, MD

Prevention of Dialysis Catheter Malfunction with Recombinant Tissue Plasminogen Activator

Hemmelgarn BR, for the Prevention of Dialysis Catheter Lumen Occlusion with rt-PA versus Heparin (PreCLOT) Study Group (Univ of Calgary, Alberta; et al)
N Engl J Med 364:303-312, 2011

Background.—The effectiveness of various solutions instilled into the central venous catheter lumens after each hemodialysis session (catheter locking solutions) to decrease the risk of catheter malfunction and bacteremia in patients undergoing hemodialysis is unknown.

Methods.—We randomly assigned 225 patients undergoing long-term hemodialysis in whom a central venous catheter had been newly inserted to a catheter-locking regimen of heparin (5000 U per milliliter) three times per week or recombinant tissue plasminogen activator (rt-PA) (1 mg in each lumen) substituted for heparin at the midweek session (with heparin used in the other two sessions). The primary outcome was catheter malfunction, and the secondary outcome was catheter-related bacteremia. The treatment period was 6 months; treatment assignments were concealed from the patients, investigators, and trial personnel.

Results.—A catheter malfunction occurred in 40 of the 115 patients assigned to heparin only (34.8%) and 22 of the 110 patients assigned to rt-PA (20.0%) — an increase in the risk of catheter malfunction by a factor of almost 2 among patients treated with heparin only as compared with those treated with rt-PA once weekly (hazard ratio, 1.91; 95% confidence interval [CI], 1.13 to 3.22; P = 0.02). Catheter-related bacteremia occurred in 15 patients (13.0%) assigned to heparin only, as compared with 5 (4.5%) assigned to rt-PA (corresponding to 1.37 and 0.40 episodes per 1000 patient-days in the heparin and rt-PA groups, respectively; P = 0.02). The risk of bacteremia from any cause was higher in the heparin group than in the rt-PA group by a factor of 3 (hazard ratio, 3.30; 95% CI, 1.18 to 9.22; P = 0.02). The risk of adverse events, including bleeding, was similar in the two groups.

Conclusions.—The use of rt-PA instead of heparin once weekly, as compared with the use of heparin three times a week, as a locking solution for central venous catheters significantly reduced the incidence of catheter malfunction and bacteremia. (Funded by Hoffmann—La Roche; Current Controlled Trials number, ISRCTN35253449.) (Figs 1 and 2).

▶ Central venous catheters are used for vascular access in the majority of patients undergoing hemodialysis. The major complications of catheters include thrombosis and infection. Approximately 50% of hemodialysis catheters fail within 1 year; up to two-thirds of the failures are because of thrombosis. Infection related to central venous catheters is also associated with adverse health outcomes and high health care costs; indeed, catheter-related sepsis is one of the most common causes of death in patients undergoing hemodialysis. The solution instilled into the central venous catheter lumens after each hemodialysis session and left in the catheter until the next session (catheter locking solution) is used to prevent thrombosis during the period between dialysis sessions and may also prevent catheter-related infection. However, evidence supporting the use of various locking solutions to achieve these objectives is limited. Heparin has been the traditional locking solution. Several small studies have assessed whether citrate and heparin are equally efficacious for maintaining catheter patency, but the interpretation of the results was limited. Recombinant tissue plasminogen activator (rt-PA) has been used primarily to treat catheter thrombosis; in one small randomized trial, it was shown to be superior to heparin as a locking solution. The relatively high cost of rt-PA and its theoretical potential to cause bleeding, as well as the morbidity and mortality associated with catheter malfunction and infection, justify the need for more definitive evidence of the efficacy of rt-PA as a locking solution.

The current study is a multicenter, randomized, blinded, controlled trial involving patients undergoing long-term hemodialysis through a newly inserted, tunneled central venous catheter to determine whether substituting rt-PA (1 mg in each lumen) for heparin once a week as a catheter locking solution, as compared with using heparin 3 times a week, would decrease the incidence of catheter malfunction and bacteremia.

Adults undergoing hemodialysis in whom a tunneled catheter had been newly inserted into the upper central venous system were eligible to be included in the study if they were being treated with hemodialysis 3 times a week and were expected to continue undergoing hemodialysis with the use of a central venous catheter for 6 months. Major exclusion criteria were long-term receipt of systemic anticoagulant therapy, a central venous catheter inserted by means of guidewire exchange, current use of antibiotics for catheter-related bacteremia, major hemorrhage or intracranial bleeding in the previous 4 weeks, intracranial or intraspinal neoplasm, pregnancy or breast-feeding, and pericarditis. Patients with known catheter-related bacteremia could be eligible for the study once the infection had been treated and the patient had not received antibiotics for a period covering 3 hemodialysis sessions. The study was conducted across 11 clinical sites. Patients were eligible for randomization after the fourth hemodialysis session if the mean blood flow was at least 300 mL per minute during sessions 3 and 4.

Eligible patients were randomly assigned, in a 1:1 ratio, by a centralized computerized service. Patients were assigned to 1 of 2 regimens for locking of

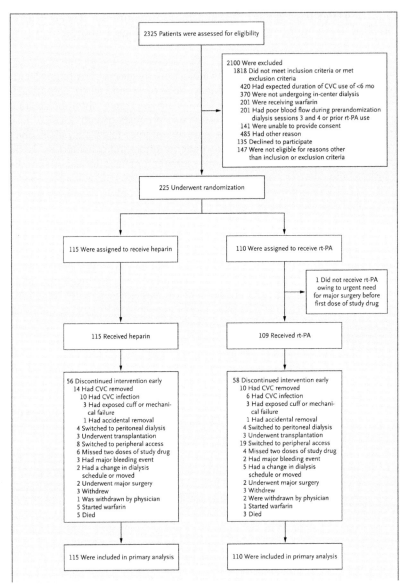

FIGURE 1.—Screening, Randomization, and Follow-up. CVC denotes central venous catheter, and rt-PA recombinant tissue plasminogen activator. (Reprinted from Hemmelgarn BR, for the Prevention of Dialysis Catheter Lumen Occlusion with rt-PA versus Heparin (PreCLOT) Study Group. Prevention of dialysis catheter malfunction with recombinant tissue plasminogen activator. *N Engl J Med.* 2011;364:303-312, copyright © 2011 Massachusetts Medical Society. All rights reserved)

the catheter after a hemodialysis session: (1) rt-PA (1 mg in each lumen) once a week, at the midweek session, with unfractionated heparin (5000 U/mL, full luminal volume) used as a locking solution for the other 2 dialysis sessions

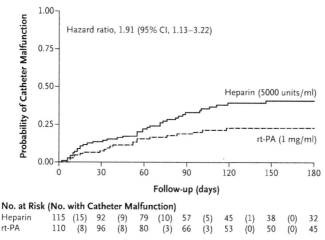

No. at Risk (No. with Catheter Malfunction)

Heparin	115	(15)	92	(9)	79	(10)	57	(5)	45	(1)	38	(0)	32
rt-PA	110	(8)	96	(8)	80	(3)	66	(3)	53	(0)	50	(0)	45

FIGURE 2.—Kaplan–Meier Curves for the Time to Catheter Malfunction, According to Study Group. The numbers in parentheses below the x axis are the numbers of patients in whom an episode of catheter malfunction occurred in the interval between follow-up assessments. The hazard ratio is for the group that received heparin as compared with the group that received recombinant tissue plasminogen activator (rt-PA). (Reprinted from Hemmelgarn BR, for the Prevention of Dialysis Catheter Lumen Occlusion with rt-PA versus Heparin (PreCLOT) Study Group. Prevention of dialysis catheter malfunction with recombinant tissue plasminogen activator. *N Engl J Med.* 2011;364:303-312, copyright © 2011 Massachusetts Medical Society. All rights reserved.)

that week or (2) 5000 U of unfractionated heparin per milliliter (full luminal volume) after each dialysis session. The rt-PA was administered in each lumen initially (1 mg in 1 mL), with saline added to fill the lock to the full luminal volume. Patients were followed up for 6 months after they underwent randomization. Patients who met the criteria for the primary outcome were followed up for at least 1 month after the primary outcome occurred and continued to be followed up until one of the following occurred: the patient underwent 6 consecutive successful hemodialysis sessions (mean blood flow ≥300 mL per minute during each treatment), 3 months elapsed, or the central venous catheter was no longer used. The follow-up period for these patients was extended so that the natural history of malfunction of the central venous catheter could be documented and the costs associated with maintaining patency could be assessed for use in the economic analysis.

The primary outcome was catheter malfunction, which was defined as the first occurrence of any of the following, after attempts to reestablish patency had been undertaken: peak blood flow of 200 mL per minute or less for 30 minutes during dialysis treatment, mean blood flow of 250 mL per minute or less during 2 consecutive dialysis treatments, or inability to initiate dialysis owing to inadequate blood flow. Catheter-related bacteremia was defined according to published criteria, with both definite and probable infections included in the outcome. Bacteremia was treated by the attending nephrologist; patients remained in the study and were followed up for the primary outcome. If a new central venous catheter was clinically indicated, the patient's data were censored at the time of removal of the initial central venous catheter. Bleeding was classified as fatal bleeding, major bleeding (bleeding at a critical site or overt bleeding with a decrease in the hemoglobin level of 20 g/L or more or requiring transfusion of 2 or more units of packed red cells), clinically important nonmajor bleeding (overt bleeding requiring admission to the hospital or a visit to a medical facility or overt bleeding leading to an intervention such as suturing), or minor bleeding (all other episodes of bleeding).

The screening, randomization, and follow-up of the study are summarized in Fig 1. The baseline characteristics of the 2 study groups were very similar. A total of 58 patients in the rt-PA group (52.7%) and 56 in the heparin group (48.7%) discontinued the study medication before the end of the 6-month study period. The median duration of follow-up was 115.5 days in the rt-PA group and 89.0 days in the heparin group. No patients were lost to follow-up.

The primary outcome occurred in 62 patients: 22 (20.0%) in the rt-PA group and 40 (34.8%) in the heparin group, as summarized in Fig 2. A total of 31 patients (50.0%) met the criteria for the primary outcome because of a peak blood flow of 200 mL per minute or less for 30 minutes, 19 patients (30.6%) because of an inability to initiate dialysis, and 12 patients (19.4%) because of a mean blood flow of 250 mL per minute or less for 2 consecutive sessions.

The results were similar in a secondary analysis that was performed according to the actual treatment received. The primary outcome occurred in 54 participants: 18 (16.4%) in the rt-PA group and 36 (31.3%) in the heparin group.

Catheter-related bacteremia (which was classified as definite, according to the published criteria used, in 45.0% of the cases) occurred in 5 patients (4.5%) assigned to receive rt-PA and 15 patients (13.0%) assigned to receive heparin alone. This corresponded to rates of 0.40 and 1.37 episodes of bacteremia per 1000 patient-days in the rt-PA and heparin groups, respectively.

Patients who met the criteria for the primary outcome were followed up for up to 3 months or until removal of the catheter, with a median follow-up period that covered 11.5 and 10.0 dialysis sessions in the rt-PA and heparin groups, respectively. Treatment with rt-PA (outside the study protocol) for repeat malfunction of the original catheter occurred in 8.8% of the sessions (32 of 364 sessions) in the rt-PA group and 12.8% of the sessions (101 of 792 sessions) in the heparin group.

Serious adverse events were reported in 23 patients (20.9%) receiving rt-PA and 34 (29.6%) receiving heparin. The rate of adverse events was similar in the 2 groups: 70.0% (77 of 110 patients) in the rt-PA group and 8.7% (79 of 115 patients) in the heparin group. Most patients had multiple events, with the result that there were a total of 454 adverse events and 68 serious adverse events. Neither the frequency nor the severity of bleeding events was greater among patients in the rt-PA group than among those in the heparin group. There were 4 intracranial bleeding episodes, all in patients in the heparin group.

For each patient who received therapy for 6 months, the mean costs (in Canadian dollars) of rt-PA and heparin were $1794 and $195, respectively; the cost of managing complications associated with catheter malfunction and catheter-related bacteremia per patient was $156 with rt-PA and $582 with heparin. Thus, the incremental cost of caring for patients with rt-PA as compared with heparin was $1173 per patient, or $13 956 per episode of catheter-related bacteremia prevented. Because management of catheter-related bacteremia is expensive and often requires replacement of central venous catheters, the finding that rt-PA reduces the risk of this complication without increasing the risk of bleeding is potentially very important.

As compared with the use of unfractionated heparin 3 times a week, the use of rt-PA as a catheter locking solution once a week (with heparin used the other 2 times) significantly decreased the incidence of catheter malfunction and bacteremia in patients with a newly inserted hemodialysis catheter. The findings were consistent between patients for whom this was the first use of a catheter and those who had used catheters previously. The frequency of bleeding or other serious adverse events was not increased with the use of rt-PA.

T. G. Walker, MD

Research

Toward an Optimal Position for Inferior Vena Cava Filters: Computational Modeling of the Impact of Renal Vein Inflow with Celect and TrapEase Filters

Wang SL, Singer MA (Kaiser Permanente Santa Clara Med Ctr; Lawrence Livermore Natl Laboratory, CA)
J Vasc Interv Radiol 21:367-374, 2010

Purpose.—To evaluate the hemodynamic effects of renal vein inflow and filter position on unoccluded and partially occluded inferior vena cava (IVC) filters with use of three-dimensional computational fluid dynamics.

Materials and Methods.—Three-dimensional models of the TrapEase and Günther Celect IVC filters, spherical thrombi, and an IVC with renal veins were constructed. Hemodynamics of steady-state flow was examined for unoccluded and partially occluded TrapEase and Günther Celect IVC filters in varying proximity to the renal veins.

Results.—Flow past the unoccluded filters demonstrated minimal disruption. Natural regions of stagnant/recirculating flow in the IVC were observed superior to the bilateral renal vein inflows. High flow velocities and elevated shear stresses were observed in the vicinity of renal inflow. Spherical thrombi induce stagnant/recirculating flow downstream of the thrombus. Placement of the TrapEase filter in the suprarenal position resulted in a large area of low shear stress/stagnant flow within the filter just downstream of thrombus trapped in the upstream trapping position.

Conclusions.—Filter position with respect to renal vein inflow influences filter trapping hemodynamics. Placement of the TrapEase filter in a suprarenal location may be thrombogenic, with redundant areas of stagnant/recirculating flow and low shear stress along the caval wall caused by the upstream trapping position and the naturally occurring region of stagnant flow from the renal veins. Infrarenal vein placement of IVC filters in a near-juxtarenal position with the downstream cone near the renal vein inflow likely confers increased levels of mechanical

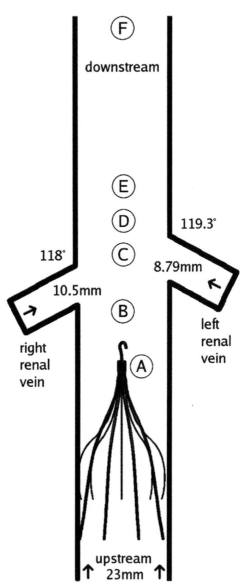

FIGURE 1.—Schematic diagram of the three-dimensional model showing the IVC, renal veins, and filter positions. Letters *A–F* correspond to positions of the downstream cone of the Celect and TrapEase filters. Positions *A* and *B* are infrarenal, *C* is just below juxtarenal position with the cone near the level of the renal vein inflow, *D* and *E* are juxtarenal, and *F* is suprarenal in position. (Reprinted from Wang SL, Singer MA. Toward an optimal position for inferior vena cava filters: computational modeling of the impact of renal vein inflow with celect and TrapEase filters. *J Vasc Interv Radiol.* 2010;21:367-374, with permission from SIR.)

lysis of trapped thrombi from increased shear stress from renal vein inflow (Fig 1).

▶ Inferior vena cava (IVC) filters play an integral role in the prevention of pulmonary embolism from deep vein thrombosis (DVT); an ideal IVC filter traps significant thrombus without significantly increasing the risk of thrombosis. However, investigators have noted that there is an increase in DVT after placement of permanent IVC filters and have suggested that this may be related to thrombosis at the filter site. A causal relationship between DVT and filters has not been established, but 2 potential theories are that (1) filters may cause progressive damage to the vein wall with secondary IVC occlusion at the filter or narrowing and eventual stenosis that contributes to DVT at or below the filter or (2) IVC filters may induce a local prothrombotic state either by their design or after trapping emboli.

Most investigators advocate filter placement in an infrarenal position, thereby decreasing the risk of renal vein thrombosis from potential filter occlusion. However, the "infrarenal" portion of the IVC is a vague term that includes the entire length of the IVC from the renal veins caudally to the common iliac venous confluence that forms the IVC. In this study, the authors attempt to determine the optimal location for filter placement in the IVC based upon computerized flow dynamic studies of the Celect and TrapEase IVC filters, with and without nonocclusive thrombus in an IVC model that incorporates anatomically correct renal vein inflows.

Three-dimensional computer models of the IVC with the renal veins, the Günther Celect filter, the TrapEase filter, and simulated thrombi were constructed to study flow dynamics with the filters in various positions. Hemodynamic properties in and around unoccluded and partially occluded filters were examined via 3-dimensional computational fluid dynamics. Fig 1 shows a schematic diagram of the IVC/renal vein model, along with 6 different IVC filter positions that were evaluated. Spherical thrombi were modeled as rigid spheres, with volumes of 0.5 mL and 1.0 mL. Simulations were performed with unoccluded and partially occluded TrapEase and Günther Celect filters. Thrombi were positioned in the upstream and downstream trapping positions of the TrapEase filter and in the single downstream position of the Günther Celect filter. Both filters were placed at the geometric center of the simulated cylindrical IVC and at varying locations in the cranial-caudal plane of the IVC to simulate infrarenal vein placement (Fig 1, positions A and B), juxtarenal vein placement (Fig 1, positions C-E), and suprarenal vein placement (Fig 1, position F).

For the unoccluded filters, there is minimal disruption to the flow upstream of the renal veins. Near the sites of renal inflow, the renal veins act as jets that introduce high-speed flow into the vena cava, and the flow downstream of the renal veins is disrupted. Immediately downstream of both renal veins, regions of low velocity and recirculating flow are observed near the wall of the IVC. The filters disrupt the renal inflow in close proximity to the renal veins; the flow must change direction to bypass the filter and flow downstream. When the filter is proximal to or downstream of the renal veins, flow inside the filter is disrupted significantly.

Partial occlusion of the filters disrupts flow downstream of the thrombus. However, when trapped thrombus is proximal to the renal veins, incoming renal flow is redirected by the thrombus and forced downstream along the vena cava wall. Consequently, flow along the vena cava wall (immediately downstream of renal inflow) is accelerated, and the volume of stagnant/recirculating flow is reduced compared with the unoccluded configuration. In addition, the renal vein inflow may be directed at the thrombus trapped downstream when the filter cones are positioned closer to the renal veins. Thus, this study indicates that renal vein inflow has significant hemodynamic effects on blood flow near IVC filters.

The authors feel that this study suggests that the ideal location for infrarenal IVC filter placement is immediately upstream of the juxtarenal position, with the downstream cone of the filter near the level of renal inflow (Fig 1, position C). The dominating high-velocity inflow from the renal veins serves as a source of higher shear stresses and flow velocities that may decrease primary and secondary hemostasis, particularly in the case of nonocclusive thrombi trapped in the downstream filter cone. True juxtarenal positioning (Fig 1, position D) confers similar higher shear stresses but also increases the risk of renal vein thrombosis from filter occlusion. In addition, the legs and centering struts of the Celect filter may become engaged in the renal veins. Suprarenal placement of IVC filters may confer a decreased risk of hemostasis as a result of much higher wall shear stress and flow velocities; however, in the event of a large occlusive thrombus, the risk of renal vein thrombosis must be considered.

T. G. Walker, MD

Tumor Ablation

Durable Oncologic Outcomes After Radiofrequency Ablation: Experience From Treating 243 Small Renal Masses Over 7.5 Years
Tracy CR, Raman JD, Donnally C, et al (Univ of Iowa; Penn State Milton S. Hershey Med Ctr, PA; Univ of Texas Southwestern Med Ctr, Dallas)
Cancer 116:3135-3142, 2010

Background.—Long-term oncologic outcomes for renal thermal ablation are limited. The authors of this report present their experience with radiofrequency ablation (RFA) therapy for 243 small renal masses (SRMs) over the past 7.5 years.

Methods.—The authors' institutional, prospectively maintained RFA database was reviewed to determine intermediate and long-term oncologic outcomes for patients with SRMs (generally <4 cm) who underwent RFA. Particular attention was placed on patients who had a minimum 3 years of follow-up. Patients were excluded from the analysis if they had received previous treatment for renal cell carcinoma (RCC) on the ipsilateral kidney or if they did not have at least 1 imaging study available for follow-up.

Results.—Two hundred eight patients (with 243 SRMs) who had no evidence of previous ipsilateral renal cancer treatment underwent RFA and had follow-up imaging studies available for review. Overall, tumor size averaged 2.4 cm, and follow-up ranged from 1.5 months to 90 months (mean, 27 months). Of the 227 tumors (93%) that underwent preablation biopsy, RCC was confirmed in 79%. The initial treatment success rate was 97%, and the overall 5-year recurrence-free survival rate was 93% (90% for 160 patients who had biopsy-proven RCC). During follow-up, 3 patients developed metastatic disease, and 1 patient died of RCC, yielding 5-year actuarial metastasis-free and cancer-specific survival rates of 95% and 99%, respectively.

Conclusions.—RFA provided successful treatment of SRMs and produced a low rate of recurrence as well as prolonged metastasisfree and cancer-specific survival rates at 5 years after treatment. Although longer term follow-up of RFA will be required to determine late recurrence rates, the current results indicated a minimal risk of disease recurrence in patients who are >3 years removed from RFA (Tables 1-3).

▶ The widespread use of abdominal cross-sectional imaging has contributed to a rise in the diagnosis of small renal masses (SRMs) with a concomitant increase in the detection of renal cell carcinoma (RCC). Although these incidentally discovered masses tend to be smaller and of lower grade than symptomatic lesions, pathologically, most of these tumors (65%-80%) are RCCs. Surveillance studies suggest that approximately 60% of these lesions will exhibit growth over time.

To prevent unnecessary removal of the entire kidney to treat an SRM, nephron-sparing surgery has replaced the gold standard of radical nephrectomy for patients in whom complete removal of the tumor is possible without

TABLE 1.—Baseline Patient and Tumor Characteristics of Patients Who Underwent Radiofrequency Ablation Separated by the Total Number of Patients and the Number of Patients With ≥3 Years of Follow-Up

Characteristic	All Ablations	≥3 Years of Follow-Up	P
No. of tumors ablated	243	84	
No. of patients	208	66	
No. of tumors in men/women[a]	156/87	54/30	.99[b]
Mean ± SD age [range], y[a]	64±12.5 [18-84]	64±13.5 [20-85]	.78[c]
No. of right-sided/left-sided tumors[a]	139/104	44/40	.16[b]
Surgical approach: No. of tumors (%)[a]			
Percutaneous	172 (71)	55 (65)	.36[b]
Laparoscopic	68 (28)	26 (31)	.36[b]
Open	3 (1)	3 (4)	.17[b]
Mean±SD tumor size [range], cm	2.4±0.8 [1.0-5.4]	2.4±0.9 [1.0-5.4]	.65[c]
Mean±SD follow-up [range], mo	27±23 [1.5-90]	53±15 [36-90]	<.001
No. of patients with hereditary conditions (%)	5 (2)	4 (6)	.005
No. of tumors in patients with hereditary conditions (%)	14 (6)	13 (15)	

SD indicates standard deviation.
[a]Surgical approach, age, sex, and side are listed by the number of tumors, not by the number of patients.
[b]Determined using the chi-square test.
[c]Determined using the Wilcoxon Mann-Whitney U test.

TABLE 2.—Biopsy Results From All Patients Who Underwent Radiofrequency Ablation and From Patients With ≥3 Years of Follow-Up

Characteristic	All Ablations	No. (%) >3 Years of Follow-Up	P
No. of masses	243	84	
Total no. of masses biopsied	227	74	.12
RCC	179 (79)	53 (72)	.09[a]
Clear cell[b]	137 (77)	38 (72)	.5[c]
Fuhrman grade 1	72	19	.93[d]
Fuhrman grade 2	50	14	.85[d]
Fuhrman grade 3	8	4	.32[d]
Unknown	3	1	.88[d]
Papillary[b]	36 (20)	13 (25)	.53[c]
Chromophobe[b]	6 (3)	2 (4)	.89[c]
Oncocytoma[e]	21 (9)	12 (16)	.14[a]
AML[e]	10 (4)	2 (3)	.47[a]
Normal parenchyma[e]	9 (4)	3 (4)	.56[a]
Nondiagnostic[e,f]	11 (5)	4 (5)	.8[a]

RCC indicates renal cell carcinoma; AML, angiomyolipoma.
[a]The chi-square test was used for comparisons between oncologic classifications of the total number biopsied.
[b]The percentage of the histologic subtype of RCC (rounded to the nearest whole number).
[c]The chi-square test was used for comparisons between subtypes of malignant tumors.
[d]The chi-square test was used for comparisons between Furman grades in patients with clear cell RCC.
[e]The percentage of totalmasses biopsied (rounded to the nearest whole number).
[f]These tumors could not be classified definitively as malignant or benign.

TABLE 3.—Recurrence Information for All Patients Who Underwent Radiofrequency Ablation and Developed Recurrent Disease After Initially Normal Postoperative Imaging Studies

Months to Recurrence	Initial Biopsy Result	Treatment of Recurrence	Final Pathology	Last Follow-Up
3	Grade 1 RCC[a]	Reablated with RFA	NA	NED at 12 mo
12	Grade 1 RCC	Laparoscopic nephrectomy	Grade 3 RCC	NED at 36 mo
12	Grade 2 RCC	Died during follow-up	NA	Died of metastatic disease
6	Grade 1 RCC	Reablated with CA	NA	Recurrence 36 mo after salvage CA
12	Grade 1 RCC	Open nephrectomy	Grade 3 RCC	NED at 42 mo
20	Grade 2 RCC	Re-ablated with RFA	NA	NED at 60 mo
24	Grade 1 RCC	Sorafenib	NA	Metastatic stabilization at 60 mo
36	Grade 2 RCC	Open nephrectomy for ESRD	Grade 3 RCC	Adrenal metastasis 12 mo after nephrectomy; adrenal glands treated with RFA
36	Grade 1 RCC	Open partial nephrectomy	Grade 3 RCC	NED at 6 mo

RCC indicates renal cell carcinoma; RFA, radiofrequency ablation; NA, not available; NED, no evidence of disease; CA, cryoablation; ESRD, end-stage renal disease.
[a]Fuhrman grade.

compromising the remnant portion of the kidney. Partial nephrectomy is associated with intermediate- and long-term cancer control rates similar to the rates produced by radical nephrectomy with the benefit of better renal preservation outcomes. However, because both open and laparoscopic partial nephrectomies are associated with significant morbidity, the use of ablative methods, such as cryoablation (CA), radiofrequency ablation (RFA), high-intensity focused ultrasound, and microwave thermotherapy, has expanded considerably. These ablation technologies offer several benefits over surgery, including a lower complication rate, shorter convalescence, absence of an ischemic insult, and the potential for outpatient surgical management.

Previously reported short-term success with RFA has been encouraging, although only 2 reports have detailed the therapeutic outcomes of patients with a defined minimum follow-up interval. Those studies, however, were limited by small patient numbers. With well-defined short-term efficacy, it is imperative that current investigations focus on intermediate- and long-term cancer control rates of this emerging technology. The current study details experience with RFA of SRMs in the management of 208 patients (with 243 tumors) over the past 7.5 years, with particular attention to 66 patients (with 84 tumors) who had a documented radiographic follow-up of at least 3 years. The authors queried a prospectively maintained renal tumor database for intermediate- and long-term oncologic outcomes of RFA treatment.

The choice of a laparoscopic or percutaneous approach was at the discretion of the treating surgeon. Tumors that were located anteriorly or medially in close proximity to bowel or adjacent organs typically were managed by laparoscopic RFA, and tumors that were oriented more posteriorly and laterally were managed by percutaneous RFA.

Follow-up for each patient included history, physical examination, chest radiograph, creatinine, and contrast-enhanced computed tomography or magnetic resonance imaging studies obtained at 6 weeks, 6 months, and at least annually thereafter. Incomplete primary ablation was defined as any evidence of contrast enhancement at the 6-week appointment. These patients were managed with repeat RFA, surgical extirpation, or active surveillance. Local disease recurrence was defined as any contrast enhancement or tumor growth within the ablation zone that occurred beyond the initial 6-week post-RFA follow-up.

Table 1 details the baseline patient and tumor characteristics of the 208 patients who had 243 tumors. There was a mean follow-up of 27 months and a mean tumor size of 2.4 cm. In this group, 66 patients (who had 84 tumors) had a minimum of 3 years of follow-up. There was no difference in sex, surgical side, surgical approach, or mean tumor size in the subgroup of patients who had > 3 years of follow-up compared with the overall cohort. However, patients who had > 3 years of follow-up had more associated hereditary RCC syndromes.

A procedural biopsy was performed on 227 tumors (93% of all tumors) and on 74 tumors (88% of tumors) in the subgroup of patients who had ≥3 years of follow-up. Table 2 summarizes the biopsy results both for all patients as well as for those with ≥3 years of follow-up. Of these, RCC was confirmed in 179 tumors (79%) and 53 tumors (72%), respectively. The distribution of RCC histologic subtypes in the treatment cohort was similar to published distributions (clear cell, 77%; papillary, 20%; and chromophobe, 3%). This distribution was unchanged in the group of patients with longer follow-up.

Of the 243 treated renal masses, 7 had an incomplete primary ablation, yielding an initial success rate of 97%. Of the 7 incomplete ablations, 5 masses underwent a repeat ablation with either RFA (4 masses) or CA (1 mass). The 4 patients who underwent RFA had no evidence of disease recurrence at a mean of 30 months of follow-up, whereas the remaining patient who was managed by CA developed a local recurrence at 36 months of follow-up. There were 9 local recurrences in the overall cohort, all of which occurred at ≤3 years of follow-up, yielding 3-year and 5-year recurrence-free survival rates of 93%. Details of RCC recurrences and subsequent management are presented in Table 3.

This study, with both a larger patient cohort and lengthier follow-up than previously reported studies, strengthens the current intermediate-term evidence of RFA efficacy. The results also appear to compare favorably with those produced by CA for SRMs.

The authors conclude that RFA provides successful treatment of SRMs with a low rate of recurrence and prolonged metastasis-free and cancer-specific survival rates at 5 years after treatment. Although longer-term follow-up of RFA ablation will be required to determine the rate of late recurrences, the current results indicate no evidence of disease recurrence in patients who are more than 3 years removed from RFA.

T. G. Walker, MD

Vascular Imaging

One hundred cases of abdominal-based free flaps in breast reconstruction. The impact of preoperative computed tomographic angiography
Ghattaura A, Henton J, Jallali N, et al (Royal Marsden Hosp, London, UK)
J Plast Reconstr Aesthet Surg 63:1597-1601, 2010

An accurate preoperative evaluation of the vascular anatomy of the abdominal wall is essential in deep inferior epigastric perforator (DIEP) flap reconstruction. We present our experience of using computed tomographic angiography (CTA) of the abdomen as part of our standard preoperative assessment of abdominal-based breast reconstruction. One hundred consecutive cases were examined retrospectively, divided equally into non-CTA and CTA periods. Following use of CTA, fewer superficial inferior epigastric artery (SIEA) flaps were performed (18% vs. 0%), although the number of DIEP and muscle-sparing transverse rectus abdominis myocutaneous (MS TRAM) flaps remained similar. There was an increased use of single perforators in the CTA group than in the non-CTA group (48% vs. 18%) as well as increased numbers of medial-row perforators (65% vs. 32%). Unilateral reconstructions were performed 1 h faster in the CTA group (489 min vs. 566 min). Finally, hernia rates decreased from 6% in the non-CTA group to 0% in the CTA group. A clear knowledge of the dominant perforator(s) to the abdominal skin prior to surgery can greatly increase the success of this procedure and reduce surgical time. In addition, by choosing the largest well-placed perforator supplying the bulk of the flap, it may be possible to reduce the overall morbidity.

▶ The use of abdominal tissue as a source of free tissue transfer in breast reconstruction is well documented. Although originally described as a musculocutaneous flap with the rectus abdominis muscle included transverse rectus abdominis myocutaneous (TRAM) flap, refinements in the flap harvest technique have led to increased use of the deep inferior epigastric perforator (DIEP) flap, the muscle-sparing (MS) TRAM flap, or the superficial inferior epigastric artery (SIEA) flap. Preservation of the rectus abdominis muscle in the DIEA and SIEA flaps has some functional advantages for the patient in terms of postoperative morbidity. As a result of these considerations, MS flaps have become increasingly popular and now represent a significant proportion of breast reconstructions.

Radiological identification of abdominal perforators prior to DIEP flap surgery has received much attention, and recent studies have shown that by locating the perforators before surgery one can improve surgical efficiency and reduce operating times considerably. Computed tomographic angiography (CTA) can assess abdominal vasculature prior to performing a DIEP flap reconstruction. Investigators have used abdominal CTA to demonstrate the course of the deep inferior epigastric artery, its perforators, and the subcutaneous branching pattern of this vessel. In addition, the accuracy of CTA has been shown to have a high sensitivity (96%-100%) and a high specificity (95%-100%). In the current study, the authors retrospectively studied 100 consecutive cases of DIEP flap breast reconstruction in a single institution, divided equally into those with CTA images and those without, in order to examine the effect of CTA imaging on breast reconstruction surgery and also to examine the process of image acquisition.

In the authors' institution, computed tomographic studies are performed using a 32-detector row scanner using energy settings that are chosen to prevent overpenetration of the deep tissues because this information is not required for this investigation (120 kVp tube voltage and 300 mA fixed tube current). Further settings included a 0.4-second gantry rotation period, collimation 20 × 0.625 mm, pitch 0.97, 19.4-mm table travel per rotation, 512 × 512 matrix, and a 180 to 240 field of view. With experience, the optimal settings to produce a good image quality with a low radiation exposure were determined (as low as reasonably achievable).

100 mL of nonionic iodinated contrast is injected at a concentration of 350 mg/mL. Depending on the flow rate, there is a 15 to 20-second delay between contrast administration and image acquisition.

We obtain images from 5 cm above the umbilicus to the lesser trochanter of the hip during a single breath hold. The radiation dose given to a patient using this technique is 6 mSv. The images obtained are then reconstructed with a slice width of 1 mm and a reconstruction interval of 0.8 mm and transferred to a computer workstation. The images produced can be reformatted in coronal, axial, and sagittal planes.

Of the 100 patients in the study, 50 each were in the non-CTA group and the CTA group.

Of these patients, 74 had unilateral breast reconstructions and 26 had bilateral reconstructions. The number of bilateral cases was greater in the non-CTA group than in the CTA group (16 patients vs 10 patients). The total number of individual flaps included in this study was 126, with 66 in the non-CTA group and 60 in the CTA group.

The type of flap used was then analyzed. With the advent of CTA imaging, the number of DIEP flap reconstructions performed increased slightly (71% in the non-CTA group vs 78% in the CTA group). In general, fewer SIEA flaps were undertaken (18% in the non-CTA group vs 0% in the CTA group) and the number of MS TRAM flaps performed remained similar. The choice of the perforator used in the flap was compared in the 2 groups. The results indicated that a far greater number of single perforators are used in the CTA group (48% vs 18%) and that the medial row is used to a much greater extent since the advent of CTA (65% vs 32%). The advantages of a medial row perforator over a lateral row are documented and these are related to improved perfusion to the contralateral abdomen. The authors further showed that since using CTA, the time taken to perform a unilateral reconstruction was reduced from 566 minutes to 489 minutes. This is a statistically significant change in operating times ($P < .001$).

The authors conclude that knowledge of the dominant perforator(s) to the abdominal skin prior to surgery can greatly increase the success of this procedure and reduce the surgical time. In addition, by choosing the largest well-placed perforator supplying the bulk of the flap, it may be possible to reduce the overall morbidity.

T. G. Walker, MD

Venous Interventions

Improving Inferior Vena Cava Filter Retrieval Rates: Impact of a Dedicated Inferior Vena Cava Filter Clinic
Minocha J, Idakoji I, Riaz A, et al (Northwestern Univ, Chicago, IL)
J Vasc Interv Radiol 21:1847-1851, 2010

Purpose.—To test the hypothesis that an inferior vena cava (IVC) filter clinic increases the retrieval rate of optional IVC filters.

Materials and Methods.—Patients who had optional IVC filters placed at the authors' institution between January 2000 and December 2008 were identified and retrospectively studied. A dedicated IVC filter clinic was established at this institution in January 2009, and there is a comprehensive database of prospectively acquired data for patients seen in the IVC filter clinic. Patients were chronologically classified into preclinic and postclinic groups. The number of optional filters retrieved and failed retrieval attempts were recorded.

Results.—In the preclinic and postclinic periods, 369 and 100 optional IVC filters were placed. Median (interquartile range) number of optional filters placed per month for preclinic and postclinic periods was 3 (range 2—5) and 10 (range 6.5—10.5) ($P < .001$). Retrieval rates in preclinic and postclinic periods were 108 of 369 (29%) and 60 of 100 (60%) (*P* < .001). The median time to filter retrieval in the postclinic group was 1.5 months (95% confidence interval 1.2−1.8). The number of failed retrieval attempts in preclinic and postclinic periods was 23 of 369 (6%) and 5 of 100 (5%) (*P* = .823).

Conclusions.—The retrieval rate of optional IVC filters at this institution was significantly increased by the establishment of a dedicated IVC filter clinic. This retrieval increase is not related to a decrease in technical failures but more likely relates to more meticulous patient management and clinical follow-up.

▶ Two basic types of inferior vena cava (IVC) filters are available in the United States, permanent and optional (or retrievable). Permanent filters are placed in patients who require long-term mechanical prophylaxis against pulmonary embolism (PE) and who have absolute contraindications to anticoagulation. Optional filters, which have been available since the late 1990s, are designed to be retrieved after the temporary risk of PE or contraindication to anticoagulation has resolved or may be left in place as a permanent filter. If retrieved, optional filters offer the theoretical benefit of fewer long-term complications associated with permanent IVC filters, such as increased risk of subsequent deep vein thrombosis. The availability of optional filters has altered the practice patterns for IVC filters, with a shift to these devices accompanied by the lowering of thresholds for filter placement. Optional filters are now placed for prophylactic indications in patients who are at increased risk for development of clinically significant PE and are unable to undergo primary prophylaxis, such as in the setting of trauma. As a result, the number of filter placements in the United States has increased steadily, with prophylactic indications now accounting for more than half of all filter placements. In clinical practice, only about 20% of optional filters are ever retrieved. The current study was designed to test the hypothesis that a dedicated IVC filter clinic increases the retrieval rate of optional IVC filters.

The authors identified and retrospectively studied patients who had optional IVC filters placed at their institution by interventional radiology between January 2000 and December 2008. They established a dedicated IVC filter clinic at their institution in January 2009. Data were collected prospectively for patients with optional IVC filters placed by interventional radiology between January 2009 and January 2010. IVC filter cases were chronologically classified into preclinic and postclinic groups.

In the preclinic period, the authors did not use a standard methodology to coordinate the removal of implanted optional devices. Referring physicians would often contact an interventional radiologist when their patients were candidates for retrieval. However, with the establishment of a dedicated IVC filter clinic, the authors maintained a comprehensive IVC filter clinic database and included a nurse coordinator working with a dedicated interventional radiologist in the clinic.

Before any filter placement, the interventional radiologist consulted with the referring physician and confirmed the indication for and type of filter to be placed (ie, permanent or optional). All optional filters were placed with the intent of their retrieval after the need for mechanical prophylaxis against PE expired. After filter placement, the nurse coordinator and interventional radiologist monitored patients with optional filters on the clinic database and coordinated filter removal with the patients' physicians when clinically indicated. Referring physicians were typically contacted 2 to 3 weeks after filter placement by the dedicated interventional radiologist to discuss the possibility of IVC filter removal or the timing of removal. This communication was repeated until the filter was removed or the decision was made to leave the filter as a permanent device.

The comparison data between the preclinic and postclinic IVC retrieval was as follows:

Preclinic period: Optional filter retrieval rate was 29% (108 of 369).

Postclinic period: Of the optional filters placed in the postclinic period, 60% were retrieved. Of 100 filters, 40 (40%) were not retrieved because of the following reasons: 33 (82.5%) were kept permanent, 5 (12.5%) had failed retrievals, 1 (2.5%) was lost to follow-up, and 1 (2.5%) is still being followed up by the IVC filter clinic. The median time to filter retrieval was 1.5 months. Failed retrieval attempts were categorized as technical failures of the retrieval procedure. The number of failed retrieval attempts in the preclinic and postclinic periods was 23 of 369 (6%) and 5 of 100 (5%), respectively.

The authors significantly increased the retrieval rate of optional IVC filters at their institution by establishing a dedicated IVC filter clinic. In the preclinic period, less than one-third of optional IVC filters placed by interventional radiology were retrieved. In the postclinic period, the retrieval rate was improved to 60%. The number of failed retrieval attempts was similar in both periods, suggesting that the improved retrieval rate was not related to a decrease in technical failures.

The authors note that although all optional filters were placed with the intent of their retrieval, the low preclinic retrieval rate was similar to rates reported in the literature. Before establishment of the clinic, there was no standard methodology to coordinate the removal of implanted optional devices. Consequently, a common reason that an optional filter was left in place as a permanent device in the preclinic group was loss to follow-up. By establishing a dedicated IVC filter clinic, many of the shortcomings associated with the management of optional IVC filters were addressed. Referring physicians were routinely contacted 2 to 3 weeks after optional filter placement to discuss the possibility of filter removal or the timing of removal, transferring all the responsibility of retrieval from the referring physicians and patients to the interventional radiologist.

These results support the establishment of an optional IVC filter clinic with a clinic database that is actively monitored by dedicated staff. Theoretically, this practice could increase the retrieval rate of optional IVC filters, reduce long-term complication rates, and result in cost savings. The higher postclinic filter retrieval rate was largely the result of improved patient follow-up, with the resultant provision of more comprehensive postprocedural care for patients.

T. G. Walker, MD

Percutaneous Mechanical and Pharmacomechanical Thrombolysis for Occlusive Deep Vein Thrombosis of the Proximal Limb in Adolescent Subjects: Findings from an Institution-based Prospective Inception Cohort Study of Pediatric Venous Thromboembolism

Goldenberg NA, Branchford B, Wang M, et al (Univ of Colorado, Aurora)
J Vasc Interv Radiol 22:121-132, 2011

Purpose.—Young individuals with occlusive, proximal-limb deep vein thrombosis (DVT) who have acutely increased plasma levels of factor VIII and D-dimer are at high risk for postthrombotic syndrome (PTS) when treated with conventional anticoagulation alone. The present report is an evaluation of experience with adjunctive percutaneous mechanical thrombolysis (PMT) and/or percutaneous pharmacomechanical thrombolysis (PPMT) in such patients.

Patients and Methods.—Among 95 children 11–21 years of age enrolled in a prospective cohort of venous thromboembolism between March 1, 2006, and November 1, 2009, 16 met eligibility criteria and underwent PMT/PPMT, typically with adjunctive catheter-directed thrombolytic infusion (CDTI) of tissue-type plasminogen activator given after the procedure.

Results.—Median age was 16 years (range, 11–19 y). Thirteen cases (81%) involved lower limbs. Underlying stenotic lesions were disclosed in 53%, with endovascular stents deployed in all cases of May–Thurner anomaly. There were no periprocedural major bleeding events and one symptomatic pulmonary embolism. Technical success rate was 94%. Early (< 30 days) locally recurrent DVT developed in 40% of cases, of which 83% were successfully treated with repeat lysis. Late recurrent DVT rate (median follow-up duration, 14 months; range, 1–42 mo) was 27%. Cumulative incidence of physically and functionally significant PTS at 1–2 years was 13%.

Conclusions.—This experience provides preliminary evidence that PMT/PPMT with adjunctive CDTI can be used safely and effectively in adolescent subjects with DVT at high risk for PTS (Fig 1, Table 3).

▶ Current consensus-based recommendations for antithrombotic therapy of deep vein thrombosis (DVT) in children suggest that thrombolytic interventions be reserved for patients with life- or limb-threatening events. However, a risk of postthrombotic syndrome (PTS) of nearly 80% was recently determined in a small cohort study evaluating young patients with completely venoocclusive proximal lower-limb DVT, managed by conventional anticoagulation according to the present standard of care. This study further observed that when intravenous tissue plasminogen activator (TPA) thrombolysis was used with salvage percutaneous mechanical thrombolysis (PMT) or percutaneous pharmacomechanical thrombolysis (PPMT) prior to conventional anticoagulation, the risk of PTS was significantly reduced, at 22%. This PTS rate is similar to the historical frequency of PTS recently defined in largely unselected children with a history of upper- or lower-extremity DVT by systematic review.

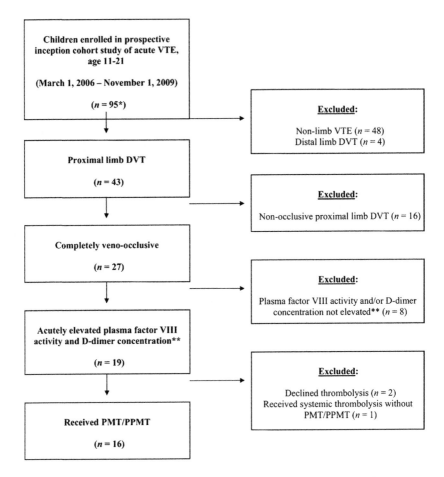

* Represents > 90% of the eligible population evaluated at The Children's Hospital, Colorado and the Mountain States Regional Hemophilia and Thrombosis Center, University of Colorado, during the study period

** As defined by previously-established prognostic thresholds of 150 U/dL for factor VIII activity and 500 ng/mL for D-dimer (2,11)

FIGURE 1.—Flowchart of subject selection from the cohort study population based on clinical and laboratory characteristics of interest for heightened a priori risk of PTS. (Reprinted from Goldenberg NA, Branchford B, Wang M, et al. Percutaneous mechanical and pharmacomechanical thrombolysis for occlusive deep vein thrombosis of the proximal limb in adolescent subjects: findings from an institution-based prospective inception cohort study of pediatric venous thromboembolism. *J Vasc Interv Radiol*. 2011;22:121-132.)

Present recommendations for management of DVT in adults suggest that thrombolysis be considered in young patients with a long anticipated life span who have a low bleeding risk and extensive and/or occlusive thrombus of recent symptomatic onset. Because most children with PTS are anticipated to endure the associated symptoms and signs for a lifetime that spans many decades, it is imperative that risk-stratified antithrombotic therapeutic strategies

TABLE 3.—Outcomes in the Study Population*

Case No.	Acute Locally Recurrent DVT†	Follow-up at Last Clinic Visit (mo)	Nonacute Recurrent VTE (Type)	Time from Procedure to Recurrent VTE Diagnosis (mo)	Any PTS at 1–2 y	Significant PTS at 1–2 y	Basic CEAP Findings	Wong–Baker Pain Findings
1	None	12	Yes (distant)	4.5	Yes	NA	C	NA‡
2	None	42	None	NA	Yes	No	None	AA, ADL
3	Yes (relysed)	36	Yes (local)	0.5	Yes	No	None	AA
4	Yes (relysed)	27	Yes (local)	14	Yes	Yes	Edema	AA, ADL
5	None	30	None	NA	Yes	No	None	AA
6	None	24	None	NA	No	NA	None	None
7	Yes (relysed)	2	None	NA	NA	No	NA	NA
8	Yes (relysed)§	14	Yes (distant)	3–12 (asymptomatic)	No‖	No	None	None
9	None	26	Yes (local)	1–3 (asymptomatic)	Yes	No	Edema	None
10	None	14	None	NA	Yes	No	Edema	None
11	None	18	Yes (local)	2	Yes	NA	None	AA, rest
12	None	6	None	NA	NA	NA	NA	NA
13	None	10	Yes (local)	9	NA	NA	NA	NA
14	None	3	None	NA	NA	NA	NA	NA
15	Yes (relysed)§	1	None	NA	NA	NA	NA	NA
16	None	6	None	NA	NA	NA	NA	NA

Note.— AA = aerobic activities; ADL = activities of daily living; C = dilated superficial venous collaterals; CEAP = Clinical, Etiologic, Anatomic, Pathophysiologic (see text); NA = not available or not applicable.

*There were no major bleeding events, and one symptomatic PE, within 7 d of the procedure.

†Acute locally recurrent DVT within 7 d of procedure, including isolated stent thrombosis; status on repeat procedure (relysed vs refractory) shown in parentheses.

‡Premorbid chronic pain.

§Recurred twice in these subjects with multiple-antibody APS with thrombotic storm. Patency was eventually maintained after mechanical/pharmacomechanical thrombectomy in each patient only after multimodal immunomodulatory therapy had been instituted and potent direct thrombin inhibition had resulted in marked decrease in D-dimer.

‖Reliability of assessment of basic CEAP component on contralateral difference in limb circumference may be limited by bilaterality of DVT at presentation.

be developed and prospectively studied in the pediatric population, with PTS risk reduction as a key aim. Rapid restoration of venous patency via thrombolysis is principal among these strategies. To date, the few studies of thrombolysis in pediatric venous thromboembolism have focused on modalities of systemic or catheter-directed thrombolytic infusion (CDTI). However, a recent survey identified PMT/PPMT as the most commonly preferred approach to thrombolysis in pediatric DVT among physician members of the American Society of Pediatric Hematology/Oncology. In this study, the authors sought to evaluate their institutional prospective cohort study experience with PMT/PPMT in adolescent subjects with acute proximal-limb DVT who were judged to be at high risk for PTS because of the combined presence of complete venoocclusion and adverse prognostic biomarkers.

Fig 1 provides details of the study population eligibility and enrollment. Of 95 children aged 11 to 21 years who were prospective subjects, 16 met eligibility criteria and were enrolled in this prospective study.

A clinical protocol was used for each component of the PMT/PPMT intervention, which permitted variability in the number of modalities used based on clinical discretion. In brief, baseline venography was performed to establish anatomy, thrombus burden, and degree of occlusion. With real-time ultrasound guidance, a 21-gauge needle was introduced into the popliteal vein for lower-limb DVT or the basilic veins for upper-limb DVT. In the setting of thrombus within 1 of these 2 venous systems, puncture was made peripheral to the thrombosed vein and an attempt at passing a wire through the thrombus was made. Via standard wire and catheter exchanges, a hydrophilic wire was advanced through the thrombus to its proximal terminus and a central venogram was obtained. An appropriately sized sheath was then placed over the guide wire. One of 3 mechanical thrombectomy devices—AngioJet (Medrad Interventional/Possis, Warrendale, Pennsylvania), Amplatz ClotBuster thrombectomy device (ev3, Plymouth, Minnesota), or Trellis (Bacchus Vascular, Santa Clara, California)—was advanced through the sheath. Mechanical thrombectomy was performed in serial passes as necessary/possible to achieve maximal patency and minimal residual clot burden. When local TPA was administered via the device during mechanical thrombectomy, this was characterized as PPMT. At the discretion of the operator (or in all cases of May-Thurner anomaly), additional percutaneous transluminal angioplasty was performed, and one or more 12- to 16-mm stents (Wallstent; Boston Scientific, Natick, Massachusetts) were deployed at sites of residual stenosis. If thrombus was noted to extend peripheral to the popliteal vein, no attempt was made to lyse this portion of the thrombus. No duplicate venous systems were identified during this study.

In most cases, CDTI was administered after the procedure directly into residual thrombus, for a period of 12 to 24 hours. CDTI uniformly used TPA at 0.5 to 1 mg/h via an infusion catheter placed in the sheath and directed at the site of PMT/PPMT or residual thrombus. During CDTI, unfractionated heparin was given at 10 U/kg/h via the sheath except in cases in which a diagnosis of severe thrombophilia or thrombotic storm was made, in which more aggressive antithrombotic therapy was maintained.

Following the thrombolytic regimen, in the absence of bleeding concerns, therapeutic anticoagulation was transitioned to low molecular weight heparin (LMWH) 24 hours after the procedure. Anticoagulation was maintained with LMWH or warfarin (goal, international normalized ratio of 2.0-3.0) for a minimum total duration of 6 months and not less than 3 months from the time of any stent placement. Radiologic imaging surveillance was performed to exclude thrombus progression/recurrence on therapy and define the extent of chronic thrombus burden of any residual thrombus. Specifically, imaging was repeated at the end of PMT intervention and at 1 to 4 weeks, 3 to 6 months, and (if persistent) 1 year. Additionally, children were evaluated for PTS at 3 to 6 months, 1 year, and annually thereafter in long-term follow-up.

Outcomes are summarized in Table 3. Technical success (grade II/III lysis) was achieved in 94% of cases. There were 5 acute local recurrences within 1 week (all of which were successfully treated with repeat lysis): 1 subacute and 4 late local recurrences. Late local recurrences were restricted in all cases to patients with severe hypercoagulability, with or without underlying stenotic venous lesions. There were no periprocedural major bleeding events and 1 case of symptomatic pulmonary embolism. Early (< 30 days) locally recurrent DVT developed in 40% of cases, of which 83% were successfully treated with repeat lysis. The late recurrent DVT rate was 27%. The cumulative incidence of physically and functionally significant PTS at 1 to 2 years was 13%.

The findings provide prospective evidence that PMT/PPMT with or without adjunctive CDTI can be used safely in children, targeting a subgroup of adolescents with DVT known to be at high risk for PTS. Despite acute locally recurrent DVT in 40% of cases, 83% of these were successfully treated with repeat lysis. Although late recurrent DVT occurred in 27% of cases overall, all were in the setting of severe hypercoagulable states. While signs and/or symptoms of PTS were still observed in some patients even when PMT/PPMT was performed within 10 days of symptom onset, functionally significant PTS occurred in only 13% of patients in this high-risk group.

A potential advantage of the PMT/PPMT approach is the reduction in total dose of thrombolytic agent administered relative to thrombolysis by systemic infusion or CDTI, with a consequent theoretical benefit of decreased bleeding risk. In addition, PMT/PPMT offers the advantage of minimizing systemic lytic exposure in particular, thereby presumably decreasing systemic bleeding risks involving critical sites such as the central nervous system.

The authors conclude that this study provides preliminary evidence that PMT/PPMT with adjunctive CDTI can be used safely and effectively in adolescent subjects with DVT at high risk for PTS.

T. G. Walker, MD

The MILLER banding procedure is an effective method for treating dialysis-associated steal syndrome
Miller GA, Goel N, Friedman A, et al (American Access Care of Brooklyn, NY; American Access Care of Florida, Plantation; et al)
Kidney Int 77:359-366, 2010

We evaluated the efficacy of the Minimally Invasive Limited Ligation Endoluminal-Assisted Revision (MILLER) banding procedure in treating dialysis-associated steal syndrome or high-flow access problems. A retrospective analysis was conducted, evaluating banding of 183 patients of which 114 presented with hand ischemia (Steal) and 69 with clinical manifestations of pathologic high access flow such as congestive heart failure. Patients were assessed for technical success and symptomatic improvement, primary and secondary access patency, and primary band patency. Overall, 183 patients underwent a combined 229 bandings with technical success achieved in 225. Complete symptomatic relief (clinical success) was attained in 109 Steal patients and in all high-flow patients. The average follow-up time was 11 months with a 6-month primary band patency of 75 and 85% for Steal and high-flow patients, respectively. At 24 months the secondary access patency was 90% and the thrombotic event rates for upper-arm fistulas, forearm fistulas, and grafts were 0.21, 0.10, and 0.92 per access-year, respectively. Hence, the minimally invasive MILLER procedure appears to be an effective and durable option for treating dialysis access-related steal syndrome and high-flow-associated symptoms (Figs 5-8).

▶ On the creation of a hemodialysis access, a low-resistance venous pathway is connected to the arterial circuit. This creates the potential for several problems, which cover a spectrum of disease from dialysis-associated steal syndrome (steal) to high-output cardiac overload. The ideal access functions with just enough pressure and flow to prevent thrombosis while maximizing hemodialysis efficiency. Steal syndrome develops in 2.7% to 4.3% of arteriovenous grafts (AVGs) and 1% of arteriovenous fistulas (AVFs). It is clinically

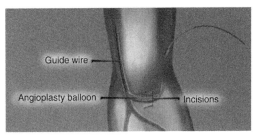

FIGURE 5.—An inflated angioplasty balloon is used as a sizing dowel inside the access. Two parallel, lateral 0.5 cm incisions are made approximately 1–3 cm from the arteriovenous anastomosis. (Reprinted with permission from Macmillan Publishers Ltd: Kidney International, Miller GA, Goel N, Friedman A, et al. The MILLER banding procedure is an effective method for treating dialysis-associated steal syndrome. *Kidney Int.* 2010;77:359-366, copyright 2010.)

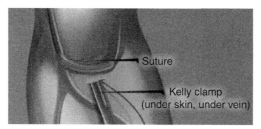

FIGURE 6.—A peri-access tunnel is dissected subcutaneously using Kelly clamp blunt dissection, and a 2-0 monofilament ligature of Prolene is pulled under the access. (Reprinted with permission from Macmillan Publishers Ltd: Kidney International, Miller GA, Goel N, Friedman A, et al. The MILLER banding procedure is an effective method for treating dialysis-associated steal syndrome. *Kidney Int.* 2010;77:359-366, copyright 2010.)

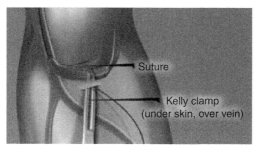

FIGURE 7.—The suture is looped over the access (under the skin) using a Kelly clamp. (Reprinted with permission from Macmillan Publishers Ltd: Kidney International, Miller GA, Goel N, Friedman A, et al. The MILLER banding procedure is an effective method for treating dialysis-associated steal syndrome. *Kidney Int.* 2010;77:359-366, copyright 2010.)

defined as hypoperfusion distal (more peripheral) to the hemodialysis access because of the access diverting an excessive amount of blood away from the distal artery. Increased resistance in the distal arteries (microvascular and macrovascular diseases) contributes to the diversion of blood into the arteriovenous (AV) access, exacerbating distal hypoperfusion and frequently resulting in ischemic symptoms. If untreated, steal can lead to debilitating neuropathy and tissue loss.

Surgical banding is a technique that has commonly been used to correct steal by reducing access flow. Various banding techniques have been described in published studies, but complexities in sizing the band and the resultant poor long-term outcomes have led to near abandonment of banding and the development of alternative treatments such as distal revascularization with interval ligation (DRIL) and proximalization of the arterial inflow (PAI).

The authors previously presented the Minimally Invasive Limited Ligation Endoluminal-Assisted Revision (MILLER) study, which included a cohort of 16 patients in which treatment was confined to patients showing steal symptoms. Since its introduction, the authors extended the use of the MILLER procedure to treat the full spectrum of low-resistance pathologic flow from steal to high flow within the access. The current paper presents the

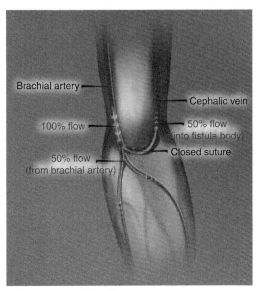

FIGURE 8.—Following the Minimally Invasive Limited Ligation Endoluminal-Assisted Revision (MILLER) banding procedure, the resistance band redirects flow, improving distal perfusion, and alleviating symptoms. (Reprinted with permission from Macmillan Publishers Ltd: Kidney International, Miller GA, Goel N, Friedman A, et al. The MILLER banding procedure is an effective method for treating dialysis-associated steal syndrome. *Kidney Int.* 2010;77:359-366, copyright 2010.)

development of a precision modification to traditional banding procedures and describes outcomes.

A total of 183 consecutive patients (100 men and 83 women) who adhered to the inclusion/exclusion criteria were treated with the MILLER banding procedure for correction of steal syndrome and high-flow fistulas during a 4-year period. Patients were evaluated and categorized as having steal or high flow according to their symptoms and physical examination. A diagnosis of steal was established on clinical grounds. Accesses were banded if they exhibited classic steal symptoms such as numbness and coldness of the hand, which were exacerbated at dialysis and alleviated by temporary shunt occlusion. Signs of steal ranged from pallor to tissue necrosis of the hand and fingers. Angiography was then performed to confirm the diagnosis. Diagnosis of a high-flow access was also established on clinical grounds. High-flow accesses were banded if the patients developed decompensated congestive heart failure directly attributable to AV access placement, visibly notable aneurysm growth, or problematic elevation of venous pressures at dialysis. Patients with simultaneous symptoms of both steal syndrome and high access flow were categorized as having high flow. All patients who underwent banding after classification into the steal and high-flow groups were included in the study. Patients with limb ischemia related to proximal arterial stenoses or arterial stenoses amenable to angioplasty were excluded from the study.

Technical success was achieved when a band was created and the patient underwent at least one successful hemodialysis treatment. Any patient who achieved complete symptomatic improvement was considered to have clinical success. Patients who experienced partial (but adequate) symptomatic improvement were classified as having partial clinical success. A thrombectomy procedure performed within 30 days of the initial banding was considered to be banding related. Primary access patency is defined as the time between the initial access intervention and any following repeat interventions. Primary patency of the MILLER band ended with balloon dilation of existing bands, rebanding, or access thrombosis. Secondary patency is defined as the time of patency from the initial intervention until the access was surgically revised or abandoned or until transplantation, death, and loss to follow-up.

Figs 5-8 illustrate the steps in the MILLER procedure.

The cohort of 183 patients had 156 upper arm accesses (78 brachiocephalic AVFs, 58 transposed brachiobasilic AVFs, and 20 AVGs) and 27 forearm accesses. A total of 114 patients were classified as having steal, and 69 patients were classified as having high flow. An access band was created (technical success) in 225 of 229 (98%) banding attempts. Overall, 89% of patients with steal and 94% of those with high flow achieved clinical success (complete symptomatic relief) with the initial banding, and 96% of patients with steal and 100% of those with high flow ultimately attained clinical success with one or more bandings. The most common first band size was a diameter of 4 mm (57%) for fistulas (range, 2.5-6 mm) and 3 mm (52%) for grafts (range, 3-4 mm).

Clinical success was not achieved in 17 (9%) of the initial bandings, with patients experiencing only partial improvement. Of the 183 (7%) patients, 12 achieved clinical success with 2 or 3 banding attempts. Of the remaining 5 patients, 3 continued to use their access with partial (but tolerable) symptomatic relief and 2 required access ligation because of persistent steal and resultant tissue loss.

The primary band patency for patients with steal and high flow was 75% and 85% at 6 months, respectively. The primary access patency for patients with steal and high flow was 52% and 63% at 3 months, with a secondary access patency of 90% and 89% at 24 months, respectively.

The authors feel that the MILLER procedure is useful for all accesses exhibiting high flow and most accesses exhibiting steal syndrome. When selecting the optimal treatment for such access dysfunctions, the primary concerns are efficacy and invasiveness. The MILLER banding procedure is the least invasive of all current treatments, and its efficacy is now well established. As most accesses exhibiting steal symptoms will likely have sufficient proximal arterial flow, the authors believe the MILLER procedure should be the initial treatment for steal. However, in cases of low-flow steal, DRIL or PAI may still be the optimal treatments. The precise sizing of MILLER banding may provide a rapid way of achieving adequate balance between access flow and distal flow without diminishing access longevity.

T. G. Walker, MD

The Safety and Effectiveness of the Retrievable Option Inferior Vena Cava Filter: A United States Prospective Multicenter Clinical Study

Johnson MS, Nemcek AA Jr, Benenati JF, et al (Indiana Univ School of Medicine, Indianapolis; Northwestern Memorial Hosp, Chicago, IL; Baptist Cardiac and Vascular Inst, Miami, FL; et al)
J Vasc Interv Radiol 21:1173-1184, 2010

Purpose.—To evaluate the safety and effectiveness of the retrievable Option inferior vena cava (IVC) filter in patients at risk for pulmonary embolism (PE).

Materials and Methods.—This was a prospective, multicenter, single-arm clinical trial. Subjects ($N = 100$) underwent implantation of the IVC filter and were followed for 180 days; subjects whose filters were later removed were followed for 30 days thereafter. The primary objective was to determine whether the one-sided lower limit of the 95% CI for the observed clinical success rate was at least 80%. Clinical success was defined as technical success (deployment of the filter such that it was judged suitable for mechanical protection from PE) without subsequent PE, significant filter migration or embolization, symptomatic caval thrombosis, or other complications.

Results.—Technical success was achieved in 100% of subjects. There were eight cases of recurrent PE, two cases of filter migration (23 mm), and three cases of symptomatic caval occlusion/thrombosis (one in a subject who also experienced filter migration). No filter embolization or fracture occurred. Clinical success was achieved in 88% of subjects; the one-sided lower limit of the 95% CI was 81%. Retrieval was successful at a mean of 67.1 days after implantation (range, 1−175 d) for 36 of 39 subjects (92.3%). All deaths ($n = 17$) and deep vein thromboses ($n = 18$) were judged to have resulted from preexisting or intercurrent illnesses or interventions and unrelated to the filter device; all deaths were judged to be unrelated to PE.

Conclusions.—Placement and retrieval of the Option IVC filter were performed safely and with high rates of clinical success.

► The Option inferior vena cava (IVC) filter (Rex Medical, Conshohocken, Pennsylvania) is among the second generation of filters specifically developed as a retrievable device. It is constructed from a single piece of nickel-titanium alloy (nitinol) tubing and has 6 expandable and collapsible struts that flare out symmetrically from a central apex. A single large hook is located at the apex. The filter is deployed through a venous sheath with the following specifications: 6.5F outer diameter, 5F internal diameter, and 70-cm length. The filter has been cleared by the Food and Drug Administration for use in caval diameters as large as 30 mm. The current study was undertaken to assess the safety and effectiveness of this filter as both a permanent and retrievable device.

This was a single-arm, prospective, multicenter, nonrandomized clinical trial conducted in patients who were 18 years and older, who were at permanent or temporary increased risk of pulmonary embolism (PE), and in whom IVC interruption was judged to be clinically indicated for 1 or more of the following 4 conditions: pulmonary thromboembolism when anticoagulant therapy was contraindicated, failure of anticoagulant therapy in thromboembolic disease, complication as a result of anticoagulant therapy in thromboembolic disease, or indication for temporary caval filtration (eg, trauma or planned operation such as bariatric or pelvic surgery). Subjects were required to have an IVC transverse diameter of no more than 32 mm and adequate venous anatomy to allow for insertion of the filter into the IVC, either from femoral or jugular access sites. At the time of the index procedure, subjects also had to have a patent jugular vein to allow potential retrieval of the filter.

Subjects were excluded from enrollment if they already had a filter in place or had undergone filter retrieval within the previous 60 days. They were also excluded if they had confirmed bacteremia, a duplication of the IVC, a life expectancy of less than 6 months, a known sensitivity to radiographic contrast medium that could not be adequately premedicated prophylactically, a known hypersensitivity to nickel or titanium alloys, or any comorbid condition that the investigator deemed might compromise the study.

One hundred subjects underwent filter placement during the study period. Of these, 36 subjects had their filter successfully retrieved and completed the full 30 days of postretrieval follow-up. No retrieved subjects died, were withdrawn, or were lost to follow-up. Of the 64 subjects who did not undergo retrieval, 17 died of preexisting or intercurrent illness before any attempted retrieval. The remaining 47 subjects completed the 180 days of follow-up with the filter still in place; 44 completed without a retrieval attempt and 3 underwent failed attempts at filter retrieval with the result that the filter remained in place.

The 2 predefined primary end points for this study were clinical success and retrieval clinical success. These primary end points combined safety and effectiveness outcomes of key interest with the placement of IVC filters. The 2 effectiveness end points were technical success and retrieval technical success. Predefined safety end points included the incidence of deep vein thrombosis (DVT), filter migration (>2 cm), filter embolization, symptomatic caval thrombosis, and recurrent PE. Adverse events were classified as serious, device related, procedure related, medication related, preexisting condition related, and/or anticipated. In addition to effectiveness and safety outcomes, the following procedural data were collected: mean filter placement time, mean filter retrieval time, and mean fluoroscopy times during both procedures.

Technical success of filter implantation was achieved in 100% of subjects. There were 8 cases of recurrent PE, 2 cases of filter migration (23 mm), and 3 cases of symptomatic caval occlusion/thrombosis. In the study, only 4 of these cases (4%) of recurrent PE were judged by the medical monitor to be related to the filter, a rate within the 5% threshold suggested by the SIR Committee and within the range of 0% to 6.0% commonly reported in the literature for various other filter designs, including retrievable filters. No filter embolization or fracture occurred. Clinical success was achieved in 88% of subjects. A total of 39 subjects underwent 42 attempted retrieval procedures. Retrieval was successful at a mean of 67.1 days after implantation (range, 1-175 days) for 36 of 39 subjects (92.3%). All deaths ($n=17$) and DVTs ($n=18$) were judged to have resulted from preexisting or intercurrent illnesses or interventions and were unrelated to the filter, and all deaths were judged to be unrelated to PE.

A number of device retrieval observations were reported that did not directly affect the primary end point of retrieval clinical success or the effectiveness end point of retrieval technical success. Difficulty snaring the filter hook was reported for 12 of the 39 subjects (30.8%) in whom it was attempted, difficulty disengaging struts from the caval wall was reported for 5 subjects (12.8%), and difficulty sheathing the filter struts was reported for 5 subjects (12.8%); retrieval success was ultimately achieved in all cases.

The authors conclude that in this population of 100 subjects at risk for PE, placement and retrieval (at a maximum of 175 days) of the Option IVC filter was performed with clinical success, was within the effectiveness and safety thresholds suggested by SIR, and had complication rates well within the limits of safety profiles reported for similarly marketed devices.

T. G. Walker, MD

Transhepatic Hemodialysis Catheters: Functional Outcome and Comparison Between Early and Late Failure
Younes HK, Pettigrew CD, Anaya-Ayala JE, et al (The Methodist Hosp, Houston, TX; et al)
J Vasc Interv Radiol 22:183-191, 2011

Purpose.—To describe the authors' experience with transhepatic placement of catheters, highlighting early and late complications, and to determine if this procedure is a viable option in patients in whom central venous occlusions present a significant challenge.

Materials and Methods.—The records of all the patients who underwent placement of transhepatic hemodialysis from January 2003 to October 2008 were retrospectively reviewed. Selected patients were dialysis-dependent, having undergone multiple access procedures and revisions. Kaplan-Meier analysis was used to estimate primary and secondary patency.

Results.—Twenty-two patients (mean age 42 years, range 22–70 years, 59% women) underwent a total of 127 transhepatic catheter placements at 24 transhepatic access sites; technical success was achieved in all cases. There were no hepatic injuries (bleeding or fistula formation). There were 105 exchanges in 14 patients, with a mean of 7.5 exchanges, a median of 5 exchanges (range 1–18 exchanges), and a catheter migration rate of 0.39 per 100 catheter-days. The sepsis rate was 0.22 per 100 catheter-days, and the catheter thrombosis rate was 0.18 per 100 catheter-days. The mean cumulative catheter duration in situ was 506.2 days, and the mean time catheter in situ was 87.7 days. The mean total access site interval was 1,046 catheter-days (range of 423–1,413 catheter-days).

Conclusions.—Transhepatic hemodialysis catheter placement is associated with low rates of morbidity. In this series, transhepatic catheters provided the possibility of long-term functionality, despite associated high rates of catheter-related maintenance, provides a potentially viable access for patients with exhausted access options (Tables 2-4).

▶ Tunneled central venous catheters are a common and fairly effective means of acquiring temporary venous access for hemodialysis. Compared with the preferred arteriovenous (AV) fistulas and grafts, these catheters are associated with higher rates of infection and line exchanges. Initially conceived as a means for temporary vascular access, tunneled transhepatic catheters have become a moderate-to long-term mode of dialysis in some patients who have exhausted traditional access sites because of widespread central venous occlusions, including the femoral veins, collateral neck veins, and renal veins, through previous catheter placements and surgeries. As a result, alternative sites have begun to be explored in patients who have become catheter dependent, including translumbar and transhepatic approaches to the inferior vena cava (IVC). Two retrospective studies regarding transhepatic hemodialysis access view this as a viable option in the short term, with considerable complications, including thrombosis and infections, limiting long-term functionality. This study describes the authors' experiences with the transhepatic hemodialysis access technique focusing on safety and functionality.

The authors retrospectively reviewed the records of patients who underwent placement of transhepatic hemodialysis catheters during a 70-month period and collected patient demographics, comorbidities, date and indication for initial placement of transhepatic catheter, procedure details, duration of catheter function, reasons for catheter exchange and removal, catheter-related complications, systemic complications, and patient survival. All identified patients were currently dialysis dependent and had undergone multiple access procedures and revisions and encountered multiple failed permanent access procedures. All patients had undergone creation of AV fistulas or graft placement (or both). In addition, these patients had routinely used internal and external jugular and femoral, with occasional subclavian and iliac, catheter access that was no longer functional for hemodialysis. The indication for transhepatic catheter placement was an inability to access the internal or external jugular, subclavian, or femoral veins, including the inability to recanalize occlusions bilaterally or attempted preservation of a final remaining peripheral site for AV access. Indications for catheter exchange included device failure and bacteremia with and without exit site infection. The translumbar approach was not routinely

TABLE 2.—Catheter-Related Complications (Total = 115)

Complication	Total Frequency (%)	Rate (Per 100 Catheter-Days)
Migration	43 (37.4)	0.39
Catheter-related sepsis	25 (21.7)	0.22
Thrombosis	20 (17.4)	0.18
Poor flow	10 (8.7)	0.05
Kinking	5 (4.3)	0.04
Bleeding	5 (4.3)	0.04
Fibrin sheath	2 (1.7)	0.02
Hematoma	1 (0.9)	0.01

TABLE 3.—Early versus Late Device Failure

Device Failure Category	Cause of Device Failure	Early Failure	Late Failure	P Value
Total overall		55	74	
Motion-related	Dislodgment	1 (1.8%)	0 (0.0%)	.42
	Migration	19 (34.5%)	34 (45.9%)	.21
	Kinking	4 (7.3%)	3 (4.1%)	.72
	Overall motion	*24 (43.6%)*	*37 (50.0%)*	*.48*
Flow-related obstruction	Occlusion	0 (0.0%)	2 (2.7%)	.51
	Thrombosis	8 (14.5%)	14 (18.9%)	.64
	Fibrin sheath	0 (0.0%)	1 (1.4%)	1
	Poor flow	7 (12.7%)	0 (0.0%)	.002
	Overall obstruction	*15 (27.3%)*	*17 (23.0%)*	*.68*
Infection-related	Site infection	2 (3.6%)	10 (13.5%)	.07
	Catheter sepsis	12 (21.8%)	10 (13.5%)	.24
	Overall infection	*14 (25.5%)*	*20 (27.0%)*	*1*
Postprocedure site complications	Bleeding	1 (1.8%)	0 (0.0%)	.43
	Intercostal pain	1 (1.8%)	0 (0.0%)	.43
	Overall site	*2 (3.6%)*	*0 (0.0%)*	*.18*

Note—The most common cause of early device failure was migration (occurring in 34.5% of patients), followed by catheter-related sepsis (21.8% of patients). There were 74 late device failures. The most common cause of late device failure was migration (45.9%), followed by thrombosis (18.9%). Kinking was seen as an early (4 patients) and a late (3 patients) complication.

TABLE 4.—Catheter Intervals and Patency

Primary service device interval	141.2 catheter-days (0−565)
Secondary service device interval	124.5 catheter-days (2−437)
Mean total access site interval	450.3 catheter-days (12−1,414)
Men	450.0 catheter-days (12−1,112)
Women	614.3 catheter-days (99−1,414)
Median total access site interval	486.5 catheter-days (12−1,414)
Mean cumulative catheter duration in situ	506.2 catheter-days
Mean time catheter in situ	87.7 catheter-days

attempted before the transhepatic approach at the authors' institution. Patients with signs and symptoms of active infection did not undergo catheter placement and were excluded from this study.

During the 70-month period, 22 patients (mean age, 42 years; range, 22-70 years; 59% women) underwent a total of 127 transhepatic catheter placements at 24 transhepatic access sites. Hypercoagulable states were found in 5 patients, including factor V Leiden deficiency, antiphospholipid antibody syndrome, and hyperhomocysteinemia. The indications for initial transhepatic dialysis catheter placement were a lack of remaining peripheral access sites in 17 patients and preservation of a single remaining venous site in 3 patients for creation of AV access. Two patients received transhepatic catheters before receiving peritoneal dialysis catheters after exhaustion of other venous access sites.

All patients underwent routine laboratory studies, including complete blood cell count, electrolyte panel, and coagulation studies, before undergoing placement of catheters. All procedures were completed in the interventional radiology suite by 4 interventional radiologists. The following catheters were used: Tesio catheter (Medcomp, Harleyville, Pennsylvania); Schon catheter (AngioDynamics, Queensbury, New York); Arrow Edge catheter (TeleFlex, Reading, Pennsylvania); and Dura-Flow catheter (AngioDynamics, Queensbury, New York). Transhepatic dialysis catheter placement was performed using the technique detailed below.

The procedures were performed under conscious sedation in 111 cases and under general anesthesia in 16 cases. Prophylactic antibiotics, typically 1 g of cefazolin, were used only when infection was the reason for the exchange. After preparing and draping the right side of the chest and abdomen in a sterile fashion, local anesthesia with lidocaine was administered, and a 21-gauge AccuStick needle (Boston Scientific, Natick, Massachusetts) was advanced into the liver from a right lateral intercostal approach under direct fluoroscopic visualization. Ultrasound guidance was not required or used in any case. The approach used involved puncture at the midaxillary line at or below the eighth intercostal space, with the needle angled toward the pedicle of the 12th thoracic vertebral body. As the needle was withdrawn, radiopaque contrast material was injected to identify a branch of the right or middle hepatic vein. When the hepatic vein was cannulated, a 0.018-in guide wire was advanced into the right atrium. Over the guide wire, the AccuStick sheath was advanced into the hepatic vein with fluoroscopic guidance. The guide wire was exchanged for a 0.035-in Amplatz Super Stiff guide wire (Boston Scientific, Natick, Massachusetts) with its tip in the right atrium. Following progressive dilations, a peel-away sheath was placed through which catheters were inserted under fluoroscopic guidance. An anteroinferior subcutaneous tunnel was created before venous access placement. An exception to this was seen in cases in which Tesio catheters were used. In these instances, the subcutaneous tunnel was created immediately after venous access placement. The venotomy site was closed using subcuticular suture. Both lumens of the catheter were flushed and aspirated and found to inject freely before the conclusion of the procedure. The catheter was locked with heparin. Postplacement images were obtained to confirm catheter position. The most common location of catheter tip placement in all catheters was the right atrium (105 catheters). Catheters were placed in the IVC in 15 cases; 4 catheters were placed in the superior vena cava (SVC). One catheter tip each was placed in the hemiazygos vein and the distal right hepatic vein.

Patients were followed up clinically in conjunction with their primary nephrologist. Follow-up visits for evaluations by the interventional radiologist were indicated if suspected catheter-related complications were found. Standard practice included guide wire exchange of the catheter in the presence of catheter malfunction, often with revision for a different type or length of catheter. In case of local infection, catheter exchange with formation of a new subcutaneous tunnel and exit site was performed. If the patient was bacteremic, the catheter was exchanged over a guide wire or the patient underwent a catheter holiday, in which case on removal of catheters, guide wires remained in place to maintain access while the patient was treated for bacteremia. On resolution of the infection, catheter exchange was completed.

Technical success was achieved in all cases without intraprocedural complications. Two instances of immediate postprocedural complications occurred, including an episode of bleeding and intercostal pain. There were a total of 105 exchanges in 14 patients, with a mean of 7.5 exchanges and a median of 5 exchanges per patient (range, 1—18 exchanges). The most common indication for exchange was device failure (63%) and catheter-related sepsis (20%). Catheter-related complications are outlined in Table 2. The most common complication was migration, seen most commonly in the SVC, IVC, and right hepatic vein. Migration occurred in 43 catheters, resulting in a catheter migration rate of 0.39 per 100 catheter-days. Other common complications were catheter-related sepsis, for which 25 catheters were exchanged with a sepsis rate of 0.22 per 100 catheter-days, and thrombosis, for which 20 catheters were exchanged with a catheter thrombosis rate of 0.18 per 100 catheter-days. The mean total access site interval was 1046.2 catheter-days (range, 423—1.413 catheter-days).

The data were analyzed further for early versus late catheter-related indications for exchange secondary to catheter-dependent complications. This is detailed in Table 3, while catheter intervals and patency are detailed in Table 4.

At the authors' institution, the transhepatic route is preferred over the translumbar route for several reasons. The transhepatic approach is possible even when the IVC is occluded. In addition, they report that the transhepatic method is associated with less risk of damage or bleeding from surrounding structures. If a bleeding complication occurs, they feel that these complications are more easily controlled with a transhepatic approach (eg, hepatic parenchymal tract embolization, if necessary). In their patient population, in which increased abdominal circumference can be a limiting factor, the transhepatic approach is an easier option for gaining access.

In contrast to previous studies that acknowledge the benefit of transhepatic catheters in short-term situations but cite high complication rates and low patency rates as reasons to for go their use in the long-term setting, the authors show in this report the complication rate to be lower than previously reported with patency rates comparable to rates seen with the translumbar approach. A prospective randomized controlled trial would provide the additional information necessary to offer recommendations on which procedure to attempt first in patients with limited access sites. The authors feel that based on their findings, transhepatic hemodialysis catheters have proven to achieve good long-term functionality. A high level of maintenance is required to preserve patency, although this approach provides remarkably durable access for patients who have otherwise exhausted access options. Finally, this method of hemodialysis access can be used as a temporary viable method that can preserve remaining venous sites and extend the time patients have to receive permanent venous access. Effective long-term functionality suggests that the transhepatic access method is a viable means to gain meaningful vascular access with good safety and functionality.

T. G. Walker, MD

7 Neuroradiology

Introduction

2010-2011 was an unusually rich year for the worldwide neuroradiology literature. Between articles in brain, spine/cord, and head and neck, we reaped a rich harvest indeed. Let's begin with what was special about articles that discussed brain pathology. I think that this was the year diffusion tensor imaging (DTI) really came of age in terms of practical applications in day-to-day clinical neuroradiology. We could title 2010-2011 something like: "DTI—not just a 'pretty face' anymore!" I've been mesmerized for several years by the gorgeous 3D color tractography images ... perhaps because neuroimaging has been pretty much black and white for decades. We haven't had much color in our neuro life! Until now. Maybe you've wondered—as did I—was there anything really useful about DTI? Pretty to look at, delightful to behold, but c'mon! And this year's articles put an emphatic "yes" answer on that question.

DTI has become part of our own day-to-day imaging of acute stroke. We use DTI in lieu of diffusion-weighted imaging (DWI) and have found it much more sensitive in depicting multiple small embolic and lacunar infarcts as well as ischemic changes in the posterior circulation. There are other growing applications of DTI as well, especially in the preoperative planning of diffusely-infiltrating gliomas. There's even a new application of DTI that measures myelin repair and axonal loss. So its use extends well beyond just tumor and stroke imaging.

So what about DWI? Does it have a future? You bet it does—and a growing one. There are a number of articles I selected for you in brain, spinal cord, head and neck applications of DWI. And the use of DWI in evaluating bone disease (skull base, vertebral end plates) is coming into its own. There's an interesting article I included on DWI that asks and nicely answers the question, "What are we REALLY seeing"?

I've included several articles on the growing importance of detecting brain "microbleeds" along with some other causes of multifocal "blooming black dots" on T2* susceptibility-weighted imaging including their prevalence in boxers. Here's another stunner for you: virtually ALL children who have cardiac bypass surgery have black brain dots afterwards. That one makes you sit up and take notice... .

Lastly, what can we look forward to in 2011-2012? All I can say is "I don't know"; but at the rate new imaging applications are growing, we will without doubt have lots of fun stuff to share with you next year!

Anne G. Osborn, MD

Brain: Aneurysms and Subarachnoid Hemorrhage

Current Imaging Assessment and Treatment of Intracranial Aneurysms
Hacein-Bey L, Provenzale JM (Radiological Associates of Sacramento Med Group, Inc, CA; Duke Univ Med Ctr, Durham, NC)
AJR Am J Roentgenol 196:32-44, 2011

Objective.—This article reviews current neuroimaging techniques used for screening, diagnosis, and follow-up of patients with intracranial aneurysms as well as neuroendovascular therapeutic options available to patients.

Conclusion.—The diagnosis and management of intracranial aneurysms have evolved dramatically in the past 20 years. MR angiography and CT angiography allow radiologists to reliably and noninvasively diagnose most intracranial aneurysms. Nonoperative endovascular techniques for treating intracranial aneurysms are now making treatment increasingly safer and more effective.

▶ Intracranial aneurysms are common, occurring in approximately 2% to 3% of the general population. Generally aneurysms remain silent, until they suddenly rupture and present with subarachnoid hemorrhage. With the increasingly wide use of brain imaging performed for unrelated reasons, unruptured aneurysms are becoming increasingly identified. The key question is whether an unruptured aneurysm should be treated (and if so, how) or can be safely left alone. And perhaps even more poignantly, what does a patient who has been told he/she has a "ticking time bomb" do?

The authors have put together a very nice topic review on the imaging assessment and treatment of intracranial aneurysm (both ruptured and unruptured). While there are lots of questions and debates about treatment, there is little doubt that endovascular treatment reduces mortality and morbidity compared with surgery even though a residual neck is more common.

If you want a quick, well-written, thorough review that covers everything from basic facts about aneurysms to imaging and treatment of unusual aneurysms, this is an excellent article for one-stop shopping! I found the figures compelling, favoring CT angiography (Fig 1 in the original article) over MR angiography (Fig 2 in the original article).

A. G. Osborn, MD

Brain: Atherosclerosis, Carotid Stenosis

Diffusion-weighted magnetic resonance imaging for the detection of lipid-rich necrotic core in carotid atheroma in vivo
Young VE, Patterson AJ, Sadat U, et al (Addenbrooke's Hosp, Cambridge, UK; et al)
Neuroradiology 52:929-936, 2010

Introduction.—Research has shown that knowing the morphology of carotid atheroma improves current risk stratification for predicting subsequent thrombo-embolic events. Previous magnetic resonance (MR) ex vivo studies have shown that diffusion-weighted imaging (DWI) can detect lipid-rich necrotic core (LR/NC) and fibrous cap. This study aims to establish if this is achievable in vivo.

Methods.—Twenty-six patients (mean age 73 years, range 54—87 years) with moderate to severe carotid stenosis confirmed on ultrasound were imaged. An echo-planar DWI sequence was performed along with standard high-resolution MR imaging. Apparent diffusion coefficient (ADC) maps were evaluated. Two independent readers reported the mean ADC values from regions of interest defining LR/NCs and fibrous caps. For subjects undergoing carotid endarterectomy ($n = 19$), carotid specimens were obtained and stained using Nile red.

Results.—The mean ADC values were 1.0×10^{-3} mm^2/s ($\pm$SD 0.3×10^{-3} mm^2/s) and 0.7×10^{-3} mm^2/s ($\pm$SD 0.2×10^{-3} mm^2/s) for fibrous cap and LR/NC, respectively; the difference was significant ($p < 0.0001$). The intra-class correlation coefficients summarising the agreement between the two independent readers were 0.84 and 0.60 for fibrous cap and LR/NC, respectively. Comparison of quantitative ADC values and histology (by subjective grading of lipid content) showed a significant correlation: heavier lipid staining matched lower ADC values ($r = -0.435$, $p = 0.005$).

Conclusions.—This study indicates that DWI can be used to distinguish LR/NC and the fibrous cap. The study also suggests that the mean ADC value may be linearly related to subjective graded LR/NC content determined by histology (Fig 3).

▶ As the authors point out in their introduction, the 2 large longitudinal studies of carotid stenosis (the American and European trials) that showed the benefit of carotid endarterectomy versus best medical treatment were based on the degree of luminal stenosis. Is that the whole story? Clearly not, as some patients with high-grade stenoses remain asymptomatic and some who have only mild or moderate stenosis have strokes.

Many investigators believe that the answer to the above conundrum lies in the nature of the atheromatous plaque itself, deeming some plaques at risk. What puts a plaque in this category is debatable, but intraplaque hemorrhage, necrosis, and a lipid core that is exposed through an ulcerated endothelium

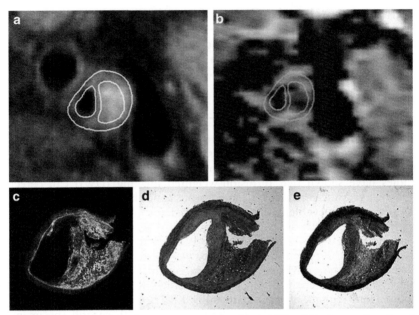

FIGURE 3.—A case study showing a symptomatic subject's MRI and histology sections through a single co-registered carotid plaque. The case is of an internal carotid plaque from a symptomatic patient who had a maximum stenosis of 70%. The figure shows MR images of a T_1-weighted image, **b** apparent diffusion coefficient (ADC) map) and stained histological sections, **c** Nile red, **d** haematoxylin and eosin and **e** elastic van Gieson. The imaging shows a hyperintense region within the plaque representing lipid-rich necrotic core with the corresponding ADC map showing the same region as hypointense i.e. low ADC values. The matched histology demonstrates the same area to be mainly blue on Nile red and yellow on elastic van Gieson staining which is consistent with the presence of lipid. (With kind permission from Springer Science and Business Media: Young VE, Patterson AJ, Sadat U, et al. Diffusion-weighted magnetic resonance imaging for the detection of lipid-rich necrotic core in carotid atheroma in vivo. *Neuroradiology.* 2010;52:929-936.)

are factors cited by many authors. A plaque with a large lipid-rich necrotic core covered by a thin fibrous cap is an at-risk plaque.

Several modalities have been explored as possible ways to image atheromatous plaques directly. Color Doppler ultrasound and high-resolution standard MR sequences have been used. This study is the first in vivo demonstration that diffusion-weighted imaging and apparent diffusion coefficient mapping may play a key role in quantitative demonstration of lipid burden in atheromatous plaques (Fig 3). As lipid burden correlates strongly with future stroke risk, this is a pretty exciting finding and—if proved correct in larger studies—could give us a wonderful addition to our diagnostic armamentarium.

A. G. Osborn, MD

Functional MR Imaging in Patients with Carotid Artery Stenosis before and after Revascularization
Schaaf M, Mommertz G, Ludolph A, et al (Aachen Univ, Germany)
AJNR Am J Neuroradiol 31:1791-1798, 2010

Background and Purpose.—Significant extracranial stenosis of the ICA is a known risk factor for future stroke and it has been shown that revascularization reduces the risk of future stroke. We applied BOLD fMRI in patients with carotid artery stenosis before and after CEA. Our purpose was to determine whether fMRI is able to demonstrate impaired CVR and to identify patient parameters that are associated with postoperative changes of cerebral hemodynamics.

Materials and Methods.—Nineteen consecutive patients with symptomatic ($n = 13$) and asymptomatic ($n = 6$) stenosis of the ICA were prospectively recruited (male/female ratio $= 16{:}3$; age, $69 \pm 8{,}1$ years). fMRI using a simple bilateral motor task was performed immediately before and after CEA.

Results.—Mean BOLD MSC was significantly increased postoperatively (MSC, 0.13 ± 0.66; $P = 0.0002$). Patients with a stenosis of <80% demonstrated an increase in MSC (MSC, 0.32 ± 0.59; $P \leq .0001$). Patients with previous ischemic stroke showed a larger MSC than patients with TIAs (stroke: MSC, 0.55 ± 0.65; $P \leq .0001$; TIA: MSC, 0.05 ± 0.26; $P = 0.054$). Patients older than 70 years had a significantly larger MSC following surgery (≤ 70 years: MSC, -0.01 ± 0.39; $P = .429$; >70 years: MSC, 0.29 ± 0.48; $P \leq .0001$).

Conclusions.—BOLD fMRI can demonstrate changes in cerebral hemodynamics before and after CEA, indicative of an ameliorated CVR. This response is dependent on the age of the patient, the degree of preoperative stenosis, and the patient's symptoms.

▶ Severe stenosis of the internal carotid artery has 2 serious consequences: (1) It is a known risk factor for future stroke, and (2) it may cause significant reductions in cerebral blood flow and cerebral perfusion pressure. Reduced oxygenation leads to acidosis and CO_2 and NO accumulation. Autoregulation results in compensatory vasodilation. An accurate method of detecting the physiologic changes before and after carotid endarterectomy (CEA) would be very valuable in answering the question: does CEA restore altered vascular hemodynamics?

The authors demonstrate that blood oxygen level—dependent (BOLD) functional MRI (fMRI) can demonstrate restoration of normal cerebrovascular reactivity after CEA. That's very useful. The authors' finding that the benefit of CEA as measured by BOLD was much more significant in patients older than 70 years (Fig 5 in the original article).

The hemodynamic changes following revascularization are complex. Something the authors didn't discuss—as it wasn't the purpose of the article—is the utility of BOLD fMRI in patients who develop cerebral hyperperfusion syndrome after CEA. It's a rare but very frightening complication that can lead to severe cerebral edema in the affected hemisphere and clinical worsening after revascularization. I've only seen a couple of cases, but the rCBV was significantly elevated compared with the contralateral hemisphere. That was a useful documentation that the clinical deterioration wasn't caused by athero-matous emboli but abnormally robust vasodilation as the formerly starved hemisphere reacted to sudden restoration of normal perfusion.

A. G. Osborn, MD

Brain: Infection, Inflammation, and Metabolic Disease

Measuring Myelin Repair and Axonal Loss with Diffusion Tensor Imaging

Fox RJ, Cronin T, Lin J, et al (Cleveland Clinic Foundation, OH)
AJNR Am J Neuroradiol 32:85-91, 2011

Background and Purpose.—DTI is an MR imaging measure of brain tissue integrity and provides an attractive metric for use in neuroprotection clinical trials. The purpose of our study was to use DTI to evaluate the longitudinal changes in brain tissue integrity in a group of patients with MS.

Materials and Methods.—Twenty-one patients with MS starting natali-zumab were imaged serially for 12 months. Gadolinium-enhancing lesions and 20 regions of interest from normal-appearing white and gray matter brain tissue were followed longitudinally. Average values within each region of interest were derived for FA, $\lambda_{||}$, $\lambda_{\perp}$, and MD. New T1 black holes were identified at 12 months. Analysis was performed by using mixed-model regression analysis with slope (ie, DTI change per month) as the dependent variable.

Results.—During 1 year, FA increased in gadolinium-enhancing lesions but decreased in NABT ($P < 0001$ for both). Changes in FA within gadolinium-enhancing lesions were driven by decreased $\lambda_{\perp}$ ($P < 001$), and within NABT, by decreased $\lambda_{||}$ ($P < 0.0001$). A higher $\lambda_{\perp}$ within gadolinium-enhancing lesions at baseline predicted conversion to T1 black holes at 12 months. MD was unchanged in both gadolinium-enhancing lesions and NABT.

Conclusions.—We observed changes in DTI measures during 1 year in both gadolinium-enhancing lesions and NABT. The DTI results may repre-sent possible remyelination within acute lesions and chronic axonal degen-eration in NAWM. These results support the use of DTI as a measure of tissue integrity for studies of neuroprotective therapies.

▶ We all know that conventional MRI in patients with multiple sclerosis (MS) is very useful in detecting lesions. Enhancement is usually associated with active inflammation and—together with the appearance of new lesions—is often used to guide therapeutic decisions. We also know that there is relatively poor correlation between imaging and clinical findings. As the authors point out, some patients with MS have progressively increasing clinical disability in the absence of new lesions.

Diffusion tensor imaging (DTI) has been touted as a novel technique for tumor imaging. Tumor cells that infiltrate fiber tracts cause displacement, deviation, and destruction of these tracts with corresponding reduction in fractional anisotropy that can be demonstrated even before changes can be seen on standard MR sequences.

Is there a role for DTI in following patients with MS? Could it detect changes in the otherwise normal-appearing white matter (NAWM)? The authors studied a relatively small group of patients starting therapy with natalizumab (better known as Tysabri). No untreated controls were studied. The authors found that changes in DTI may represent remyelination within acute lesions as well as chronic axonal degeneration in the NAWM. That might just make DTI a better way to monitor response to MS therapy than our standard imaging sequences. Only time—and a larger study group—will tell, but this looks like a promising development. Stay tuned!

A. G. Osborn, MD

Neuroimaging Findings in Alcohol-Related Encephalopathies

Zuccoli G, Siddiqui N, Cravo I, et al (Univ of Pittsburgh Med Ctr, PA; Hosp Fernando Fonseca, Lisboa, Portugal; et al)
AJR Am J Roentgenol 195:1378-1384, 2010

Objective.—Our aim was to review the emergent neuroimaging findings of alcohol-related CNS nontraumatic disorders. Alcohol (ethanol) promotes inflammatory processes, increases DNA damage, and creates oxidative stress. In addition, the accompanying thiamine deficiency may lead to Wernicke encephalopathy. Associated changes in serum osmolarity may lead to acute demyelination.

Conclusion.—Alcohol-related encephalopathies can be life-threatening conditions but can be prevented or treated, if recognized (Fig 1).

▶ Worldwide, alcohol probably ranks just about at the top as the most commonly abused substance. Ethanol causes different effects on different organs. Ethanol easily crosses the blood-brain barrier and is a potent neurotoxin.

Excessive alcohol consumption can result in chronic brain changes as well as acute, life-threatening neurologic diseases. One of the problems in sorting out alcoholic encephalopathy is that there are a number of comorbid diseases that complicate both the clinical evaluation and the imaging diagnosis of alcohol-related central nervous system disorders.

The authors do an excellent job in updating the important neuroimaging findings that are helpful in diagnosing alcohol-related encephalopathies. Among these, perhaps the most important are the immediately treatable diseases such as Wernicke encephalopathy (WE). WE is caused by thiamine (vitamin B_1) deficiency. Imaging may provide the first clues to the presence of WE. Rapid intravenous thiamine replacement is imperative to avoid the most serious sequelae of WE (Korsakoff psychosis).

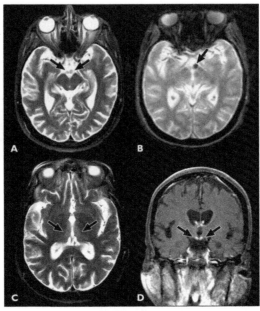

FIGURE 1.—61-year-old alcoholic man with Wernicke encephalopathy during acute phase of disease. **A,** Axial T2-weighted image shows asymmetric edema of mamillary bodies (*arrows*). **B,** Multiplanar gradient-recalled image shows blooming consistent with hemorrhage (*arrow*) in left mamillary body. **C,** Symmetric involvement of medial thalami (*arrows*) is seen on T2-weighted image. **D,** Contrast enhancement of mamillary bodies (*arrows*) is seen on T1-weighted image. (Reprinted from Zuccoli G, Siddiqui N, Cravo I, et al. Neuroimaging findings in alcohol-related encephalopathies. *AJR Am J Roentgenol.* 2010;195:1378-1384, with permission from the American Journal of Roentgenology.)

One thing the authors didn't emphasize that is worth mentioning is that almost half the cases of WE are nonalcohol related. Children (yes, children) can develop WE if thiamine replacement in parenteral nutrition isn't adequate.

Bottom line: if it looks like WE (Fig 1), it probably is. Don't be dissuaded by a lack of history of alcoholism or young patient age.

A. G. Osborn, MD

Brain: Miscellaneous

Imaging and clinical characteristics of children with multiple foci of microsusceptibility changes in the brain on susceptibility-weighted MRI

Niwa T, Aida N, Takahara T, et al (Kanagawa Children's Med Ctr, Yokohama, Japan; Univ Med Ctr Utrecht, The Netherlands; et al)
Pediatr Radiol 40:1657-1662, 2010

Background.—Microsusceptibility changes in the brain are well known to correspond with microbleeds or micrometal fragments in adults, but this phenomenon has not been explored well in children.

Objective.—To assess imaging and clinical characteristics of children with multiple foci of microsusceptibility changes using susceptibility-weighted imaging (SWI).

Materials and Methods.—Between 2006 and 2008, 12 children with multiple foci of microsusceptibility on SWI without corresponding abnormal signal on conventional MRI were identified and were retrospectively assessed.

Results.—The locations of foci of microsusceptibility included the cerebral white matter, basal ganglia, brainstem and cerebellar white matter, without any clear systematic anatomic distribution. CT ($n = 5$) showed no calcification at the locations corresponding to the microsusceptibility on SWI. Conventional MR imaging showed white matter volume loss ($n = 5$), delayed myelination ($n = 2$), acute infarction ($n = 1$), chronic infarction ($n = 1$), meningitis ($n = 1$), slight signal abnormality in the white matter ($n = 1$) and no abnormal findings ($n = 1$). Follow-up SWI ($n = 3$) showed no change of the microsusceptibility foci. Interestingly, all children had a history of heart surgery under extracorporeal circulation for congenital heart disease.

Conclusion.—Multiple foci of microsusceptibility can be seen in the brain on SWI in children with congenital heart disease who underwent heart surgery with extracorporeal circulation (Fig 1).

▶ I totally LOVE it when I learn something completely new from an article, as I did from this one. Niwa and colleagues report 12 cases of children who had multiple foci of microsusceptibility (black dots) on susceptibility-weighted imaging (SWI) with normal imaging on other sequences.

While they didn't give total numbers of patients who had MR with SWI, they looked at all cases collected over a 2-year period. They identified all cases in which foci of microsusceptibility were noted only on SWI. Interestingly enough,

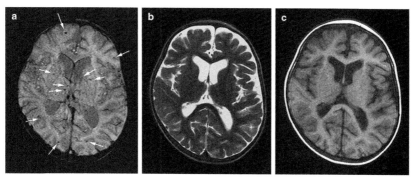

FIGURE 1.—Two-year-old boy with hypoplastic left heart syndrome who underwent Fontan and Norwood surgery with extracorporeal circulation. **a** Axial SWI shows multiple foci of dotted signal loss (*arrows*). **b** T2- and **c** T1-W images show no abnormal signal at the location corresponding to the area of signal loss on SWI. (With kind permission from Springer Science and Business Media: Niwa T, Aida N, Takahara T, et al. Imaging and clinical characteristics of children with multiple foci of microsusceptibility changes in the brain on susceptibility-weighted MRI. *Pediatr Radiol.* 2010;40:1657-1662.)

all 12 cases were in children who had congenital heart disease (CHD) and had extracorporeal circulation during surgery (Fig 1). While the authors carefully noted the exact type of CHD for each patient, they didn't state what (if any) prosthetic devices might have been used. So we don't know whether the black dots were from metallic microfragments or small microbleeds.

Multiple black dots on T2* scans in older adults are fairly common and usually related to chronic hypertension or amyloid angiopathy. Other than diffuse axonal injury and (possibly) Zabramski type 4 multiple cavernous malformations, I'm not aware of many other causes of microsusceptibility lesions in kids. This was a new one—on me!

A. G. Osborn, MD

Hypertension and Cerebral Diffusion Tensor Imaging in Small Vessel Disease

Gons RAR, de Laat KF, van Norden AGW, et al (Radboud Univ Nijmegen Med Ctr, The Netherlands; et al)
Stroke 41:2801-2806, 2010

Background and Purpose.—Hypertension is a risk factor for cerebral small vessel disease, which includes white matter lesions (WML) and lacunar infarcts. These lesions are frequently observed on MRI scans of elderly people and play a role in cognitive decline. Preferably, one would like to evaluate the effect of hypertension before fluid-attenuated inversion recovery visible macrostructural lesions occur, possibly by investigating its effect on the microstructural integrity of the white matter. Diffusion tensor imaging provides measures of structural integrity.

Methods.—In 503 patients with small vessel disease, aged between 50 and 85 years, we cross-sectionally studied the relation between blood pressure, hypertension, and hypertension treatment status and diffusion tensor imaging parameters in both normal-appearing white matter (NAWM) and WMLs. All of the subjects underwent 1.5-T MRI and diffusion tensor imaging scanning. Fractional anisotropy and mean diffusivity were calculated in both NAWM and WMLs.

Results.—Increased blood pressure and hypertension were significantly related to lower fractional anisotropy in both NAWM and WMLs and to higher mean diffusivity in WMLs. For hypertensives, odds ratios for the risk of impaired microstructural integrity (fractional anisotropy) were 3.1 (95% CI: 1.8 to 5.7) and 2.1 (95% CI: 1.2 to 3.5) in NAWM and WMLs, respectively, compared with normotensives. Fractional anisotropy odds ratios for treated uncontrolled subjects were 6.5 (95% CI: 3.3 to 12.7) and 2.7 (95% CI: 1.5 to 5.1) in NAWM and WMLs, respectively, compared with normotensives.

Conclusions.—Our data show that diffusion tensor imaging may be an appropriate tool to monitor the effect of blood pressure and the response to treatment on white matter integrity, probably even before the development of WMLs on fluid-attenuated inversion recovery.

▶ The growing utility of diffusion tensor imaging (DTI) in depicting a broad spectrum of brain lesions is an exciting development. I think we were all enchanted by the gorgeous 3-dimensional color fiber maps generated with 3-T MR. But is DTI more than just a pretty face? Its initial clinical use was the attempt to demonstrate tumor infiltration rather than displacement in glioma imaging. The authors of this nice study show that DTI may show changes in microstructural white matter integrity even before the development of frank lacunar infarcts and T2/FLAIR hyperintensities, which we associate with small vessel vascular disease (more accurately, arteriolosclerosis and lipohyalinosis).

As hypertension remains a worldwide health problem and a significant factor in the development of cognitive impairment, it would be pretty cool to have an imaging method of assessing damaged white matter integrity in the early stages of development. Even better would be a method to monitor the effectiveness of hypertension treatment. DTI may just be the answer. Score another one for this new technique!

A. G. Osborn, MD

Brain: Neoplasms

Correlation of Diffusion and Perfusion MRI With Ki-67 in High-Grade Meningiomas
Ginat DT, Mangla R, Yeaney G, et al (Univ of Rochester Med Ctr, NY)
AJR Am J Roentgenol 195:1391-1395, 2010

Objective.—Atypical and anaplastic meningiomas have a greater likelihood of recurrence than benign meningiomas. The risk for recurrence is often estimated using the Ki-67 labeling index. The purpose of this study was to determine the correlation between Ki-67 and regional cerebral blood volume (rCBV) and between Ki-67 and apparent diffusion coefficient (ADC) in atypical and anaplastic meningiomas.

Materials and Methods.—A retrospective review of the advanced imaging and immunohistochemical characteristics of atypical and anaplastic meningiomas was performed. The relative minimum ADC, relative maximum rCBV, and specimen Ki-67 index were measured. Pearson's correlation was used to compare these parameters.

Results.—There were 23 cases with available ADC maps and 20 cases with available rCBV maps. The average Ki-67 among the cases with ADC maps and rCBV maps was 17.6% (range, 5−38%) and 16.7% (range, 3−38%), respectively. The mean minimum ADC ratio was 0.91 (SD, 0.26) and the mean maximum rCBV ratio was 22.5 (SD, 7.9). There was a significant positive correlation between maximum rCBV and Ki-67 (Pearson's correlation, 0.69; $p = 0.00038$). However, there was no significant correlation between minimum ADC and Ki-67 (Pearson's correlation, -0.051; $p = 0.70$).

MRI in High-Grade Meningiomas

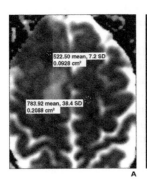
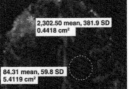
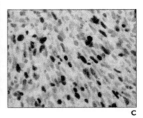

A   B   C

FIGURE 2.—52-year-old man with right frontal anaplastic meningioma. **A,** Apparent diffusion coefficient (ADC) map shows relatively low diffusivity in right frontal anaplastic meningioma with minimum relative ADC of 0.67. Regions of interest (*circles*) are included over tumor and contralateral white matter. **B,** Regional cerebral blood volume (rCBV) map shows a highly hypervascular anaplastic tumor with maximum relative rCBV of 27.3. Regions of interest (*circles*) are included over tumor and contralateral white matter. **C,** Ki-67 labeling index was estimated to be 38% on corresponding immunohistochemical stain. (×20). (Reprinted from Ginat DT, Mangla R, Yeaney G, et al. Correlation of diffusion and perfusion MRI with Ki-67 in high-grade meningiomas. *AJR Am J Roentgenol.* 2010;195:1391-1395, with permission from the American Journal of Roentgenology.)

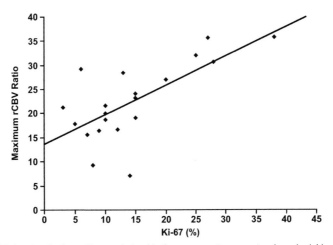

FIGURE 4.—Graph shows linear relationship between maximum regional cerebral blood volume (rCBV) ratios and Ki-67. There is significant positive correlation between these parameters for both atypical and anaplastic meningiomas. (Reprinted from Ginat DT, Mangla R, Yeaney G, et al. Correlation of diffusion and perfusion MRI with Ki-67 in high-grade meningiomas. *AJR Am J Roentgenol.* 2010;195:1391-1395, with permission from the American Journal of Roentgenology.)

Conclusion.—Maximum rCBV correlated significantly with Ki-67 in high-grade meningiomas (Figs 2 and 4).

▶ So speaking of meningiomas, there are 3 World Health Organization grades of them: I, II, and III. More than 90% are grade I, which is the benign garden variety meningioma with which we are all familiar...not least because they are common incidental findings on imaging studies (and what to do with these so-called incidental meningiomas is another story).

I've seen malignant meningiomas that looked totally innocent. And I've seen what I thought was a perfectly typical benign meningioma that turned out to be anaplastic or malignant. I write, and believe, that we radiologists can't tell the grade of a meningioma on standard imaging sequences. The pathologists are the ones who make the call based on both microscopic features and immuno-histochemistry proliferation indices. As the authors point out, proliferation indices (Ki-67, MIB-1) are very good predictors of recurrence and survival.

Can we do better? The authors say yes and make a convincing case. Anaplastic meningiomas are highly hypervascular tumors with elevated maximum regional cerebral blood volume (rCBV) (Fig 2). There is a pretty nice correlation between rCBV and Ki-67 (Fig 4). Some of their data points were widely scattered, so this won't always hold true. But it adds one more potential arrow to our diagnostic quiver.

A. G. Osborn, MD

Distinction between postoperative recurrent glioma and radiation injury using MR diffusion tensor imaging
Xu J-L, Li Y-L, Lian J-M, et al (Henan Provincial People's Hosp, Zhengzhou, China; et al)
Neuroradiology 52:1193-1199, 2010

Introduction.—This study aims to evaluate the differentiated effectiveness of MR diffusion tensor imaging (DTI) to postoperative recurrent glioma and radiation injury.

Methods.—Conventional MRI and DTI examination were performed using Siemens 3.0 T MR System for patients with new contrast-enhancing lesions at the site of treated tumor with postoperative radiotherapy. The region of interest was manually drawn on ADC and FA maps at contrast-enhancing lesion area, peri-lesion edema, and the contra-lateral normal white matter. Then ADC and FA values were measured and, the ADC ratio and FA ratio were calculated. Twenty patients with recurrent tumor and 15 with radiation injury were confirmed by histopathologic examination (23 patients) and clinical imaging follow-up (12 patients), respectively. The mean ADC ratio and FA ratio were compared between the two lesion types.

Results.—The mean ADC ratio at contrast-enhancing lesion area was significantly lower in patients with recurrent tumor (1.34 ± 0.15) compared to that with radiation injury (1.62 ± 0.17; $P<0.01$). The mean FA ratio at contrast-enhancing lesion area was significantly higher in patients with recurrent tumor (0.45 ± 0.03) compared to that with radiation injury (0.32 ± 0.03; $P<0.01$). Neither mean ADC ratio nor FA ratio in edema areas had statistical difference between the two groups. A recurrent tumor was suggested when either ADC ratio <1.65 or/and FA ratio >0.36 at contrast-enhancing lesion area according to the receiver operating characteristics curve analysis. Three patients with recurrent tumor and two with radiation injury were misclassified.

Conclusion.—DTI is a valuable method to distinguish postoperative recurrent glioma and radiation injury (Figs 1 and 2).

▶ One of the dilemmas that both neuro-oncologists and neuroradiologists face in the posttreatment follow-up of malignant gliomas is telling the difference between tumor recurrence and radiation injury. Delayed radiation-induced brain injury is the most common complication of radiation therapy and needs to be differentiated from tumor recurrence, as patient management for each is quite different.

Some modalities such as perfusion MRI (pMRI) and positron emission tomography (PET) or PET-CT have been used to help distinguish these 2 entities that may look quite similar on standard MR sequences. Radiation necrosis is generally cold, and tumor recurrence is generally hot. We use both pMRI and PET to assess for radiation-induced pseudoprogression. But both require additional imaging and may not be available in many institutions.

The authors show that diffusion tensor imaging, which many if not most MR scanners now have available, can be helpful. Apparent diffusion coefficient is

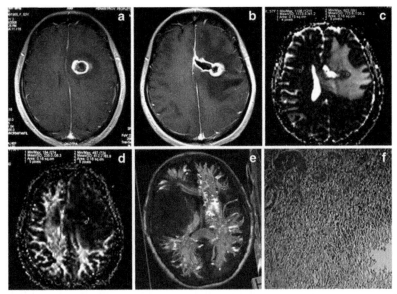

FIGURE 1.—Recurrent pleomorphic glioblastoma in the left frontal lobe after postoperative radiotherapy. a The preoperative contrast-enhanced MRI; b a new contrast-enhancing lesion on the contrast-enhanced MRI image when 7 months after postoperative radiotherapy; c the low ADC value in the contrast-enhancing lesion on ADC map, the ADC ratio of 1.55; d the damaged white matter with low FA value on FA map, the FA ratio of 0.38; e 3D white matter tractography demonstrated the damaged corticospinal tracts and corpus callosum; f the pathological section from brain biopsy (HE staining; magnification ×120) showed many intensive pleomorphic astrocytoma cells in the lesion. (With kind permission from Springer Science and Business Media: Xu J-L, Li Y-L, Lian J-M, et al. Distinction between postoperative recurrent glioma and radiation injury using MR diffusion tensor imaging. *Neuroradiology.* 2010;52:1193-1199.)

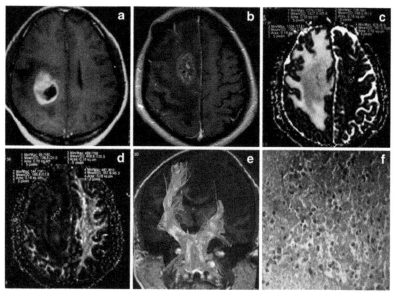

FIGURE 2.—Right parietal lobe radiation injury after postoperative radiotherapy for an anaplastic astrocytoma. (a) The preoperative contrast-enhanced MRI. (b) A new contrast-enhancing lesion on the contrast-enhanced MRI image when 14 months after postoperative radiotherapy. (c) The slightly high ADC value in the contrast-enhancing lesion on ADC map, the ADC ratio of 1.8. (d) The damaged white matter with low FA value on FA map, the FA ratio of 0.29. (e) The 3D white matter tractography map demonstrated the damaged corticospinal tracts (f) The pathological section from the brain biopsy (HE staining, magnification: ×160) showed gliosis and necrosis in the lesion. (With kind permission from Springer Science and Business Media: Xu J-L, Li Y-L, Lian J-M, et al. Distinction between postoperative recurrent glioma and radiation injury using MR diffusion tensor imaging. *Neuroradiology.* 2010;52:1193-1199.)

generally lower and fractional anisotropy (FA) is higher in patients with a new contrast-enhancing focus caused by tumor recurrence (Fig 1), while damaged (necrotic) white matter has low FA value (Fig 2). Their series was small, but if this holds up in larger studies, it's a really valuable addition to tumor follow-up imaging.

A. G. Osborn, MD

Fiber Density Mapping of Gliomas: Histopathologic Evaluation of a Diffusion-Tensor Imaging Data Processing Method

Stadlbauer A, Buchfelder M, Salomonowitz E, et al (Univ of Erlangen-Nuremberg, Schwabachanlage, Germany)
Radiology 257:846-853, 2010

Purpose.—To evaluate fiber density mapping (FDM) in the quantification of the extent of destruction of white matter (WM) structures in the center, transition zone, and border zone of intracranial gliomas.

Materials and Methods.—This retrospective study was approved by the institutional review board. Diffusion-tensor imaging (DTI) and magnetic resonance (MR) imaging—guided biopsies were performed in 20 patients with glioma. FDM is a three-step approach that includes diagonalization of the diffusion tensor, fiber reconstruction for the whole brain, and calculation of fiber density values. Coregistration of FDM data with MR imaging data used for stereotactic biopsy guidance enabled us to correlate these results with histopathologic findings. Data were analyzed by using regression analyses and Hoetelling-Williams and Wilcoxon signed rank tests.

Results.—Histopathologic correlation revealed strong negative correlations with both the logarithm of tumor cell number (CN) ($R = -0.825$) and the percentage of tumor infiltration (TI) ($R = -0.909$). Complete destruction of WM structures was found when the percentage of TI was 60% or greater and when the tumor CN was 150 or greater. We estimated a fiber density value of 18 as a limit in the identification of fiber structures that are infiltrated with tumor yet are still potentially functional.

Conclusion.—FDM provides histologic insight into the structure of WM; therefore, it may help prevent posttreatment neurologic deficits when planning therapy of brain tumors.

▶ We've known for some years that there are viable tumor cells in the nonenhancing edema that surrounds diffusely infiltrating astrocytomas. We've also recognized that tumor cells can be found in brain parenchyma far beyond any detectable hyperintensity seen on fluid-attenuated inversion recovery or T2-weighted MR images. Microscopic tumor infiltration in white matter tracts may not be visible on standard MR sequences, but, as the authors beautifully demonstrate, using diffusion tensor imaging and fiber tract mapping is very helpful in assessing the border zone around gliomas. Further, they demonstrate that fiber density mapping provides a quantitative assessment that is superior to standard fiber tracking and fractional anisotropy maps (Fig 2 in the original article).

Does it really matter? Does it affect patient management and (even more important) outcome? It interested me that the authors excluded the most malignant astrocytoma (glioblastoma multiforme [GBM], a World Health Organization [WHO] grade IV tumor) from their study, looking only at low-grade (WHO grade II) and anaplastic (WHO grade III) astrocytomas. That may be because the prognosis of GBM is so dismal that it wouldn't have made any difference regardless of imaging findings. I teach our residents and fellows that a GBM should essentially be considered a holobrain lesion with malignant tumor cells extending *way* beyond what we can detect with even our most sensitive imaging studies. So far, there isn't much that significantly improves survival (let alone quality of life) in these unfortunate patients.

A. G. Osborn, MD

Diffusion Tensor MR Imaging of Cerebral Gliomas: Evaluating Fractional Anisotropy Characteristics

White ML, Zhang Y, Yu F, et al (Univ of Nebraska Med Ctr, Omaha)
AJNR Am J Neuroradiol 32:374-381, 2011

Background and Purpose.—FA correlation to glioma tumor grade has been mixed if not disappointing. There are several potential underlying fundamental issues that have contributed to these results. In an attempt to overcome these past shortfalls, we evaluated characteristics of FA of the solid tissue components of gliomas, including whether high-grade gliomas have a greater variation of FA than low-grade gliomas.

Materials and Methods.—Thirty-four patients with gliomas (9 grade II, 8 grade III, and 17 grade IV) underwent diffusion tensor imaging at 3T. Mean FA, maximum FA, and minimum FA values were measured within the solid tissue components of the tumors. The variations of FA were evaluated by determining the range of FA values and the maximum SDs of FA. The variations of FA values among different tumor grades were compared statistically. We also correlated FA variations with minimum FA and maximum FA.

Results.—The maximum FA, FA range, and maximum SD for grade II tumors were significantly lower than those for grade III and IV tumors ($P < .0001 \sim P = .0164$). A very good correlation of maximum FA to FA range ($r = 0.931$) and maximum SD ($r = 0.889$) was observed.

Conclusions.—The FA range and maximum SD appear useful for differentiating low- and high-grade gliomas. This analysis added value to the findings on conventional MR imaging. In addition, focal maximum FA is a key factor contributing to the larger FA variation within high-grade gliomas.

▶ As a neuroradiologist, my toughest problem in brain tumor imaging isn't identifying glioblastoma multiforme (GBM), a World Health Organization (WHO) grade IV tumor. The histologic hallmarks of GBM are necrosis and neo-vascularity. Over 95% of GBMs demonstrate detectable necrosis and contrast enhancement on MR. Hemorrhage is also very common, and even relatively small foci can be detected with T2* (GRE or—even better—SWI).

The real challenge is differentiating an anaplastic astrocytoma (WHO grade III) from a low-grade diffusely infiltrating astrocytoma (WHO grade II). I don't really worry much about oligodendroglioma, as the key factor affecting treatment is whether the tumor shows 1p19q deletion (favorable prognosis).

An elevated rCBV in an otherwise relatively low-grade—appearing glioma may herald malignant degeneration and should therefore be the biopsy target.

The authors of this interesting article demonstrate that diffusion tensor imaging (DTI) with fractional anisotropy (FA) maps can differentiate low-(WHO II) from high (WHO IV)-grade gliomas. They remarked that 5 of the 8 grade III gliomas were diagnosed preoperatively as grade II gliomas because of benign imaging features (supposedly, no enhancement, edema, or necrosis, although the imaging example of a grade II tumor they illustrated showed strong uniform enhancement in a tumor that looks like a hypothalamic pilocytic astrocytoma in a child). It was only the maximum (not the mean or minimal) FA of grade III and IV gliomas (Fig 2 in the original article) that seemed to distinguish them from grade II (low grade) tumors (Fig 3 in the original article).

Is this a useful application of DTI? Their study had relatively small numbers (especially of the low-grade gliomas, which are much less common), so it's hard to tell. Stay tuned.

A. G. Osborn, MD

Brain: Stroke and Intracranial Hemorrhage

Diffusion weighted imaging and estimation of prognosis using apparent diffusion coefficient measurements in ischemic stroke
Gonen KA, Simsek MM (State Hosp, Tekirdag, Turkey; Haydarpasa Numune Training and Res Hosp, Uskudar, Istanbul, Turkey)
Eur J Radiol 76:157-161, 2010

Objective.—Estimation of the prognosis of infarction by using diffusion weighted imaging (DWI) and quantitative apparent diffusion coefficient (ADC) measurements.

Methods.—23 patients having acute stroke symptoms with verified infarction in magnetic resonance imaging (MRI) were included in this study. Their MRI studies were performed between 6 and 12 h after the onset of their symptoms and were repeated on the fifth day. The infarction volumes were calculated by using DWI and the patients were divided into two groups as the ones having an expansion in the infarction area (group 1, $n = 16$) and the others having no expansion in the infarction area (group 2, $n = 7$). Quantitative ADC values were estimated. The groups were compared in terms of the ADC values on ADC maps obtained from DWI, performed during the between 6 and 12 h from the onset of the symptoms, referring to the core of the infarction (ADC_{IC}), ischemic penumbra (ADC_P) and the nonischemic parenchymal tissue (ADC_N). P values < 0.05 were accepted to be statistically significant.

Results.—During the between 6 and 12 h mean infarction volume calculated by DWI was 23.3 cm^3 for group 1 patients (ranging from 1.1 to 68.6) and this was found to be 40.3 cm^3 (ranging from 1.8 to 91.5) on the fifth day. For the group 2 patients these values were found to be 42.1 cm^3 (ranging from 1 to 94.7) and 41.9 (ranging from 1 to 94.7) for the same intervals respectively. A significant statistical result was failed to be demonstrated between the mean ADC_{IC} and ADC_N values ($p = 0.350$ and $p = 0.229$ respectively). However the comparison of the ADC_P values between the groups was found to be highly significant ($p < 0.001$). When the differences between the ADC_P and ADC_{IC} and ADC_N and ADC_P were compared the results proved to be statistically significant ($p = 0.038$ and $p < 0.001$ respectively).

Conclusions.—We believe that ADC results that would be obtained from the core and the penumbra of the infarction area will be beneficial in the estimation of the infarction prognosis and in the planning of a treatment protocol (Figs 1 and 2).

▶ The Holy Grail of stroke imaging is an accessible, reproducible, quick, accurate (anything else?) way to determine the densely ischemic core of an infarct (dead, doomed brain) from the theoretically salvageable brain in the ischemic penumbra surrounding the core. According to the well-known stroke researcher Gilberto Gonzalez, we should go from saying, "Time is Brain" to "Time is Penumbra."

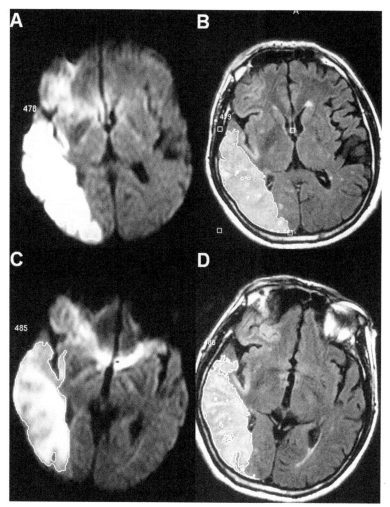

FIGURE 1.—Area calculations in the DWI and FLAIR images of a patient in whom infarction did not show an expansion. Area measurements in the DWI (A) and FLAIR (B) between 6 and 12 h; area calculations in the DWI (C) and FLAIR images (D) on the fifth day. (Reprinted from Gonen KA, Simsek MM. Diffusion weighted imaging and estimation of prognosis using apparent diffusion coefficient measurements in ischemic stroke. *Eur J Radiol.* 2010;76:157-161, with permission from Elsevier.)

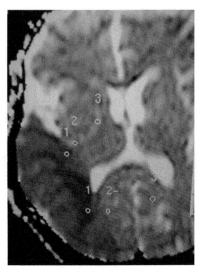

FIGURE 2.—ADC measurement points in ADC maps. 1: infarction core (IC), 2: penumbra (P), 3: non-ischemic brain parenchyma (N). (Reprinted from Gonen KA, Simsek MM. Diffusion weighted imaging and estimation of prognosis using apparent diffusion coefficient measurements in ischemic stroke. *Eur J Radiol.* 2010;76:157-161, with permission from Elsevier.)

If penumbra is the thing, it's a big thing. Viability of ischemic brain seems to vary from patient to patient, and the treatment window in some cases may stretch beyond the golden 6-hour limit. Infarction prognosis is very important in determining patient triage for possible thrombolysis.

Perfusion MR (pMR) has been touted as the most accurate portrayal of core versus penumbra. The difficulty is that pMR is time consuming and not as widely available as standard MR with diffusion-weighted imaging (Fig 1). The authors, in great technical detail, show that taking apparent diffusion coefficient measurements from different points in the affected brain (Fig 2) is strongly correlated with core infarct and ischemic penumbra.

A. G. Osborn, MD

Diffusion Weighted Imaging: What Are We Really Seeing?

Zenonos G, Friedlander RM (Congress of Neurological Surgeons)
Neurosurgery 67:N26-N29, 2010

Background.—The diagnostic investigation and workup of individuals suspected to have ischemic stroke have benefited from the use of diffusion-weighted magnetic resonance imaging (DWI). The apparent diffusion coefficient (ADC) is believed to reflect the diffusibility of protons attached to water molecules in brain tissues. The ADC values fall within minutes of an ischemic insult, producing high intensity signal on DWI. It has been believed that decreased blood flow rapidly produces dysfunction of the sodium-potassium ion pump, and cytotoxic edema occurs because of fluid shifts from the extracellular to the intracellular space. Diminished water diffusibility and ADC values result from the more complex intracellular environment and the restricted and more tortuous extracellular space after edematous cell expansion. Various less plausible explanations have also been offered to describe the effect, but none have been substantiated scientifically. A new hypothesis suggests that reduced expression of aquaporin-4 (AQP4) in the astrocytic processes may contribute to diminished ADC values. Aquaporins are transmembrane proteins that function as water channels, facilitating bidirectional selective water transport in and out of cells. More than 10 families of aquaporins are known, but AQP4 is the most abundant one in brain parenchyma and is preferentially expressed in astrocytic cell membranes that contact blood vessels. Reduced expression of AQP4 in rat models of ischemia-hypoxia have correlated with reduced ADC values. It was hypothesized that diminished astrocytic AQP4 expression associated with hypoxia-ischemia causes a fall in transcellular, extracellular, and intracellular water diffusibility and lowers ADC values. This was tested using selective inhibition of AQP4 expression by targeting it with small interfering RNAs (siRNAs) in normal brains in vivo. The effects on ADC values were noted.

Methods and Results.—An in vitro experiment was conducted to confirm that AQP4 expression was effectively inhibited in cultured astrocytes after AQP4-siRNA (siAQP4) treatment. Such inhibition did not affect the cells' morphological integrity or produce signs of toxicity. In vivo, an intracerebral infusion of the same siAQP4 showed that siRNAs diffused widely from the injection site, reaching the entire brain. Treatment with siAQP4 for 3 days significantly reduced AQP4 expression compared to controls, who were treated with scrambled siRNA (siGLO). The reduction was most apparent in astrocyte endfeet in contact with blood vessels, in the neuropil, and in the glia limitans. Again, no changes in normal tissue histology, no disruption in the blood brain barrier (BBB), no neuronal cell death, and no significantly altered astrocyte morphology resulted. Acute AQP4 silencing with siAPQ4 confirmed the hypothesis and showed a decline in ADC values by an order of 50% compared to controls. The lower ADC values corresponded histologically with the initial siAPQ4 diffusion and AQP4 reduction.

Analysis.—There is now evidence that AQP4 may modulate ADC values in the normal brain while producing no disruption of brain histology. At least part of the decrease in ADC values seen in stroke patients is caused by reduced water diffusibility as a result of lower levels of astrocytic AQP4 rather than by cytotoxic edema. Additionally, these experiments showed that the needle used to introduce the siRNAs into the brain naturally induced a mild mechanical lesion that disrupted the BBB and caused reactive gliosis. AQP4 silencing prevented the reactive gliosis and BBB disruption, suggesting that AQP4 inhibition may be protective after mechanical trauma. The absence of AQP4 was protective against edema-related cell death. Thus siAQP4 and AQP4 silencing may offer

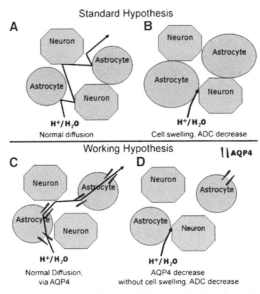

FIGURE 1.—Hypothesis for apparent diffusion coefficient (ADC) value changes in brain tissue. Schema depicting the standard (A, B) and the Loma Linda University group's working hypothesis (C, D) to explain decreased brain ADC values following decreased AQP4 expression. Classically, decreased ADC is associated with decreased extracellular space due to cellular swelling (B). The water channel, AQP4, is expressed in astrocyte membranes and can facilitate water movement (C). When APQ4 is decreased, they hypothesize that lower ADC values are caused by decreased water permeability in and out of the cells caused by the absence of these water channels (D). (Adapted from Badaut J, Ashwal S, Adami A, et al. *Brain water mobility decreases after astrocytic aquaporin-4 inhibition using RNA interference.* J Cereb Blood Flow Metab. September 29, 2010.) (Reprinted from Zenonos G, Friedlander RM. Diffusion weighted imaging: what are we really seeing? *Neurosurgery.* 2010;67:N26-N29.)

a therapeutic effect in preventing edema after acute brain injury. This will be especially helpful if improved methods of drug delivery are developed, such as an intranasal route (Fig 1).

▶ I don't often (if ever) review a letter or commentary on an article. But in this case, I made an exception to my general rule. The reason? Many of this year's selections focus on the use of diffusion-weighted and diffusion tensor MRI. So a report in the Science Times section of *Neurosurgery* (one of my favorite journals) caught my eye. The title—"Diffusion weighted imaging: what are we really seeing?"—was fascinating.

The authors, George Zenonos and Robert M. Friedlander, discuss an article on aquaporins by Badaut et al that was recently published in the *Journal of Cerebral Blood Flow & Metabolism*, September 29, 2010. I have to say I would have missed the article and its importance, had the authors of the commentary not pointed it out.

Their conclusion is that it is reduced expression of aquaporin-4 in astrocytic processes that may cause the reduction of water diffusibility, not cytotoxic edema (Fig 1). Who knew? Try that idea on the next time your stroke neurologists drop by your reading room ...

A. G. Osborn, MD

Imaging the Future of Stroke: II. Hemorrhage

Liebeskind DS (Univ of California, Los Angeles)
Ann Neurol 68:581-592, 2010

Bleeding into the brain or adjacent structures is one of the most devastating neurological conditions, incurring tremendous emotional, financial, and societal costs. Imaging is essential to differentiate variants of hemorrhage, as the clinical features may be insufficient. A comprehensive approach to hemorrhage therefore relies on imaging to disclose pathophysiology, elucidate mechanisms, and thereby open further avenues to effective treatment. Hemorrhage patterns from superficial to deep locations in the brain are surveyed in this work, noting myriad potential causes and the influential pathophysiology of arterial ischemia, venous hypertension, and microvascular dysfunction. Recent progress of imaging studies and novel techniques to evaluate hemorrhage are explored. For decades, only computed tomography was available to define a hematoma without corroborating evidence of other pathology whereas multimodal computed tomography and magnetic resonance imaging, including noninvasive imaging of brain tissue, vessels, and perfusion, have now radically altered clinical practice. Imaging of the blood-brain barrier, cerebral microbleeds, coexistent ischemia, associated vascular lesions, and markers of hemorrhage expansion is possible with routine protocols akin to diagnostic strategies for ischemic stroke. Imaging applications for hemorrhagic transformation, venous thrombosis, and microvascular disorders are considered with a perspective that balances concern for hemorrhage with prevention of ischemia as these processes are often intertwined and clinical conundrums arise. Imminent imaging advances are anticipated with increased use of detailed imaging for hemorrhage and overlap with cerebral ischemia. Numerous questions abound regarding optimal management of hemorrhage and definitive treatments are lacking, yet imaging of pivotal pathophysiology offers tremendous opportunity for future progress in combating this debilitating condition (Fig 11).

▶ Brain hemorrhages are among the most devastating neurologic conditions. Even in 2011, hypertensive (HTN) intracranial hemorrhage is the second most common cause of stroke. My grandfather died 50 years ago from what I now know was almost certainly an HTN basal ganglionic hemorrhage (he had high blood pressure and wasn't very consistent about taking his medications). More than a half-century later, people still die from HTN brain bleeds. Survivors often have serious neurologic sequelae. And patients with chronic HTN don't have to have big brain bleeds to become impaired; we now know HTN is probably the single most common cause of silent brain microbleeds that are often associated with general cognitive decline.

Probably the most important contribution this article makes is the reminder that ALL brain bleeds, including epi- and subdural hematomas, may be nontraumatic and spontaneous (or medication related). The emphasis on the

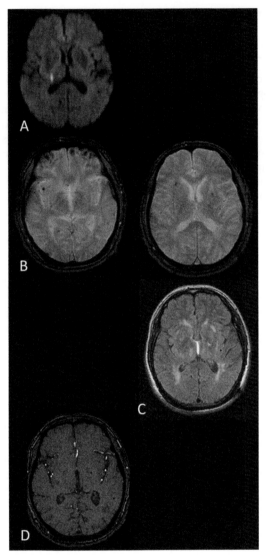

FIGURE 11.—Signal characteristics of CMBs across other MRI sequences may indicate pathogenic potential and hemorrhage risk. (A) Lacunar infarction is noted on DWI with contralateral CMBs. (B) GRE reveals scattered CMBs in various locations. (C) FLAIR shows only a subpopulation of the CMBs; and (D) MRA source images reveal others due to the relative T1-weighted properties of this acquisition. (Reprinted from Liebeskind DS. Imaging the future of stroke: II. Hemorrhage. *Ann Neurol.* 2010;68:581-592. Copyright 2010 and the American Neurological Association. Reprinted with permission of John Wiley & Sons, Inc.)

much underrecognized venous side of the circulation and the relatively common pattern of microbleeds is also well put (Fig 11). One minor disappointment is the lack of any discussion of the newest T2* technique for detecting brain microbleeds, susceptibility-weighted imaging (SWI). SWI can be positive when gradient recalled echo is negative.

A. G. Osborn, MD

Posterior versus anterior circulation strokes: comparison of clinical, radiological and outcome characteristics
De Marchis GM, Kohler A, Renz N, et al (Univ of Bern, Switzerland)
J Neurol Neurosurg Psychiatry 82:33-37, 2011

Background and Purpose.—Physicians treating patients with posterior circulation strokes (PCS) tended to debate more on whether or not to introduce anticoagulation rather than performing investigations to identify stroke aetiology, as in patients with anterior circulation strokes (ACS). Recent findings suggest that stroke aetiologies of PCS and ACS are more alike than dissimilar, suggesting that PCS deserve the same investigations as ACS. The characteristics and current diagnostic evaluation between patients with PCS and ACS were compared.

Methods.—312 consecutive patients with first ever ACS and 93 patients with first ever PCS were prospectively analysed.

Results.—Patients with ACS and PCS did not differ in terms of demographic characteristics, prevalence of vascular risk factors, diagnostic evaluation or stroke aetiology. The median National Institutes of Health Stroke Scale score was 8 in ACS and 4 in PCS (p=0.004). Brain imaging revealed more often pathological findings in ACS than PCS. The proportion of non-thrombolysed patients with a favourable clinical outcome (modified Rankin score 0—2) was similar in ACS and PCS (67.0% vs 78.4%; p=0.08). In non-thrombolysed patients, stroke severity was an independent predictor of clinical outcome both in ACS (OR 1.60, 95% CI 1.2 to 2.1; p<0.0001) and in PCS (OR 1.22, 95% CI 1.03 to 1.44; p=0.02) while age predicted poor outcome only in ACS (OR 1.11, 95% CI 1.01 to 1.22; p=0.007). In thrombolysed patients, stroke severity was the only outcome predictor in ACS (OR 1.14, 95% CI 1.04 to 1.25; p=0.004) while we identified no statistically relevant predictor of PCS outcome.

Conclusions.—In PCS and ACS, baseline variables, aetiology and outcome are more alike than different.

▶ Despite a lot of evidence in the literature to the contrary, some physicians still believe that posterior circulation (vertebrobasilar) strokes (PCSs) should be managed differently from anterior circulation stroke (ACS) events. The old outdated concept is that PCSs are mostly hemodynamic in origin, whereas ACSs are mostly embolic. The practical result of this is that patients with PCSs often were empirically anticoagulated without further investigation for possible cardiac sources of emboli.

This study demonstrated that the prevalence of a demonstrable cardioembolic source was equal in patients with PCS (35%) and ACS (31%). The outcome of patients with PCS and ACS was also similar. So that's that.

But, and this is a big but, as the authors point out, unlike carotid stenoses, to date we still don't know the optimal management of patients with vertebral and basilar artery stenoses. There is no equivalent of the American and European trials that demonstrated the efficacy of endarterectomy. That's been a hugely useful study in managing patients with carotid stenosis. But what do we do with patients who have demonstrable posterior circulation stenosis on digital subtraction angiography? That's a study that remains to be done.

In the meantime, this study shows that patients with PCS should undergo the same cardiac investigations (transthoracic echocardiography, transesophageal echocardiography, and 24-hour electrocardiogram) that patients with ACS routinely undergo.

A. G. Osborn, MD

Stunned brain syndrome: serial diffusion perfusion MRI of delayed recovery following revascularisation for acute ischaemic stroke
Bang OY, for the UCLA-Samsung Stroke Collaborators (Sungkyunkwan Univ, Seoul, South Korea; et al)
J Neurol Neurosurg Psychiatry 82:27-32, 2011

Background.—Clinical response immediately after revascularisation therapy differs among patients. Although reperfusion is the deciding factor with respect to this dramatic response to revascularisation therapy, the influence of pre- and post-treatment diffusion—perfusion status on the speed and degree of recovery are unknown.

Methods.—Consecutive stroke patients who were eligible for revascularisation therapy underwent serial diffusion—perfusion MRI. Tmax perfusion maps were generated, and stroke severity and recovery were assessed up to day 90. The relationship of diffusion and perfusion lesion indices with the speed and degree of recovery were evaluated.

Results.—69 patients (42 men; aged 66.3 ± 15.9 years) were included; National Institutes of Health Stroke Scale (NIHSS) score was 13.3 ± 6.4 points. 19 received intravenous tissue plasminogen activator (tPA) and 50 received endovascular therapy with/without intravenous tPA. Early dramatic improvement (NIHSS score reduction of $\geq 40\%$ within 24 h) was observed in 24 (34.8%) patients. Among the other 45 patients, 18 (40%) showed good outcomes (modified Rankin score 0–2 at day 90), suggesting delayed recovery. The volume of post-treatment perfusion delay was similar between the early and delayed recovery groups (p=0.329) but smaller than in the non-responders group (p<0.05). Multivariate testing revealed that smaller post-treatment perfusion delay volumes were independently associated with both early dramatic improvement and delayed recovery. In addition, initial diffusion weighted imaging lesion volume was smaller in the former than in the latter (p=0.029) and was independently associated with early dramatic recovery.

Conclusions.—A significant proportion of patients with a lack of early dramatic improvement (40%) showed delayed recovery. Both pretreatment

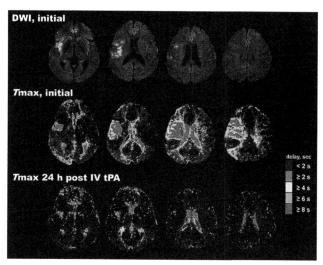

FIGURE 1.—Serial MRI findings of a 60-year-old right-handed woman with left hemiparesis and neglect. On arrival at the hospital, her National Institutes of Health Stroke Scale (NIHSS) score was 13 (consciousness 1, gaze 1, face 2, arm 4, leg 1, dysarthria 2 and neglect 2). Pretreatment MRI disclosed multiple acute cortical infarcts on diffusion weighted imaging (DWI) and a more extensive perfusion delay was noted throughout the right middle cerebral artery distribution. After 24 h of treatment with intravenous tissue plasminogen activator (tPA), clinical improvement was noted with a decrease in the NIHSS to 2 points at 24 h (face 1 and dysarthria 1). Perfusion weighted imaging PWI showed a marked improvement in perfusion delay. (Reprinted with permission of the BMJ Publishing Group Ltd from Bang OY, for the UCLA-Samsung Stroke Collaborators. Stunned brain syndrome: serial diffusion perfusion MRI of delayed recovery following revascularisation for acute ischaemic stroke. *J Neurol Neurosurg Psychiatry.* 2011;82:27-32.)

infarct volume and post-treatment reperfusion correlated with the degree and speed of recovery (Fig 1).

▶ If for no other reason, I'd select this article as one I'd want to read just for its title. Stunned brain? Never heard of such a thing. So my curiosity was aroused. Just what is a stunned brain? Turns out, it is patients who have an acute ischemic stroke and undergo revascularization therapy but don't show dramatic improvement. What I hadn't realized until I read this article is that some patients lack early clinical improvement after 24 hours of thrombolysis, yet some still achieve good outcomes at 3 months. Hence the term stunned brain syndrome. That simply means delayed recovery. It may represent between one-third and 40% of patients who don't demonstrate initial improvement.

The authors allowed up to an 8-hour window for revascularization therapy. Speed of recovery wasn't associated with the extent and severity of perfusion delay or ischemic penumbra. However, pretreatment infarct volume and post-treatment reperfusion were associated with improved outcome.

The bottom line seems to be that a stunned brain is not necessarily a dead brain. Delayed improvement occurs in up to 40% of patients (Fig 1). While their series is small, it does suggest that serial diffusion-perfusion MR (not just a single immediate posttreatment study) may identify patients with stunned brain syndrome.

A. G. Osborn, MD

The Hidden Mismatch: An Explanation for Infarct Growth Without Perfusion-Weighted Imaging/Diffusion-Weighted Imaging Mismatch in Patients With Acute Ischemic Stroke
Ma HK, Zavala JA, Churilov L, et al (Univ of Melbourne, Victoria, Australia; et al)
Stroke 42:662-668, 2011

Background and Purpose.—In ischemic stroke, MR perfusion-weighted imaging (PWI) and diffusion-weighted imaging (DWI) mismatch represents tissue at risk for infarction. Infarct growth should only take place in the presence of mismatch, although there have been reports of this occurring. We hypothesized that this observation may be attributable to the presence of undetected "hidden mismatch," which may become obvious when coregistration techniques are used.

Methods.—MR PWI/DWI was performed within 48 hours of stroke onset and a final T2-weighted image at ≈3 months. Volumetric-subtraction mismatch volume was defined as PWI minus DWI volume and infarct growth was defined as T2 minus DWI volume. Coregistration mismatch volume was PWI not overlapped by DWI. Mismatch salvage was the proportion of coregistered mismatch tissue that had not progressed to infarction.

Results.—Thirty-four patients were studied with MR at a median of 4.9 hours (interquartile range, 2.9−21.1 hours). With the volumetric-subtraction technique, 5 patients (14.7%; 95% CI, 0.05%−0.31%) had infarct growth exceeding mismatch volume, 11 patients (32.0%) had no mismatch and, among these, 3 (27.3%) had infarct growth (median volume, 2.2 mL; interquartile range, 1.0−6.5 mL). All patients had mismatch volume identified by coregistration method that was greater than infarct growth volume. The proportion of this volume salvaged was 77.7% (interquartile range, 63.0%−98.9%).

Conclusions.—The illogical finding of infarct growth volume being greater than the presence of mismatch volume can be explained by the presence of "hidden mismatch," which may be detected by coregistration methods.

▶ The authors deal with the perplexing issue of why some infarcts seem to become larger with time (grow) when there is no mismatch between perfusion-weighted imaging (PWI) and diffusion-weighted imaging (DWI). Theoretically, only if there is an at-risk area, that is, the perfusion area of abnormality is larger than the abnormal area delineated by DWI, would an infarct have the potential to extend with time. Yet we have all seen cases where this happens.

The authors examined why this might happen. The traditional way of determining mismatch volume has been to subtract the DWI from PWI volume (volumetric-subtraction method). The authors used both the traditional methodology and a coregistration technique that incorporated precise topographical details. Approximately 15% of the patients they examined had infarct growth that exceeded mismatch volume. Coregistration virtually eliminated this, indicating that the problem is an artifact of the volumetric-subtraction method (Fig 2 in the original article). Hence their term, hidden mismatch.

A. G. Osborn, MD

Brain: Trauma

Cerebral Microhemorrhages Detected by Susceptibility-Weighted Imaging in Amateur Boxers

Hasiloglu ZI, Albayram S, Selcuk H, et al (Istanbul Univ, Turkey; Bakirkoy Dr. Sadi Konuk Training and Res Hosp, Istanbul, Turkey; et al)
AJNR Am J Neuroradiol 32:99-102, 2011

Background and Purpose.—SWI is a new technique for evaluating diffuse axonal injury associated with punctate hemorrhages. The aim of our study was to determine the prevalence of cerebral microhemorrhages in amateur boxers compared with nonboxers by using SWI and to evaluate the sensitivity of SWI compared with T2 FSE and T2*GE sequences.

Materials and Methods.—We performed cranial MR imaging with a 1.5 T scanner in 21 amateur boxers and 21 control subjects. The study protocol included conventional MR images, T2 FSE, T2*GE, and SWI sequences. The proportions of boxers and controls having CSP, DPVS, cerebral atrophy, cerebellar atrophy, ventricular dilation, PSWMD, and microhemorrhages were computed and were compared by using the χ^2 test of proportions. The relationship between microhemorrhages and boxing-related covariates was assessed by using the Wilcoxon rank sum test. The association between the categories was tested by using the Fisher exact test.

Results.—Using SWI, microhemorrhages were found in 2 (9.52%) of 21 boxers. The microhemorrhages were not visible on T2 FSE or T2*GE images. The proportion of subjects with microhemorrhages did not differ significantly between the boxers and control subjects ($\chi^2 = 0.525$, $df = 1$, $P = .4688$). The prevalence of CSP and DPVS was significantly higher in the boxers than in the control subjects.

Conclusions.—More microhemorrhages were detected in amateur boxers than in controls, but this difference was not statistically significant.

▶ Chronic traumatic encephalopathy (CTE) is much in the news these days. Getting your bell rung during a football, soccer, or rugby match isn't a joking matter. Repeated concussions from sequential head blows are a real cause for concern in contact sports (even in putatively noncontact sports like basketball).

CTE has most typically been discussed in terms of its long-term consequences, ie, brain volume loss, in retired professional athletes who develop
cognitive impairment.

The use of susceptibility-weighted imaging (SWI), a T2* sequence that is
significantly more sensitive than the more commonly used gradient-refocused
scan, is growing. Black dots in the brain often (but not invariably) represent
cerebral microhemorrhages. The most common cause in middle-aged and
older adults is chronic hypertension, followed by amyloid angiopathy.

Trauma is another cause of punctate microbleeds, which can result from
axonal stretch injury or contusion. In this study, microbleeds were more
common in boxers than the control group, but this did not reach statistical
significance.

I feel instinctively that microbleeds are probably part of the CTE syndrome
but can't yet prove it. Bottom line: If you are scanning an athlete in a contact
sport who just got his/her "bell rung," add an SWI sequence to the scan.
You might pick up microhemorrhages that can't be seen any other way. And
you might save a life, or prevent long-lasting disability, if the patient can be
persuaded to give up contact sports.

A. G. Osborn, MD

Head and Neck

An Evidence-Based Approach to Zygomatic Fractures
Evans GRD, Daniels M, Hewell L (Univ of California, Irvine, Orange)
Plast Reconstr Surg 127:891-897, 2011

The Maintenance of Certification module series is designed to help the
clinician structure his or her study in specific areas appropriate to his or
her clinical practice. This article is prepared to accompany practice-
based assessment of preoperative assessment, anesthesia, surgical treatment plan, perioperative management, and outcomes. In this format, the
clinician is invited to compare his or her methods of patient assessment
and treatment, outcomes, and complications, with authoritative,
information-based references.

This information base is then used for self-assessment and bench-
marking in parts II and IV of the Maintenance of Certification process
of the American Board of Plastic Surgery. This article is not intended to
be an exhaustive treatise on the subject. Rather, it is designed to serve as
a reference point for further in-depth study by review of the reference articles presented (Fig 3).

▶ I loved this article for a number of reasons: (1) It's evidence based; (2) it's
a great review on a common topic (facial fractures); and (3) it's a Maintenance
of Certification article. I wish more pithy review articles were based on best
available evidence in the literature.

While much of this article is oriented toward preoperative assessment,
surgical planning, and discussion of postoperative outcomes, it has one of

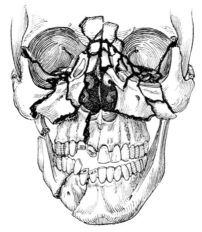

FIGURE 3.—Complex comminuted zygomatic injury. (Reprinted from Evans GRD, Daniels M, Hewell L. An evidence-based approach to zygomatic fractures. *Plast Reconstr Surg.* 2011;127:891-897, with permission from the American Society of Plastic Surgeons.)

the best discussions of complex comminuted zygomatic injury that I've come across. The only radiology image they show is a postoperative 3-dimensional reconstruction but that's a minor point.

If we as radiologists are to be of maximum utility to our clinical colleagues, we need to understand not just how to diagnose pathology but comprehend what the surgeons want and need to know. This article scores high on both points. I highly recommend reading this one. Once you do, you'll not only have a better understanding of complex facial fractures (Fig 3) but also be better positioned to help your referring clinicians.

A. G. Osborn, MD

Diffusion MR Imaging Features of Skull Base Osteomyelitis Compared with Skull Base Malignancy

Ozgen B, Oguz KK, Cila A (Hacettepe Univ, Ankara, Turkey)
AJNR Am J Neuroradiol 32:179-184, 2011

Background and Purpose.—SBO is a life-threatening infection that may have radiologic features similar to those of the neoplastic processes. The purpose of this study was to evaluate the DWI findings in SBO to facilitate the differential diagnosis.

Materials and Methods.—The MR imaging findings of 9 patients with SBO were retrospectively evaluated and compared with MR imaging studies from 9 patients with NPC, 9 with lymphoma, and 9 with metastatic disease of the skull base. ADC measurements were performed from the ADC_{ST} and the ADC_{NST} in all 4 groups.

Results.—The mean ADC_{ST} values were $1.26 \pm 0.19 \times 10^{-3}$ mm^2/s for SBO, $0.74 \pm 0.18 \times 10^{-3}$ mm^2/s for NPC, $0.59 \pm 0.11 \times 10^{-3}$ mm^2/s for lymphoma, and $0.99 \pm 0.34 \times 10^{-3}$ mm^2/s for metastatic disease, respectively. The mean ADC value of SBO was significantly higher than those of NPC and lymphoma ($P < .0001$). There was no significant difference for

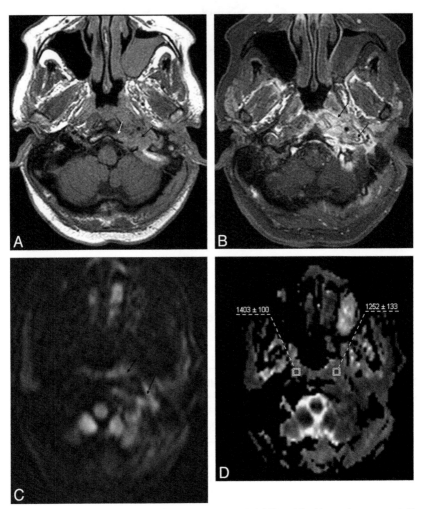

FIGURE 1.—MR images in a case of SBO (patient 8). *A,* Axial T1-weighted image demonstrates infiltration with decreased T1 signal intensity of the left jugular foramen (*black arrow*) extending to the poststyloid parapharyngeal space with loss of the cortical margin of the clivus on the left (*white arrow*). *B,* Axial postcontrast and fat-suppressed T1-weighted image reveals extensive enhancement of the affected region (*arrows*). *C,* Diffusion TRACE image of the same region shows increased signal intensity (*arrows*). *D,* Corresponding ADC map with the regions of interest placed to measure the ADC values from the abnormal soft tissues (on the left) and normal-appearing soft tissues (on the right). (Reprinted from Ozgen B, Oguz KK, Cila A. Diffusion MR imaging features of skull base osteomyelitis compared with skull base malignancy. *AJNR Am J Neuroradiol.* 2011;32:179-184.)

the comparison of SBO and metastatic lesions. When an ADC value equal to or higher than 1.08×10^{-3} mm^2/s was used to rule out lymphoma and NPC, the accuracy was 96%.

Conclusions.—Although SBO is a relatively rare condition, its differential diagnosis from neoplastic processes of the skull base is essential to start appropriate treatment promptly. ADC values may help to distinguish patients with SBO from those with malignant lesions (Fig 1).

▶ Skull base osteomyelitis (SBO) is much less common than skull base malignancy (SBM). SBO is usually seen in the setting of elderly patients with diabetes as well as in immunocompromised patients. SBM occurs with invasive nasopharyngeal carcinomas (most commonly squamous cell) as well as lymphoma and metastases.

Both diseases are serious and may be life threatening. General imaging features, permeative destruction of the skull base with or without associated soft tissue mass, are similar. The treatment is very different. Especially with SBO, early recognition and accurate diagnosis are vital in this potentially fatal disease.

The score is 1 for diffusion imaging. Having a high apparent diffusion coefficient (ADC) value is most consistent with SBO, significantly higher than nasopharyngeal carcinoma and lymphoma (Fig 1). That's the good news. The bad news is that the authors found no significant difference in ADC value between SBO and metastatic disease. However, the clinical history is very helpful, as patients with skull base metastases usually have a history of known malignancy.

A. G. Osborn, MD

Diffusion-Weighted Magnetic Resonance Imaging of Head and Neck

Razek AAKA (Mansoura Faculty of Medicine, Egypt)
J Comput Assist Tomogr 34:808-815, 2010

Our aim was to review the clinical applications of diffusion-weighted magnetic resonance imaging in the head and neck. Diffusion-weighted magnetic resonance imaging plays a role in the differentiation of benign from malignant head and neck tumors, squamous cell carcinoma from lymphoma, and metastatic from benign lymphadenopathy as well as in the selection of the biopsy site. It can be used for the differentiation of recurrent tumors from posttreatment changes and in monitoring the patient after radiotherapy. It helps in the differentiation of necrotic tumors from abscesses. Additionally, it can be used for the diagnosis and grading of diffuse autoimmune diseases, such as Sjogren and Graves diseases.

▶ Maybe you remember how excited many of us were when the use of fat-suppressed T2-weighted imaging came into general use for detecting cervical lymphadenopathy. It was a huge help and a useful addition to the standard procedure for imaging head and neck cancer, that is, thin-section contrast-enhanced CT.

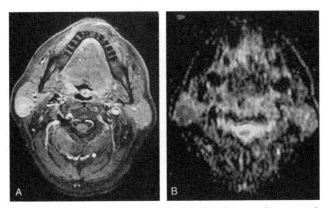

FIGURE 2.—Acinar cell carcinoma. A, Contrast T1-weighted image shows an enhanced lesion involving the right parotid mass. B, ADC map shows restricted diffusion with a low ADC value for the mass (1.03×10^{-3} mm^2/s). (Reprinted from Razek AAKA. Diffusion-weighted magnetic resonance imaging of head and neck. *J Comput Assist Tomogr.* 2010;34:808-815.)

Here's another score for diffusion-weighted imaging (DWI). We are all highly aware of the utility of DWI in brain imaging. Hyperacute stroke? Check! Differentiating between arachnoid and epidermoid cyst? Check! The author reviews the emerging utility of DWI in head and neck imaging. Clinical applications ranging from differentiating malignant from benign lesions, squamous cell carcinoma from lymphoma, and metastatic from benign lymphadenopathy are reviewed. The numbers aren't large yet, and most reported studies are preliminary at best. But it looks as though apparent diffusion coefficient values are a worthwhile contribution in assessing disease in this anatomically difficult area (Fig 2).

A. G. Osborn, MD

The ongoing dilemma of residual cholesteatoma detection: are current magnetic resonance imaging techniques good enough?
Clark MPA, Westerberg BD, Fenton DM (Univ of British Columbia, Vancouver, Canada)
J Laryngol Otol 124:1300-1304, 2010

Introduction.—There is a clear clinical need to reliably detect residual cholesteatoma after canal wall up mastoid surgery. Ideally, this would be achieved through non-invasive radiological means rather than second-look surgery, thus preventing morbidity in those patients in whom no residual disease is found.

Case Report.—We describe a case in which non-echo-planar, diffusion-weighted magnetic resonance imaging sequences were used preoperatively, and compared with subsequent surgical findings. This case highlights both the potential of this increasingly popular magnetic resonance technique and also its current limitations.

Discussion.—Various magnetic resonance sequencing types have been employed to try to reliably detect residual cholesteatoma, each with varying success. Non-echo-planar, fast-spin echo, diffusion-weighted

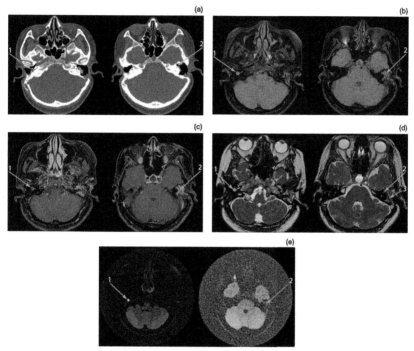

FIGURE 1.—(a) Pre-operative, axial computed tomography scan (bone algorithm, slice thickness 0.625 mm): a soft tissue mass is seen in the right middle ear, corresponding to the sinus tympani, where residual cholesteatoma was found (arrow 1); on the left side, the anterior limb of the superior semicircular canal is dehiscent with some loss of attenuation (arrow 2), corresponding to the location of the subsequently discovered residual cholesteatoma, possibly represented by an adjacent soft tissue mass visible in the middle-ear space. (b) Axial, T1-weighted, fat-saturated magnetic resonance imaging (MRI) scan (echo train = 3, repetition time = 500 ms, echo time = 31.12 ms; 2 mm contiguous slices): the right ear lesion shows some hyperintensity with patches of more central isointensity (arrow 1); on the left side, hyperintense signal is seen lateral to the void left by the retained Silastic sheet which represents the pus and infected tissue found at re-exploration (arrow 2), while the soft tissue adjacent to the superior semicircular canal is isointense. (c) Axial, T1-weighted, post-gadolinium, fat-saturated MRI: the soft tissue mass in the right ear does not enhance, excluding granulation tissue (arrow 1), but does show rim enhancement, suggestive of cholesteatoma; on the left side, the soft tissue lateral and medial to the Silastic sheet is hyperintense, more indicative of inflammatory tissue (arrow 2). (d) Axial, T2-weighted, fast imaging employing steady-state acquisition (FIESTA) MRI (echo train = 1, repetition time = 5.3 ms, echo time = 1.98 ms; 1.4 mm slices, interpolated to 0.7 mm): there is a hyperintense signal for the right middle-ear mass (arrow 1); in the left ear (at the site of the now known residual cholesteatoma and superior semicircular canal fistula), the soft tissue mass fails to show the hyperintensity expected in residual cholesteatoma (arrow 2), there is some loss of signal within the anterior limb of the canal but no hyperintensity, and the void left by the Silastic sheet can be seen (arrow 3) with a lateral hyperintense signal where pus was subsequently found. (e) Axial, propeller, diffusion-weighted MRI (echo train = 24, repetition time = 8000 ms, echo time = 131.32 ms; b-value 1500): the right ear mass shows a high signal which, when taken in context with the signal characteristics described above, makes this lesion highly likely to be residual cholesteatoma (subsequently confirmed at surgery) (arrow 1); no such signal change is seen on the left side, at the other known site of residual cholesteatoma (arrow 2). (Reprinted from Clark MPA, Westerberg BD, Fenton DM. The ongoing dilemma of residual cholesteatoma detection: are current magnetic resonance imaging techniques good enough? *J Laryngol Otol.* 2010;124:1300-1304, with permission of Cambridge University Press.)

sequences currently appear to be the most reliable at detecting even the smallest pearl of cholesteatoma, down to 2 mm in diameter. In our unit, a propeller, diffusion-weighted image sequence is employed on a GE Signa scanner. However, both this case study and other reports show that the accuracy of the technique is not 100 per cent. This begs the question of how much one can rely on the findings of such techniques when deciding whether second-look surgery is indicated. Scan-negative patients will require continued follow up as, at the time of imaging, residual disease may not have reached a detectable size (Fig 1).

▶ Cholesteatoma is a common ear, nose, and throat (ENT) disorder. The so-called canal wall up mastoidectomy is the common treatment. ENT surgeons have blind spots such as the facial nerve recess in which it is difficult to detect residual or recurrent cholesteatoma.

In recent years, MRI has been used extensively, and touted enthusiastically, as *the* imaging procedure of choice, with diffusion-weighted sequences being the most reliable at detecting small pearls of cholesteatoma.

This single case report shows that the accuracy of even the best techniques isn't 100%, and scan-negative patients need continued follow-up to avoid second-look surgery and detect residual disease that hasn't yet reached detectable size (Fig 1).

A. G. Osborn, MD

Spine and Spinal Cord

Ankylosing Spondylitis: Patterns of Radiographic Involvement—A Re-examination of Accepted Principles in a Cohort of 769 Patients

Jang JH, Ward MM, Rucker AN, et al (Cedars-Sinai Med Ctr, Los Angeles, CA; Natl Insts of Health, Bethesda, MD; et al)
Radiology 258:192-198, 2010

Purpose.—To re-examine the patterns of radiographic involvement in ankylosing spondylitis (AS).

Materials and Methods.—This prospective study had institutional review board approval, and 769 patients with AS (556 men, 213 women; mean age, 47.1 years; age range, 18—87 years) provided written informed consent. Radiographs of the cervical spine, lumbar spine, pelvis, and hips were scored by using the Bath Ankylosing Spondylitis Radiology Index (BASRI) by an experienced radiologist. Differences in sacroiliitis grade between right and left sacroiliac joints, frequency of cervical-and lumbar-predominant involvement by sex, frequency of progression to complete spinal fusion, and association between hip arthritis and spinal involvement were computed for the cohort overall and for subgroups defined according to duration of AS in 10-year increments.

Results.—Symmetric sacroiliitis was seen in 86.1% of patients. Lumbar predominance was more common during the first 20 years of the disease, after which the cervical spine and lumbar spine were equally involved.

Men and women were equally likely to have cervical-predominant involvement. Complete spinal fusion was observed in 27.9% of patients with AS for more than 30 years and in 42.6% of patients with AS for more than 40 years. Patients with BASRI hip scores of 2 or greater had significantly higher BASRI spine scores.

Conclusion.—There were no sex differences in cervical-predominant involvement in AS. Hip arthritis was strongly associated with worse spinal involvement (Fig 3, Table 2).

▶ Ankylosing spondylitis (AS) is a disease that our musculoskeletal colleagues are generally more familiar with than neuroradiologists. While the pelvis is an essential part of the spinal axis, we tend to look more at the vertebrae than the rest of the spine, not to mention the hips. As one of my body imaging colleagues is fond of reminding us, "There *is* life outside the neural foramina!"

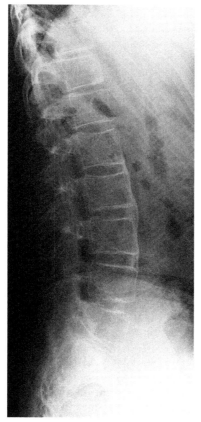

FIGURE 3.—Lateral radiograph of lumbar spine in a patient with AS and a BASRI lumbar spine score of 4 shows bridging syndesmophytes at multiple levels. (Reprinted from Jang JH, Ward MM, Rucker AN, et al. Ankylosing spondylitis: patterns of radiographic involvement—a re-examination of accepted principles in a cohort of 769 patients. *Radiology*. 2010;258:192-198. Copyright by the Radiological Society of North America.)

TABLE 2.—Cervical- and Lumbar-Predominant Disease According to Decade of AS

Disease Duration (y)	Equal Disease	Cervical-Predominant Disease	Lumbar-Predominant Disease
0–9.9	117 (75.5)	8 (5.2)	30 (19.4)
10–19.9	70 (57.4)	16 (13.1)	36 (29.5)
20–29.9	116 (64.4)	36 (20.0)	28 (15.6)
30–39.9	58 (60)	24 (25)	14 (15)
≥40	66 (76)	9 (10)	12 (14)
All	427 (66.7)	93 (14.5)	120 (18.8)

Note.—Data are numbers of patients, with percentages in parentheses. Cervical and lumbar BASRI scores that differed by one grade were excluded from this analysis.

In this excellent study, the authors report some expected and unexpected findings. We all know about symmetric sacroiliitis, which they observed in more than 85% of the patients. What may come as a surprise is that while lumbar predominance is more common during the first 2 decades of AS, the cervical spine and lumbar spine are equally involved afterward (Table 2). Not surprising was the progressive increase in prevalence of complete spinal fusion with longer term AS (Fig 3).

Something this article reminds us is to look at the hips, as hip arthritis is strongly associated with worse spinal involvement.

A. G. Osborn, MD

Combined diffusion-weighted and dynamic contrast-enhanced imaging of patients with acute osteoporotic vertebral fractures

Biffar A, Sourbron S, Dietrich O, et al (LMU Ludwig Maximilian Univ of Munich, Germany; et al)
Eur J Radiol 76:298-303, 2010

Objectives.—To evaluate the potential and to analyze parameter correlations of combined quantitative diffusion-weighted MRI (DWI) and high-temporal-resolution dynamic contrast-enhanced MRI (DCE-MRI) in vertebral bone marrow (vBM) of patients with osteoporosis and acute vertebral compression fractures, providing additional information for a better understanding of the physiological background of parameter changes.

Materials and Methods.—20 patients with acute osteoporotic fractures were examined with DWI and DCE-MRI at 1.5 T. DCE-MRI was performed with a 2D saturation-recovery turbo-FLASH sequence, acquiring 300 dynamics with a temporal resolution of 1 s. For DWI measurements, a DW HASTE sequence with *b*-values from 100 to 600 s/mm^2 was applied. In each patient, ROIs were drawn manually in the fractures and in normal appearing vertebrae. For DCE-MRI, the concentration–time curves of these ROIs were analyzed using a two-compartment tracer-kinetic model in the lesions, providing separate estimates of perfusion and permeability, and a one-compartment model in normal vBM, providing only a mixed representation of perfusion and permeability in terms of a mixed flow parameter K^{trans} and the extracellular volume (ECV). In the case of DWI, attenuation curves were fitted to

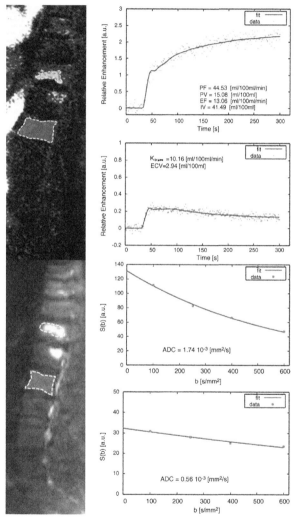

FIGURE 2.—The first image shows the PF-map of a patient with an osteoporotic fracture in T12. Manually drawn regions in T12 and in a normal appearing vertebral body L2 are shown. On the right, the fit of an exchange model to the ROI in the fracture (upper plot) and of a 1-compartment model to normal appearing vBM are shown (lower plot). In the second image, the diffusion-weighted image with b = 100 s/mm² is shown and the selected ROIs in the lesion in T12 and L2. On the right, the fit of the ROI-curve to the monoexponential decay model are shown for the fracture (upper plot) and for the normal appearing vertebral body (lower plot). (Reprinted from Biffar A, Sourbron S, Dietrich O, et al. Combined diffusion-weighted and dynamic contrast-enhanced imaging of patients with acute osteoporotic vertebral fractures. *Eur J Radiol.* 2010;76:298-303, with permission from Elsevier.)

a monoexponential decay model to determine the apparent diffusion coefficient (ADC).

Results.—Mean perfusion parameters and ADCs were significantly ($p < 0.001$) different in the fractures compared to adjacent normal appearing vertebrae (K^{trans}: 7.81 mL/100 mL/min vs. 14.61 mL/100 mL/min, ECV: 52.84 mL/100 mL vs. 4.61 mL/100 mL, ADC: 1.71×10^{-3} mm^2/s vs. 0.57×10^{-3} mm^2/s). ADCs showed a significant correlation with the ECV.

Conclusion.—The quantitative analysis of DWI and DCE-MRI could distinguish osteoporotic fractures from normal appearing vertebrae. A significant correlation found between ECV and ADCs might be able to explain the cause for the increased diffusivity in osteoporotic fractures. Since the other perfusion parameters do not correlate with the ADC, they provide additional pathophysiological information not accessible with DWI (Fig 2).

▶ A challenge faced by radiologists in interpreting spine MRs in elderly patients with compression fracture is whether the fracture is benign (osteoporotic) or malignant (metastatic). In the case of chronic fractures, it's not so difficult. Signal intensity in the affected vertebral body is the same as the other vertebral bodies (ie, usually fatty). Chronic osteoporotic fractures were suppressed on short-tau inversion recovery or fat-saturated T2-weighted images.

But, and this is a big *but*, if an osteoporotic fracture is acute, it may hemorrhage, incite edema, enhance after contrast administration, and look fairly nasty. In such cases, our task becomes more difficult. The growing use of diffusion-weighted imaging (DWI) in the spine has been shown to be helpful, with apparent diffusion coefficients in osteoporotic vertebral compression fractures helping to differentiate these benign fractures from malignant infiltration of the vertebral body with pathologic fracture.

This article takes the utility of spine DWI one step further. The authors show that DWI and dynamic contrast-enhanced MR can distinguish osteoporotic from normal vertebrae (Fig 2). They looked at fractured osteoporotic vertebrae. An intriguing next step would be to see if DWI could differentiate normal-appearing but vulnerable (prefracture) osteoporotic vertebrae. Now wouldn't that be great!

A. G. Osborn, MD

Diffusion Magnetic Resonance Imaging to Differentiate Degenerative From Infectious Endplate Abnormalities in the Lumbar Spine
Eguchi Y, Ohtori S, Yamashita M, et al (Chiba Univ, Chuo-ku, Japan; et al)
Spine 36:E198-E202, 2011

Study Design.—A retrospective observational study of healthy volunteers and patients with degenerative and infectious endplate abnormalities in the lumbar spine.

Objectives.—Our purpose was to evaluate the usefulness of diffusion-weighted imaging (DWI) for the differentiation of degenerative and infectious endplate abnormalities using 1.5-T magnetic resonance imaging (MRI).

Summary of Background Data.—DWI can provide valuable structural information about tissues that may be useful for clinical applications in differentiation between degenerative and infectious endplate abnormalities.

Methods.—Sixteen consecutive patients with endplate abnormalities that was detected by MRI of the lumbar spine, and 15 healthy volunteers were studied. DWI was performed using whole-body imaging with background body signal suppression with a b value of 1000 s/mm^2. Apparent diffusion coefficient values of normal and abnormal vertebral bone marrow were calculated.

Results.—Twenty-nine vertebral abnormalities were found in 16 patients. Nine vertebral abnormalities in 5 patients were because of infections and 20 vertebral abnormalities in 11 patients were because of degenerative changes; 7 levels were classified as Modic type 1, 7 levels as type 2, and 6 levels as type 3. DWI showed hyperintensity in all patients with infection, similar to that used in positron emission tomography, but not in the intervertebral spaces of any patients with degenerative disease. Apparent diffusion coefficient values of infectious bone marrowwere significantly higher than normal and degenerative bone marrow.

Conclusion.—DWI is useful for differentiation of degenerative and infectious endplate abnormalities. Moreover, MRI is widely used clinically because of the lack of ionizing radiation, low cost, and fast imaging time as compared with positron emission tomography. Therefore, DWI has the potential to be used as a screening tool.

▶ I really loved this article. Even though it's a retrospective review (as most imaging articles are) and thus has some limitations, it addresses one of the most perplexing problems in spine imaging: how can we reliably distinguish (or if we can) between aggressive discogenic disease and infection? The 2 processes can look quite similar on standard imaging studies. Widespread end plate disruption, enhancement, and signal abnormalities can be seen in both noninfectious degenerative disease and discitis/osteomyelitis.

Is there an MR sequence that might be helpful—like REALLY helpful—in making this distinction? The answer seems to be a resounding yes! Diffusion-weighted imaging (DWI)! If it works in the brain, it should work in the spine. We have been using DWI and diffusion tensor imaging of the spine for about a year and have found it very useful. FDG-PET also works in detecting both tumors and infections, which both show increased uptake. However, that's an expensive additional procedure. Adding DWI takes just a few minutes and adds highly useful information. In this series, the authors found hyperintensity on DWI in all patients with infectious end plate abnormalities (Fig 3 in the original article) and none in degenerative disease (Fig 2 in the original article).

A. G. Osborn, MD

Surgical Technique and Outcomes in the Treatment of Spinal Cord Ependymomas, Part 1: Intramedullary Ependymomas

Kucia EJ, Bambakidis NC, Chang SW, et al (St Joseph's Hosp and Med Ctr, Phoenix, AZ; Univ Hosps Case Med Ctr, Cleveland, OH)

Neurosurgery 68:ons57-ons63, 2011

Background.—Intramedullary spinal ependymomas are rare tumors.

Objective.—To provide a large retrospective review in the modern neuroimaging era from a tertiary center where aggressive surgical resection is favored.

Methods.—Charts of intramedullary spinal ependymomas treated between 1983 and 2006 were reviewed.

Results.—Sixty-seven cases were reviewed. The mean age was 45.6 years (range, 11-78 years) with a male-to-female ratio of 2:1. The most common location was the cervical spine, followed by the thoracic and lumbar spine. The average duration of symptoms was 33 months, with the most common symptom being pain and/or dysesthesias, followed by weakness, numbness, and urinary or sexual symptoms. Gross total resection was achieved in 55 patients and a subtotal resection was performed in 12 patients; 9 patients were treated with adjuvant radiation therapy. Mean follow-up was 32 months. The mean McCormick neurological grade at last follow-up was 2.0. The preoperative outcome correlated significantly with postoperative outcome ($P < .001$). A significant number of patients who initially worsened improved at their 3-month follow-up examination. Outcomes were significantly worse in patients undergoing subtotal resection with or without radiation therapy ($P < .05$). There were 3 recurrences. The overall complication rate was 34%. The primary complications were wound infections or cerebrospinal fluid leaks.

Conclusion.—Spinal cord ependymomas are difficult lesions to treat. Aggressive surgical resection is associated with a high overall complication rate. However, when gross total resection can be achieved, overall outcomes are excellent and the recurrence rate is low.

▶ This is one of those good news/bad news kind of articles. The authors present 67 cases of intramedullary ependymomas, which is an enormous number of cases—one of the largest series ever published. Their demographics document some useful statistics, that is, the mean age is 45 years. While intracranial ependymomas are common in children, spinal cord ependymomas are rare. Their youngest patient was 11 years old (the most common intramedullary neoplasm in children is astrocytoma).

Intracranial ependymomas are not nice tumors. Their intramedullary counterparts are even worse. In both instances, gross total resection is the goal. Again, operating in the posterior fossa isn't easy, but operating in a much smaller space—the spinal cord—is even more challenging. The complication rate, which the authors frankly discuss, is high with aggressive surgical resection. Between 15% and 20% of their patients worsened significantly after operation.

On the other hand, if gross total resection can be achieved, outcomes overall are excellent and recurrence risk is low.

They make the important point that early diagnosis is part of improving outcome. Of interest, most of their patients had symptoms (pain being the most common) for nearly 3 years before their tumors were diagnosed. They don't really mention imaging, except briefly in passing.

A. G. Osborn, MD

8 Cardiac Imaging

Introduction

Many of this year's publications in the cardiovascular field revolve around the appropriate use of imaging. The past year's research has helped establish the accuracy of cardiac MRI and CT for various clinical applications in numerous single-center trials, meta-analyses, and more recently in multicenter trials with independent core laboratory analyses of the imaging data. One may argue that, for example, the accuracy of cardiac CT for detection of significant obstructive coronary artery disease is now established. Several recent publications have also shown the prognostic value of MRI and CT imaging findings using Kaplan-Meyer analysis and hard outcomes, such as all-cause mortality or major adverse cardiac events (MACE).

Another strong focus recently has been on research revolving around the ALARA (as low as reasonably achievable) principle, which has resulted in dramatic radiation dose reduction in CT imaging. Cardiac CT is now used by national organizations as the "poster child" for radiation reduction strategies, as it has driven the vendors' research and development efforts and has evolved from one of the "worst offenders" in the CT arena to the test with some of the lowest radiation doses. Now that these huge leaps have been made, the focus is shifting toward appropriate utilization of the tests. Accuracy and prognostic value alone may not justify the use of a test, and therefore some payers still refuse to cover CT even today. Is there a benefit that can be measured (eg, improved mortality) when adding these tests to the workup/management or by replacing other tests? These questions are the focus of recent and ongoing large-scale multicenter trials.

A multisociety guideline is included in this issue of the YEAR BOOK because it provides appropriateness ranking based on the currently available published data. This document allows cardiac imagers to advise our referring physicians as to "appropriate utilization." I have also included an article written by cardiologists that explains their use of current technology. Understanding how our referring physicians use the information we can provide is important, and this article gives us a neat insight. There are also several articles included here that discuss some of the imaging findings that we may stumble on unexpectedly but that may have great clinical impact. For example, one article nicely reviews the various potential cardiovascular sources of embolic stroke. This is certainly something to be on the lookout for when reading CT, whether gated or routine non-gated chest CT.

Another hot topic today is adenosine stress-rest myocardial perfusion CT. We had highlighted one of the first articles in last year's YEAR BOOK. This has triggered numerous studies that are still under way or submitted for publication—hence, not much to include in this edition. However, I have the feeling that next year's YEAR BOOK will be all about stress-rest myocardial CT perfusion—stay tuned! I truly hope you will enjoy reading this selection of articles.

Suhny Abbara, MD

ACCF/SCCT/ACR/AHA/ASE/ASNC/NASCI/SCAI/SCMR 2010 Appropriate Use Criteria for Cardiac Computed Tomography

Taylor AJ, Cerqueira M, Hodgson JM, et al (Washington Hosp Ctr, Washington, DC; Cleveland Clinic Foundation, OH; Geisinger Health System, Danville, PA; et al)

J Cardiovasc Comput Tomogr 4:407.e1-407.e33, 2010

The American College of Cardiology Foundation (ACCF), along with key specialty and subspecialty societies, conducted an appropriate use review of common clinical scenarios where cardiac computed tomography (CCT) is frequently considered. The present document is an update to the original CCT/cardiac magnetic resonance (CMR) appropriateness criteria published in 2006, written to reflect changes in test utilization, to incorporate new clinical data, and to clarify CCT use where omissions or lack of clarity existed in the original criteria (1). The indications for this review were drawn from common applications or anticipated uses, as well as from current clinical practice guidelines. Ninety-three clinical scenarios were developed by a writing group and scored by a separate technical panel on a scale of 1 to 9 to designate appropriate use, inappropriate use, or uncertain use. In general, use of CCT angiography for diagnosis and risk assessment in patients with low or intermediate risk or pretest probability for coronary artery disease (CAD) was viewed favorably, whereas testing in high-risk patients, routine repeat testing, and general screening in certain clinical scenarios were viewed less favorably. Use of noncontrast computed tomography (CT) for calcium scoring was rated as appropriate within intermediate- and selected low-risk patients. Appropriate applications of CCT are also within the category of cardiac structural and functional evaluation. It is anticipated that these results will have an impact on physician decision making, performance, and reimbursement policy, and that they will help guide future research.

▶ This publication is a consensus document generated by writing panel members from multiple societies. The published versions are abbreviated summaries that appeared in 3 journals simultaneously in electronic form.[1-3]

The full version is available on the society Web pages and the journal Web pages for download and contains several helpful flowcharts that address patient management in specific clinical settings. An example is "Use of CT angiography in the setting of prior test results" that has 12 end points resulting from the various combinations of the prior test results. Each end point is assigned an inappropriate, uncertain, or appropriate rating.

This article or at least the information that is summarized in the appropriateness tables is a must have for all physicians who perform cardiac CT. It will make it easy for imagers to advise our referring physicians about appropriate utilization—a hot topic these days on the national level.

S. Abbara, MD

References

1. Taylor AJ, Cerqueira M, Hodgson JM, et al. ACCF/SCCT/ACR/AHA/ASE/ASNC/NASCI/SCAI/SCMR 2010 appropriate use criteria for cardiac computed tomography. A report of the American College of Cardiology Foundation Appropriate Use Criteria Task Force, the Society of Cardiovascular Computed Tomography, the American College of Radiology, the American Heart Association, the American Society of Echocardiography, the American Society of Nuclear Cardiology, the North American Society for Cardiovascular Imaging, the Society for Cardiovascular Angiography and Interventions, and the Society for Cardiovascular Magnetic Resonance. *J Am Coll Cardiol.* 2010;56:1864-1894.
2. Taylor AJ, Cerqueira M, Hodgson JM, et al. ACCF/SCCT/ACR/AHA/ASE/ASNC/NASCI/SCAI/SCMR 2010 Appropriate Use Criteria for Cardiac Computed Tomography. A Report of the American College of Cardiology Foundation Appropriate Use Criteria Task Force, the Society of Cardiovascular Computed Tomography, the American College of Radiology, the American Heart Association, the American Society of Echocardiography, the American Society of Nuclear Cardiology, the North American Society for Cardiovascular Imaging, the Society for Cardiovascular Angiography and Interventions, and the Society for Cardiovascular Magnetic Resonance. *Circulation.* 2010;122:e525-e555.
3. Greenland P, Alpert JS, Beller GA, et al. 2010 ACCF/AHA guideline for assessment of cardiovascular risk in asymptomatic adults: a report of the American College of Cardiology Foundation/American Heart Association Task Force on Practice Guidelines. *Circulation.* 2010;122:e584-e636.

Cardiac computed tomography and magnetic resonance imaging: the clinical use from a cardiologist's perspective
Townsend JC, Gregg D 4th (Med Univ of South Carolina, Charleston)
J Thorac Imaging 25:194-203, 2010

The introduction and continued evolution of cardiac computed tomography and magnetic resonance imaging have added considerable noninvasive diagnostic insight into a wide range of frequently encountered clinical cardiology scenarios. With an increasing range of imaging modalities, and multiple methods of image acquisition in each, a detailed understanding of the clinical question at hand is often necessary to select the proper study and make optimal use of imaging data. We review common cardiac issues from a clinician's perspective, along with the unique role to be played by computed tomography and magnetic resonance imaging in each condition. This review will hopefully facilitate a strong dialogue between imagers and managing clinicians, creating a shared knowledge of both the capabilities of imaging and the management challenges that treating clinicians face.

▶ This is a high-level overview article about the role of cardiac imaging modalities as tools within the tool boxes that are available to the clinicians who manage cardiac patients. This article will be particularly valuable to those of us who wear many hats and perform cardiac imaging as a part of a complex practice. To know how best to help our patients, we need to understand the management decision that our referring physicians have to make and the evidence that support use of cardiac MRI or CT to aid in this decision making. This article furnishes the reader with that kind of insight. Naturally, instead of discussing one imaging modality after the other (coronary calcium scoring, CT angiography, MRI, MR angiography, etc), the article is divided into disease process sections, such as ischemic heart disease that is then subdivided into the relevant scenarios (detection of coronary atherosclerosis, direct coronary imaging, myocardial perfusion imaging, and assessment of myocardial viability).

S. Abbara, MD

Atrial and ventricular functional and structural adaptations of the heart in elite triathletes assessed with cardiac MR imaging
Scharf M, Brem MH, Wilhelm M, et al (Univ of Erlangen-Nuremberg, Germany)
Radiology 257:71-79, 2010

Purpose.—To assess cardiac morphologic and functional adaptations in elite triathletes with magnetic resonance (MR) imaging and to compare findings to those in recreationally active control subjects.

Materials and Methods.—The institutional review board approved the study, and written informed consent was obtained from all subjects. Twenty-six male triathletes (mean age ± standard deviation, 27.9 years ± 3.5; age range, 18-35 years) and 27 nonathletic male control subjects (mean age, 27.3 years ± 3.7; age range, 20-34 years) underwent cardiac MR imaging. Electrocardiographically gated steady-state free-precession cine MR imaging was used to measure indexed left ventricular (LV) and right ventricular (RV) myocardial mass, end-diastolic and endsystolic volumes, stroke volume, ejection fraction (EF), and cardiac index at rest. The ventricular remodeling index, which is indicative of the pattern of cardiac hypertrophy, was calculated. The maximum left atrial (LA) volume was calculated according to the biplane area-length method. Differences between means of athletes and control subjects were assessed by using the Student t test for independent samples.

Results.—The atrial and ventricular volume and mass indexes in triathletes were significantly greater than those in control subjects (P < .001). In 25 of the 26 athletes, the LV and RV end-diastolic volumes were greater than the normal ranges reported in the literature for healthy, male, nonathletic control subjects (47-92 mL/m(2) and 55-105 mL/m(2), respectively). There was a strong positive correlation between end-diastolic volume and myocardial mass (P < .01). The mean LV and RV remodeling indexes of the athletes (0.73 g/mL ± 0.1 and 0.22 g/mL ± 0.01, respectively) were similar to those of the control subjects (0.71 g/mL ± 0.1 [P = .290] and 0.22 g/mL ± 0.01 [P = .614], respectively). There was a negative correlation between LA end-systolic volume and heart rate (P < .01).

Conclusion.—Changes in cardiac morphologic characteristics and function in elite triathletes, as measured with cardiac MR imaging, reflect a combination of eccentric and concentric remodeling with regulative enlargement of atrial and ventricular chambers. These findings are different from what has been observed in previous studies in other types of elite athletes.

▶ Ok, here is a scenario that you may have encountered—I certainly have:
You are very excited because that famous athlete comes to your hospital for a medical workup. After meeting the guy (he will be bigger than he seems to be on TV), you will have to read his cardiac MRI. Unfortunately, all his numbers are borderline or abnormal, and the diseases that this normally would indicate come with the risk of sudden cardiac death (eg, a dilated right ventricle [RV], especially in the setting of arrhythmias, and the referring clinician wants to rule out arrhythmogenic RV dysplasia). But then you think—he is an athlete. Aren't they entitled to an enlarged heart? This article is included here because it addresses exactly this issue. It provides us with solid quotable data that allow us to use more appropriate normal ranges for myocardial mass index, chamber volumes, and end-diastolic wall thickness. The study found statistically significant differences in virtually all parameters, except the ejection fraction, which is unchanged at rest.

S. Abbara, MD

Prevalence of fat deposition within the right ventricular myocardium in asymptomatic young patients without ventricular arrhythmias
Kirsch J, Johansen CK, Araoz PA, et al (Mayo Clinic, Rochester, MN)
J Thorac Imaging 25:173-178, 2010

Purpose.—Variable amounts of intramyocardial fat can be found within the right ventricular muscle fibers. We aimed to determine the prevalence of intramyocardial fat deposition within the right ventricle (RV) in asymptomatic patients aged 40 years and younger who underwent imaging of the heart for coronary artery disease screening.

Materials and Methods.—Retrospective review of 540 consecutive patients aged 40 years or younger referred for coronary calcium scoring.

Results.—The images were reviewed by 2 dedicated cardiac radiologists, and the following specific observations were made: presence or absence of macroscopic fat in the RV by location, RV size as normal or enlarged, and presence of additional foci of fat deposition in the visualized thorax. The clinical data were reviewed from the patients' medical record, and the following information was recorded: age, sex, body mass index, and the presence of cardiac risk factors. The electrocardiographic examinations were reviewed as well. The study cohort included 398 males (73%) and 142 females (27%), with a mean age of 36.2+/−4.3 years and a range of 12 to 40 years. Sixty-two patients (11.5%) had macroscopic fatty deposition of the RV myocardium.

Conclusions.—Fatty replacement of the free wall of the RV is common, occurring in up to 11% of asymptomatic patients younger than 40 years of age undergoing cardiac screening examinations. No statistically significant association with cardiac risk factors or body mass index was found.

▶ Imagine that today you perform an MRI to rule out arrhythmogenic right ventricular dysplasia/cardiomyopathy (ARVD/C). You run dedicated pulse sequences to detect fat within the right ventricle (RV) (which is the equivalent of a major criterion for ARVD, equivalent because the criteria ask for pathology). Tomorrow you find 2 patients who have fat in the RV on CT. The problem is that ARVD is extremely rare, but fat in the RV is apparently quite common, and your CT patients were sent for completely unrelated reasons. This article is included because it gives us good prevalence data in case we need to argue with, say, a referring physician (or a resident who just read about ARVD) that fat in the RV incidentally detected on chest or cardiac CT is common and does NOT mean we need to be concerned about ARVD or send the patient for MRI or to a cardiologist. Because of the recent realization that fat is common, some sites have advocated that cardiac MRI to rule out ARVD does not need to include sequences searching for fat. The interobserver variability with MRI is high anyway, and false positives are expected. The more robust criteria that MRI can deliver are global RV dilatation and function and regional abnormalities such as presence of RV aneurysms (a major criterion for ARVD).

S. Abbara, MD

Improved Detection of Subendocardial Hyperenhancement in Myocardial Infarction Using Dark Blood—Pool Delayed Enhancement MRI
Farrelly C, Rehwald W, Salerno M, et al (Northwestern Univ, Chicago, IL)
AJR Am J Roentgenol 196:339-348, 2011

Objective.—Delayed enhancement MRI using fast segmented k-space inversion recovery (IR) gradient-echo imaging is a well established "bright-blood" technique for identifying myocardial infarction and is used as the reference standard sequence in this study. The purpose of this study was to validate a recently developed dark blood—pool delayed enhancement technique in a porcine animal model, evaluate its performance in human patients, and quantify its performance compared with the reference standard in both.

Subjects and Methods.—In an animal study, the reference standard and dark blood–pool delayed enhancement were assessed in three pigs with induced myocardial infarction. In a human study, 26 patients, 31–81 years old (19 men and seven women), with a known history of myocardial infarction were imaged using the reference standard and dark blood–pool delayed enhancement. Contrast-to-noise ratio (CNR), signal intensity ratio, signal-to-noise ratio (SNR), and qualitative scores of hyperenhancement were recorded. Measurements were compared using paired samples *t* test and Wilcoxon's signed rank test.

Results.—In the animal study, the mean CNR of infarct to blood pool was 11 times higher for dark blood–pool delayed enhancement than for the reference standard. The mean SNR was 4.4 times higher for the reference standard. In the human study, the mean CNR and signal intensity ratio of hyperenhancing myocardium to the blood pool were 1.9 ($p = 0.04$) and 5.5 ($p < 0.01$) times higher, respectively, for dark blood–pool delayed enhancement compared with reference standard. The mean CNR and signal intensity ratio of hyperenhancing myocardium to normal myocardium and SNR were 2.8 ($p < 0.01$), 1.3 ($p = 0.07$), and 2.8 ($p < 0.01$) higher, respectively, for the reference standard. Qualitative analysis identified seven extra segments with grade 1 scars using dark blood–pool delayed enhancement ($p < 0.01$).

Conclusion.—Dark blood–pool delayed enhancement is complementary to the reference standard. It can detect more subendocardial foci of hyperenhancement, thus potentially identifying more infarcts and changing patient management.

▶ An occasional problem with MR delayed enhancement imaging is the following: We are supposed to find the infarct, which is a bright signal on a background of normal black or a dark ring of myocardium. Infarcts occur in the subendocardial myocardium—immediately adjacent to the lumen of the ventricle. The lumen is usually bright because there is some contrast still circulating. So if you have a small nontransmural infarct, it may be completely missed because it can easily be misinterpreted as the beginning of the lumen. This article describes a novel approach to make the blood pool in the left ventricular lumen black. So now normal myocardium is dark, the lumen will be dark, and the infarcts—even if small—will stand out as a rim of subendocardial high signal intensity. The authors show nice examples in 26 cases and demonstrate not only markedly improved contrast-to-noise ratios between infarct and lumen (expected) but also to a lesser degree between normal and abnormal myocardium. We have to keep in mind that these are preliminary results, and further study is needed to determine accuracy values of the novel dark blood–pool delayed enhancement method. In my eyes, this is another big step forward for myocardial viability MRI, and we will probably see more about this new pulse sequence in the future.

S. Abbara, MD

Embryology and Developmental Defects of the Interatrial Septum

Rojas CA, El-Sherief A, Medina HM, et al (Harvard Med School and Massachusetts General Hosp, Boston)
AJR Am J Roentgenol 195:1100-1104, 2010

Objective.—The various types of atrial septal defects (ASDs) can be differentiated on the basis of their imaging appearance on MDCT.

Conclusion.—It is fundamental for the cardiac imager to understand the embryologic development of the interatrial septum and the morphogenic differences of ASDs.

▶ This article is a nice review of the normal development of the interatrial septum and the defects that result from various abnormal courses of development. Don't worry—although embryology can be overwhelming, at least for me, this article boils it down to what matters, and it provides simple drawings that make the matter understandable. Moreover, the reason why we get the different types of atrial septal defects (ASDs) becomes clearer, which makes it easier to remember.

In addition to the flap valve mechanism responsible for patent foramen ovale, the article reviews the mechanisms, locations, associations, and imaging appearance of primum ASD, secundum ASD, sinus venosus ASDs, endocardial cushion defects or atrioventricular canals and unroofing of the coronary sinus. The latter is oddly not a defect within the atrial septum itself but because of the similar physiologic consequences is considered (the rarest type of) an ASD. A very nice article that focuses on just the imaging appearance of atrial and ventricular septum was published by Rajiah and Kanne.[1]

S. Abbara, MD

Reference

1. Rajiah P, Kanne JP. Computed tomography of septal defects. *J Cardiovasc Comput Tomogr.* 2010;4:231-245.

Cardioembolic Origin in Patients With Embolic Stroke: Spectrum of Imaging Findings on Cardiac MDCT

Jin KN, Chun EJ, Choi SI, et al (Seoul Natl Univ Bundang Hosp, Korea)
AJR Am J Roentgenol 195:W38-W44, 2010

Objective.—The purpose of this article is to show various cardiac MDCT findings of a cardioembolic origin in patients with embolic stroke.

Conclusion.—Cardiac MDCT is an emerging technique for the identification and assessment of a cardioembolic origin in patients with embolic stroke. In the near future, it will play an increasing role in the assessment of patients with a suspected embolic stroke.

▶ This is a beautiful review article that comprehensively reviews the various cardiac sources for cardiogenic, embolic, cerebral infarcts, which account for up to 20% of all ischemic infarcts. The authors did a fine job in adding illustrative high-quality figures demonstrating not only the cardiac source of the embolus but also the corresponding brain imaging in the same patients. The authors nicely review and illustrate abnormalities, including atrial fibrillation and resulting left atrial appendage thrombosis, other left atrial thrombi, myocardial infarcts with resulting aneurysms and mural thrombus, cardiac valve disease with vegetation/thrombus formation of native or bioprosthetic valves, and masses such as left atrial myxoma. They also address some differential diagnostic considerations and mimickers of cardiac thrombi, namely slow mixing of contrast that can be seen in a left atrial appendage in atrial fibrillation and mimic a filling defect on early arterial phase CTs. An example of how to differentiate the 2 entities by applying a delayed scan to allow more time for contrast/blood mixing is given.

S. Abbara, MD

Article Index

Chapter 1: Thoracic Radiology

Chapter 2: Breast Imaging

Chapter 3: Musculoskeletal System

Chapter 5: Economics, Research, Education, and Quality

Chapter 6: Interventional Radiology

Chapter 7: Neuroradiology

Chapter 8: Cardiac Imaging

Author Index

Printed and bound by CPI Group (UK) Ltd, Croydon, CR0 4YY

08/05/2025

01864677-0012